Family Health Care Nursing:
Theory, Practice, and Research

Family Health Care Nursing:
Theory, Practice, and Research

Shirley May Harmon Hanson,
Professor, School of Nursing
Oregon Health Sciences Universit
and
Private Practice
Licensed Child, Marriage, and Fam
Portland, OR

Sheryl Thalman Boyd, RN, PhD
Associate Professor
School of Nursing
Oregon Health Sciences University
Portland, OR

 F. A. DAVIS COMPANY • Philadelphia

F. A. Davis Company
1915 Arch Street
Philadelphia, PA 19103

Cover Art: Wassily Kandinsky
Improvisation No. 29 (The Swan)
Philadelphia Museum of Art: The Louise and Walter Arensberg Collection
Accession number: '50-134-102

Inside front cover: The Jung Family Collection, 1915
Philadelphia, Jung Family Photo Collection
Balch Institute for Ethnic Studies Library

Inside back cover: John Paul Scott (born 1859 in Harrisburg, PA)
Pictured here with his children in 1916 "when mother died"
Philadelphia, Scott-Johnson Family Photo Collection
Balch Institute for Ethnic Studies Library

Printed in the United States of America

Last digit indicates print number: 10 9 8 7 6 5

As new scientific information becomes available through basic and clinical research, recommended treatments and drug therapies undergo changes. The author(s) and publisher have done everything possible to make this book accurate, up to date, and in accord with accepted standards at the time of publication. The authors, editors, and publisher are not responsible for errors or omissions or for consequences from application of the book, and make no warranty, expressed or implied, in regard to the contents of the book. Any practice described in this book should be applied by the reader in accordance with professional standards of care used in regard to the unique circumstances that may apply in each situation. The reader is advised always to check product information (package inserts) for changes and new information regarding dose and contraindications before administering any drug. Caution is especially urged when using new or infrequently ordered drugs.

Library of Congress Cataloging-in-Publication Data

Family health care nursing: theory, practice, and research   /   [edited by]
Shirley May Harmon Hanson, Sheryl Thalman Boyd.
p. cm.
Includes bibliographical references and index.
ISBN 0-8036-0022-4 (alk. paper)
1. Family nursing.   2. Family—Health and hygiene.   3. Sick—
Family relationships.   I. Boyd, Sheryl Thalman.
[DNLM: 1. Nursing Care.   2. Family Practice.   3. Health Promotion.
4. Nursing Process.   5. Child Health Services.   6. Hanson, Shirley
M. H., 1938–   WY 100 F198 1995]
RT120.F34F35   1996
610.73 — dc20
DNLM/DLC
for Library of Congress   95-38702

To the fond memories I have with my family of origin:

> Betty and Kenny Harmon, my parents
> and to my siblings Albert Jr., Bill, Marj, Peggy, and Kathy

And to the memorable times I have with family of procreation:

> my in-laws Ralph and Louise Hanson, their sons Larry and Neal, and especially to my children Derek Harmon and Gwen Louise. Gwen will carry on the family tradition of "family nurse" for the next generation.

Shirley May Harmon Hanson

With my love and appreciation, I dedicate my contributions to my parents, John and Pauline Thalman, and to my children, Nathan, Aaron, and Kasi and to my husband, Douglas.

Sheryl Thalman Boyd

Foreword

Nursing as a profession has a close alignment with the family because nursing shares many of the responsibilities families have for the care and protection of their family members. It is therefore from this aligned perspective that the profession has an obligation to advance the capacity of families, to provide security, and to promote growth of both individuals and the family unit itself. Whereas in the past an important role of the family was for economic support of all family members, this is not the case today. In fact governmental support of women and children with "no man in the house" and the increasing participation of women in the work force have contributed to the economic independence of adult female members of families. Today the affiliative/relationship and socialization roles of the family are being demonstrated as the most vital roles for the well-being of family members and determining their capacity to be adaptive and successful adults in the society.

There is abundant evidence that the affiliative role of the family is critical to the society. It is within the emotional connections family members have with each other that commitment to others, the capacity for shared intimacy, and personal well-being are nurtured. There are alarming statistics about emotional connections within families that suggest all is not well. The increasing rate of divorce, violence within the family, and increasing frequency of mental illness in adults and children all attest to the failures in communication, bonding, and commitment among family members. Freud once asserted that the family was the one and only social unit in society that was able to maintain itself in spite of the expression of strong emotions and conflicts. A sense of being important, a sense of caring for others, and guidance about how to live life are developed within the family system. Today's "youth gangs" are attributed to the strong need that young people have for belonging and recreating the family ties they find lacking in their own families. A sense of well-being comes from being cared for; from this sense comes committed relationships.

As societies have evolved the collective group has taken on the role of supporting the family in promoting the well-being of individuals and in providing protection for those families unable to care for their own. For example, most communities provide a process for the education of children and adults, whereas in more primitive societies this function fell to the family. Likewise the creation of hospitals, prisons, systems of public health, social welfare programs, child care, and nursing homes are all examples of institutionalizing the roles of families on a broader scale. Most of these institutionalized systems are regulated to be complementary to the family as the basic caregiving system and the system of most sustained affiliative commitments. Recently we have experienced the cost of these extensions of the family roles. It is very expensive to provide for the care of individuals by means other than family members. Care of children outside their family home is costly. Hospital care has become too expensive to afford, except for the most acutely ill. Prisons cost more to run per individual than the annual average family income. We are questioning our support for women and children on welfare. Technology has brought us to a point where the demand for material goods such as televisions, computers, cars, communication systems, travel opportunities, convenience machines, and the highest level of illness care threaten resources for human relationships and caregiving. At a time when families are stretched to adequately maintain the style of living they desire, there is a trend toward curtailing these substitute family roles. We are experiencing a reappraisal of our basic value and belief systems.

There is a need to reorganize our approach in nursing to be more oriented to working in partnerships with the family about the nurture and care of individual family members as well as to strengthen the family as a system of affiliation, commitment, and care. This textbook provides an orientation to working in partnerships with families. The models promoted illustrate the complexity of working within the dynamic family system and orient the learner to theories that can be used to understand how families are structured and most importantly how they work to accomplish their role in society. The earliest inclusion of families in nursing care has come from maternity, pediatric, and community health nurses; their guidance and example provides historical evidence of the strength contained within a partnership with families. In this volume clinical examples are successfully used to illustrate both the family, health care, and nursing partnership issues. These illustrations clarify the need to focus our nursing assessment beyond the individual and incorporate the family system. The family is a partner in the care that nurses and other clinicians provide. I find viewing my role as an advocate and consultatant to the family puts a perspective on my relationship and role that creates an effective collaboration with the family about the health of both individual members and the family system itself.

Kathryn E. Barnard, RN, PhD
Professor of Nursing and Pyschology
University of Washington
Seattle, WA

Preface

Family health care nursing is a specialty whose time has come. For some time we in the health care professions, particularly nursing, have recognized a relationship between the interaction within families and their health status. Much has evolved in family nursing since the early thinkers and writers started 20 years ago. We are grateful to stand on the shoulders of some of the early scholars in the field: Kathryn Barnard, Martha Barnard, Imelda Clements, Suzanne Feetham, Marie-Luise Friedemann, Marilyn Friedman, Catherine Gillis, JoAnne Hall, Debra Hymovich, Ellen Janosik, Maureen Leahey, Maribelle Leavitt, Jean Miller, Florence Roberts, Grayce Sills, Lorraine Wright, and of course Florence Nightingale, just to name a few.

The purpose of this book is to provide a foundation in the concepts and theories of family health care nursing and to demonstrate how they are practiced in the traditional nursing specialities. We believe that family nursing is *the umbrella* under which all nursing specialties could practice, although each specialty may draw on different theories and research. How family nursing is practiced today seems to be a matter of whether nurses have been schooled in a family nursing paradigm as part of a formal undergraduate/graduate education or are self taught by experience. We believe this book moves the art and science of family nursing forward by integrating the theory, practice, and research (TPR) of family nursing theory with that of family social science and family therapy and by providing the insights that help students and practitioners make the connection between assessment and intervention.

As teachers of undergraduate and graduate family nursing core courses, we identified a need for literature in this specialty that focused on family health care nursing and its application in a variety of health care settings by different levels of practitioners. It was evident at the graduate level that many students had not received a family nursing foundation in their original associate, diploma, or baccalaureate programs. Indeed they were being exposed to these ideas for the first time. This book was created to be a comprehensive textbook for these student nurses and practitioners at the undergraduate and graduate levels.

Family Health Care Nursing: Theory, Practice, and Research is organized so that it can be used early in a nursing program by focusing on Unit I, "Foundations of Family Health," and then during specialty rotations focusing on Unit II, "Family Nursing Practice."

Concerning the contributors for this textbook, great efforts were made to garner the best talent available in family nursing from across the country, nurses who were sound clinicians and academicians. Congratulations to our contributors for hanging in during a long process.

The book is divided into two sections. Unit I consists of "Foundations of Family Health Care Nursing." There are eight chapters in this section. Chapter 1, "Family Nursing: An Overview" gives a broad overview of the subject. Family, family health, and family nursing are defined and the reasons for learning about family nursing are discussed. Next, the history of families in America and the history of family nursing care are reviewed. The roles of family nurses and some of the contemporary issues pertaining to family nursing practice, research, and education are presented.

Chapter 2, "Theoretical and Research Foundations of Family Nursing" provides an overview of the development of family nursing theory and the state of family nursing research. Students are introduced to theoretical frameworks that are used by family health care nurses to guide theory in practice, research, and education. In addition, this chapter summarizes design and measurement issues in family nursing research.

Chapter 3, "Family Structure, Function and Process" addresses core issues pertaining to sociologic aspects of families in America. The relationship between family function and structure and the health status of families is explored. A discussion of family process includes an overview of familial roles and the effects of communication, power, and decision making on the enactment of these roles.

Chapter 4, "Sociocultural Influences on Family Health" focuses on how sociocultural dimensions influence both individual family members' health, and family systems' health, as well as implications for family nursing practice. These authors differentiate among culture, ethnicity, social class, acculturation, and ethclass. Incorporating a cultural assessment while working with families is emphasized.

Chapter 5, "Factors Influencing Family Functioning and the Health of Family Members" examines the relationship between family systems and health status. This chapter looks at how health factors within families influence the health of individual members and, conversely, how health factors within an individual family member influence the health of the family as a whole. The factors they specify are physical and psychological health, spirituality and religion, and legal and ethical issues and how these factors impact family policy. The resiliency model of family stress, adjustment, and adaptation is used to provide insight into factors that are important for evaluating how families adjust and adapt when faced with a member's illness.

Chapter 6, "Nursing Process and Family Health Care" summarizes the systematic steps of the nursing process and demonstrates how these ideas fit the paradigm of family nursing. In addition, two classification systems (NANDA and Omaha) are reviewed and used to define family health problems and concerns. Families' involvement in each step of the nursing process is emphasized.

Chapter 7, "Family Assessment and Intervention" expands on the concept of assessment as the first and essential ingredient to provide comprehensive family health care. It differentiates between assessment and measurement and then presents three different family nursing assessment models that can be used by clinicians in the field. These models are followed by a case example that demonstrates the different levels and scope of information that can be derived from using the various models and instruments.

Chapter 8, "Family Health Promotion" provides an overview of family health promotion, highlighting family health and illness cycles and models of family health and health promotion. The author points out that the nursing process is used as an approach to empower families to achieve optimum wellness and includes such activities as assessment, contracting, health teaching, and anticipatory guidance. Finally the implications for practice, education, family policy, and research are discussed in relation to family health promotion.

Unit II of this book contains eight chapters that examine family nursing practice. Following a general orientation, a chapter is devoted to each of the mainstream specialty areas within nursing.

Chapter 9, "Family Nursing and Health Care Settings" is an orientation to the various settings in which family nursing can be practiced. The multiple settings discussed in this chapter represent a cross section of health resources used by individuals and families.

Chapter 10, "Family Nursing with Childbearing Families" includes a brief history of family nursing with selected theories and an overview of nursing process; health promotion; threats to health; and implications for education, research, and policy. Emphasis is on health promotion in relation to developmental tasks of childbearing families. A case study of a family experiencing preterm birth is used to illustrate the impact of threat to health on childbearing families. Throughout the chapter, nursing interventions with childbearing families are emphasized.

Chapter 11, "Family Child Health Nursing" presents a history of family child-centered nursing and a family interaction model that includes concepts that guide nursing practice in the care of families with children. Application of this interactional model to four areas of practice is examined: health promotion, acute illness, chronic illness, and life-threatening illness. In addition, practice, education, research, and health care policy that are relevant to family child health nursing care is reviewed.

Chapter 12, "Family Nursing in Medical-Surgical Settings" describes factors and issues for nurses to consider as they plan care for families in medical-surgical settings. The topics addressed include: history of medical-surgical family nursing; families' stressors during hospitalization; the therapeutic quadrangle; application of family theoretical models; family needs during the pre-illness; acute, chronic, and terminal phases of care; and family nursing interventions.

Chapter 13, "Family Mental Health Nursing" provides a historical overview of trends in family mental health nursing, relating conceptual models to the practice of family mental health nursing. The focus is on acute and chronic mental illness as well as a section on health promotion. Strategies are identified that assist nurses in creating a healthy environment for families within any health care setting. Implications for practice, research, and health policy are discussed.

Chapter 14, "Gerontological Family Nursing" describes the partnership that nurses create with families to maintain optimal functioning, restore health, and prevent/reduce the negative effects of illness in its older members. A broad scope of practice is discussed including the multiple roles of family nurses and the variety of settings in which this practice occurs.

Chapter 15, "Families and Community Health Nursing" describes the practice of community health nursing and its interface with family nursing. This chapter includes a discussion of the historical roots of the care of families in the community; common theoretical perspectives in community family nursing; and nursing interventions that promote health, prevent disease, and provide care for acute and chronic illness within families. Implications for family community health nursing practice, education, research, and social policy are reviewed.

Chapter 16, "Family Nursing Practice in the Twenty-First Century" provides a brief overview of the American family and projects future demographic trends. The impact of health technology and the influence of health care reform on family nursing practice is explored. The implications of changing families and environments are discussed in relation to the practice of family nursing, research, and the development of theory.

The editors are grateful for the help and encouragement of the publisher, F. A. Davis Company, especially Melanie Freely, who stayed patient and brought her expertise to this project. We encourage anyone to write with critiques and ideas that could be included in the next edition of this textbook. We hope this book will serve as a catalyst that will encourage family nurses in thinking and doing.

Best wishes and happy reading.

Shirley May Harmon Hanson

Sheryl Thalman Boyd

Acknowledgments

The editors would like to acknowledge the many people who have contributed to this textbook on family health care nursing. First, we would like to thank the authors of the various chapters. They were hand picked to write because of their expertise in their respective areas. Second, we would like to thank various colleagues for their assistance in critiquing, editing, or offering expertise of a special nature—Naomi Ballard, Julia Brown, Marion Hemstrom, Jane Kirschling, Sheila Kodadek, Karen Mischke, Marie Napolitano, and Elizabeth Tornquist. Third, this book would not have become a reality without F. A. Davis Company and Melanie Freely. We have enjoyed working with each and every one of you and we believe we have moved the science and art of family nursing forward. Thank you all.

Shirley May Harmon Hanson

Sheryl Thalman Boyd

Consultants

Terry Allor, MPH, RN
University of Michigan
Ann Arbor, MI

Kathryn Anderson, RN, PhD
2335 Trilliam Drive
Eau Claire, WI

Kay Avant, RN, PhD, FAAN
University of Texas at Austin
7601 Tallahassee
Waco, TX

Sharon Beck, RN, MSN, EdM
LaSalle University
Philadelphia, PA

Elizabeth Dietz, RN, CS, EdD
San Jose State
605 Princeton Drive
Sunnyvale, CA

Jacqueline Fawcett, RN, PhD
University of Pennsylvania
720 Middle Turnpike
Storrs, CT

Margaret Frainier, RN, PhD
Niagara University
32 Elm Avenue
Buffalo, NY

Debra Hymovich, RN, PhD, FAAN
University of Southern Florida
Tampa, FL

Theresa Julian, RN, C, PhD
Ohio State University
Columbus, OH

Barbara Logan, RN, PhD, FAAN
University of Illinois at Chicago
Chicago, IL

Kay Lundy, RN, PhD
University of Southern Mississippi
89 J. Switzer Road
Purvis, MS

Ida Martinson, RN, PhD
University of California
Department of Family Health Care Nursing
Rm 411Y
San Francisco, CA

Sandy Mott, MS, RN, C
Boston College
11 Miller Road
Beverly, MA

Elizabeth Rudolph, MSC, RN
University of Nebraska Medical Center
College of Nursing
600 South 42nd Street
Omaha, NE

Janet Widell, MSN, RN, C
Auburn University
1011 Sanders Street
Auburn, AL

Judy Winterhalter, DNSc, RN, CS
Gwyned Mercy
461 Tailer Way
Lansdale, PA

Contributors

Nancy Trygar Artinian, PhD, RN
Associate Professor
Wayne State University
College of Nursing
Detroit, MI

Naomi R. Ballard, RN, MA, MS, CNRN
Oregon Health Sciences University
Individuals With Complex Illness
School of Nursing
Portland, OR

Perri J. Bomar, PhD, RN
Professor
East Carolina University
School of Nursing
Parent-Child Nursing Department
Greenville, NC

Sheryl Thalman Boyd, RN, PhD, FAAN
Associate Professor
School of Nursing
Oregon Health Sciences University
Portland, OR

Cecelia Capuzzi, RN, PhD
Oregon Health Sciences University
School of Nursing
Community Health Care
Portland, OR

Eleanor G. Ferguson-Marshalleck, RN, MPH
Professor of Nursing
California State University
Los Angeles, CA

Marilyn M. Friedman, RN, PhD
Professor of Nursing
Director, Pediatric Nurse Practitioner
   Program
California State University
Los Angeles, CA

Vivian Gedaly-Duff, RN, DNSc
Associate Professor
Oregon Health Sciences University
Family Nursing
School of Nursing
Portland, OR

Shirley May Harmon Hanson, RN, PMHNP,
   PhD, FAAN
Professor, School of Nursing
Oregon Health Sciences University
and
Private Practice
Licensed Child, Marriage, and Family
   Therapist
Portland, OR

Marsha L. Heims, RN, EdD
Associate Professor
Oregon Health Sciences University
School of Nursing
Portland, OR

Margaret A. Imle, RN, PhD
School of Nursing
Oregon Health Sciencies University
Portland, OR

Doris Julian, RN, EdD
Associate Professor, Emeritus
Oregon Health Sciences University
School of Nursing
Portland, OR

Louise Kelly Martell, RN, PhD
School of Nursing
University of Washington
Seattle, WA

Marilyn McCubbin, RN, PhD
Associate Professor
University of Wisconsin — Madison
School of Nursing
Madison, WI

Karen B. Mischke, PhD, OGNP/WHCNP, CFLE
Hillsboro Women's Health Clinic
Hillsboro, OR

Helene J. Moriarty, PhD, RN, CS
Assistant Professor
Villanova University
College of Nursing
Villanova, PA
and
Nurse Researcher
Veterans Affairs Medical Center
Philadelphia, PA

Beverly S. Richards, RN, DNS
Associate Professor
School of Nursing
Department of Psychiatric Mental Health
    Nursing
Indiana University
Indianapolis, IN

Beverly J. Ross, RN, MANEd, MSEd
Assistant Professor of Nursing
Indiana University
School of Nursing
Indianapolis, IN

Margaret P. Shepard, PhD, RN
Assistant Professor
University of Rochester
School of Nursing
Rochester, NY

Marcia Van Riper, RN, PhD
Assistant Professor
Ohio State University
College of Nursing
Columbus, OH

Special material contributed by

Marion Hemstrom, RN, DNSc
Drake University
Family Health Department
Des Moines, IA

Contents

Credits for Photographs

U N I T

I

Foundations of Family Health Care Nursing

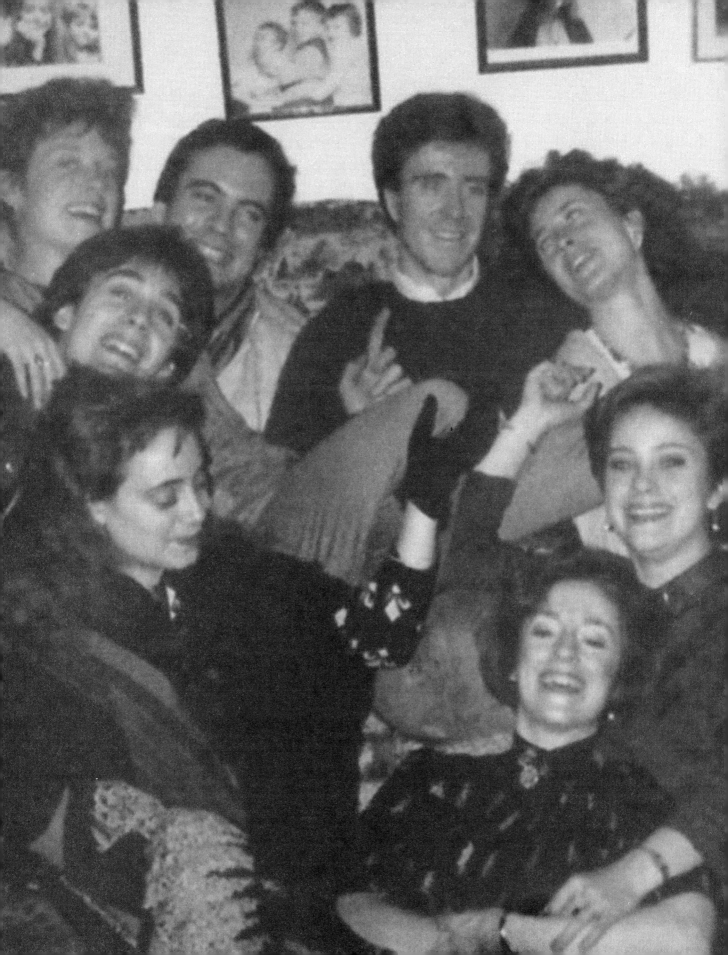

Family Nursing: An Overview

This chapter introduces you to one of the most important clients in nursing practice today, the human family. If you are a typical nursing student, the focus of your education has been the practice of nursing with individual clients. In this chapter you will get to know the family client, the first of many aggregate clients you will encounter in professional nursing practice.

Because we all have families, many of you may question the need for special study in this area of nursing. You may have assumed that nursing practice is uniform for individuals with similar nursing diagnoses. You are reminded, however, that nursing is an interpersonal profession, and that just as nurses' personal characteristics affect individual client relationships, so too nurses' experiences and assumptions from their families of origin influence their interaction with the family client. For this reason professional nursing demands an objective, as well as a personal, basis for family practice.

In addition to the curiosity and energy characteristic of most nursing students, the authors expect that you bring to this textbook a background in natural sciences, social sciences, and humanities, all of which will assist you to understand the complex family client.

We begin with a broad overview of family nursing, which will provide you with the "big picture" regarding this important area of nursing. A thorough discussion of the history of the family and family health will help you to appreciate the complexity of this client. The chapter proceeds with an examination of the development of family nursing and of the roles of family nurses and closes with a discussion of the state of the art, and of family nursing practice, research, and education. At this point we hope that your questions regarding the need to study family nursing will have been answered, and that you will discover challenging new insights as you study this book.

CHAPTER 1

Family Nursing: An Overview

Shirley May Harmon Hanson, RN, PMHNP, PhD, FAAN ■
Sheryl Thalman Boyd, RN, PhD, FAAN

OUTLINE

FAMILY NURSING
What Is the Family?
What Is Family Health Care Nursing?
Why Learn About Family Health Care Nursing?

HISTORY OF THE FAMILY
Prehistoric Family Life
European History
Industrialization to Present Day
American Families
Families Today

CHANGING DEMOGRAPHICS OF AMERICAN FAMILIES
Family Variation
Marriages
Singleness
Divorces
Remarriages and Stepparenting
Skip-Generation Families
Single-Parent Families

FUNCTIONS OF FAMILY
Traditional Functions
Contemporary Functions

FAMILY HEALTH
What Is Family Health?
Healthy Families

FAMILY HEALTH PERSPECTIVES
The Family Health and Illness Cycle
Levels of Family Care
When to Assemble the Family in Health Care
The Therapeutic Triangle in Health Care

DEVELOPMENT OF FAMILY NURSING
Conceptual Models for Family Nursing
Interventions in Family Nursing
Approaches to Family Nursing
Variables Influencing Family Nursing
Obstacles to Family Nursing Practice

FAMILY NURSING ROLES

STATE OF THE ART AND SCIENCE OF FAMILY NURSING
Family Nursing Practice
Family Nursing Research
Family Nursing Education

LEVELS OF PREPARATION FOR FAMILY NURSING

OBJECTIVES *Upon completion of this chapter, the reader will be able to:*

1. Explain why it is important for nurses to focus on the family.
2. Define family, family health, and family healthcare nursing.
3. Describe the changing demographics of American families and the implications of these changes for the future of family nursing.
4. Describe the interactions between families and the health/illness continuum.
5. Compare and contrast four different views of families.
6. Summarize the history of the modern family and family nursing.
7. Differentiate between family theory, family therapy, and family nursing.
8. Name the various health professionals involved in family health care and describe the roles of the family nurse.

FAMILY NURSING

Family nursing is an emerging field, upon which great talent and effort have been expended during the last 10 years. There are now a number of textbooks that focus on family nursing, and family content is included in both undergraduate and graduate curricula. Renowned family nursing scholars all over the world, particularly in the United States and Canada, publish articles in an array of scientific journals, including a journal called the *Journal of Family Nursing*. Though family nursing has come a long way, we must continue to (1) classify and describe the elements in family nursing, (2) build the science of family nursing, and (3) develop theories from clinical practice to explain and guide nursing and family interactions in health and illness (Gilliss, 1990). We will begin this examination of family nursing by identifying the meaning of the much-used term, "family."

What Is the Family?

"Family" is a word that conjures up different images for different individuals. Depending on the discipline, some definitions focus on a specific aspect of the family. For example, the legal definition of family emphasizes relationships through blood ties, adoption, guardianship, or marriage, whereas the biological definition focuses on genetic biological networks among people. Sociologists define the family as a group of people living together; psychologists define it as a group with strong emotional ties.

The US Bureau of the Census has used the same definition for years: the family is a group of two or more persons related by blood, marriage, or adoption and residing together. Taking a similar approach, early family social science theorists (Burgess & Locke, 1953) adopted the following definition: "The family is a group of persons united by ties of marriage, blood, or adoption, constituting a single household; interacting and communicating with each other in their respective social roles of husband and wife, mother and father, son and daughter, brother and sister; and creating and maintaining a common culture" (pp. 7–8). The early *family nursing* scholars also used a similar definition.

It was not until the 1980s that the definitions of family moved beyond the traditional ties of blood, marriage, or legal adoption. In 1985, one of the first family nursing departments in the country adopted this definition: "The family is a social *system* composed of two or more persons who coexist within the context of some expectations of reciprocal affection, mutual responsibility, and temporal duration. The family is characterized by commitment, mutual decision making and shared goals" (Department of Family Nursing, Oregon Health Sciences University, 1985).

The definition of the family used in this book is even broader: *Family refers to two or more individuals who depend on one another for emotional, physical, and/or economic support. The members of the family are self-defined.*

Nurses working with families should first ask their clients whom they consider to be their family and then include those people in health care planning. The family may range from the traditional nuclear and extended family to such postmodern family structures as single-parent families, blended families, and same-gender families. In a recent study, Ford (1994) asked people what they thought "family" meant. She found that young people's definitions of family included a variety of possibilities such as cohabitating couples without children, same-gender partners, and certain extended groups. Interestingly, the women Ford questioned were more likely than men to consider nontraditional groups as families. Ford suggests that there will be even more alternative family forms in the future and advises professionals to explore their own perceptions and definitions of families so that they can work more effectively with alternative family structures.

What Is Family Health Care Nursing?

Family nursing cuts across the various other specialty areas of nursing, but there is still some disagreement about how it differs from other specialties that involve families, such as maternal/child health nursing, community health nursing, or mental health nursing. In this book family healthcare nursing is defined as: *the process of providing for the health care needs of families that are within the scope of nursing practice. Family nursing can be aimed at the family as context, the family as a whole, the family as a system, or the family as a component of society.*

Why Learn About Family Health Care Nursing?

Why should nurses learn about families? Most people believe they are already experts in the family, having had personal experience with their own family of origin. Unfortunately, based on such limited experience, nurses may make erroneous assumptions and judgments about the families they work with. This is because when nurses operate only from their own family experience, they have a view of families that is ethnocentric — based on their own socialization, culture, and value systems. The goal of this book is to provide students with a broad understanding of families and useful information on theory, practice, and research in the nursing care of families.

Why is it important for nurses to focus on the family? Because research shows that (1) health and illness behaviors are learned within the context of the family (Pratt, 1976); (2) family units are affected when one or more members experience health problems, and the family is a significant factor in the health and well-being of individuals (Gilliss, 1993); (3) families affect an individual's health, and an individual's health and health practices affect the family (Doherty, 1985a; Doherty & McCubbin, 1985; Doherty & Campbell, 1988); (4) health care is more effective when it emphasizes the family rather than the individual alone (Gilliss & Davis, 1993); and (5) promotion, maintenance, and restoration of the health of families are important to society's survival (Anderson & Tomlinson, 1992). Also there is growing recognition that health crises are critical events in the life of a family. When such crises occur, the mental and physical health of family members may deteriorate and the family's functioning may deteriorate as well; however, families also have opportunities to increase their adaptive capacity and mental health during a crisis, and family nurses can provide supportive interventions to help them during these critical events.

Although families have been recipients of nursing care for many years, the family is now widely perceived to be the unit of care or the context of care. The centrality of the family in health care delivery is emphasized by the American Nurses' Association (ANA,

1995) and by the legal definitions of nursing in many states, which mandate that nurses provide family as well as individual care.

HISTORY OF THE FAMILY

Understanding the history of families is important for understanding family nursing. The past helps to explain the present realities of family life; also, understanding of family history helps to enlighten or dispel preferences for those forms that are personally familiar and can thus broaden the nurse's view of the world of families.

Prehistoric Family Life

Archaeologists and anthropologists have found evidence of family life before the time of written history. Ancient family forms varied from those of the present but the functions of the family have remained more or less constant. Families have always constituted the basic unit of society and family structure, process, and function have always been a response to everyday needs. As communities grew and civilization developed, families became more institutionalized and homogeneous, reflecting the culture, that is, the shared values and attitudes derived from membership in a particular group.

The earliest human matings tended to be permanent and monogamous. Indeed, men and women dyads are the oldest and most tenacious unit in history, which is perhaps why the "nuclear" family has dominated modern experience. Biologically immature humans need care and protection longer than other animals, and this necessity has led humans to long-term relationships. The necessity for care does not dictate family structure, but family structure is essential for the activity of parenting.

In most societies, reproductive pairing led to the creation of a nurturing pair, the economic unit, gender role differentiation, and ultimately, socialization. Early in history, children became part of the family economic unit. A variety of skills were needed for living and no single person could perform all of them, so male and female role differentiation began.

As small groups of conjugal families formed communities, the complexity of the social order increased. This in turn changed the family.

European History

Many Americans are of European ancestry. In the European social structure of the past, authority was concentrated in a few individuals (almost all men) at the top of a hierarchical structure (kings, lords, fathers). Families emphasized consanguineous (genetic) bonds; the heads of families were always men; family property was transferred through the male line; and in the eyes of the law women and children were considered property. Marriage was a contract between families, not individuals, and because women left home to join their husband's family, the establishment of a strong mother-daughter bond was not prevalent. These patriarchal family characteristics prevailed until the advent of industrialism.

Industrialization to Present Day

The Industrial Revolution began in England about 1750 and then spread to Western Europe and North America. Until this time, multigenerational families living in close proximity had always been the norm. But now families left farms to move into the cities and men went to work in the factories, leaving women at home to maintain the house and care for the children. At the same time, the Protestant ethic promoted the idea that the individual, not the family, was paramount; that is, salvation became an individual decision by choice rather than automatically guaranteed by church or family affiliation.

When more factories began to be built, people began to move about. The state began to provide services that families had once performed for their members. At the same time, the state codified into law a man's power and authority over their families, and in exchange men gave the state their loyalty and service. Women were not expected to love their husbands, but to obey them. Some feminists suggest that it is hard to separate love and submission and think that the introduction of love into human consciousness served as a powerful force to limit female activity.

Society today is still struggling with the remnants of patriarchal family life. Women are still struggling to escape from the rules and expectations of the state, of men, and of themselves. The women's movement in general, and the National Organization for Women (NOW) in particular, have improved the lives of women in present-day America. However, more work needs to be done to make all Americans equal.

In recent years, men have begun to identify the bondage they experience. They cannot meet all the needs of their families and therefore feel inadequate. This is especially true of men who do not have access to money and occupational status through education (e.g., African-American men). A men's movement is now promoting male causes, although this movement is not yet very dynamic. One of the organizations supporting this work is the National Congress for Men.

American Families

America did not share the history of Europe's preindustrialized age, and English patriarchy was not transplanted in its pure form to America. Instead, American society and families were molded from the beginning by economic logic. In the new world, both women and men had to labor and this fact gave women new power. Moreover, in the United States, status was achieved rather than inherited through familial lines.

Children also experienced a new status in American families. Originally, they were part of the family economic unit and worked on farms. Then in the early 1900s, parents began to think they could create a better world for their children through education. So each generation of children obtained more education and income than their parents, and most left the family farms and moved to faraway cities. This change, which has now occurred in other Westernized countries as well, is currently taking place in developing countries. For example, in Korea, Seoul has grown from 2 to 14 million people in one decade, largely due to the migration of young people to the cities for work and education. In these circumstances, parents no longer have any assurance that their children will take care of them during their old age.

Accompanying these developments have been changes in the functions of families in American society. For example, with the burgeoning of cities, adolescents who had previously worked on family farms lost their productive function. Because teenagers could not hold jobs in the cities, due to labor laws pertaining to children, the public school system was created, largely to help keep adolescents off the streets. This development is an example of how societal institutions have taken over many of the traditional roles of families, particularly their socialization functions. Although these institutions (churches, schools, social agencies) attempt to strengthen families, many of them are a source of strain on the families.

Families Today

Families cannot be viewed separately from the larger system of which they are a part, nor can they be separated from their history. For example, today's employers (military or civilian) move families around for the sake of optimizing production. This reduces social support and security, so that people turn to their immediate families for support instead of feeling a part of a larger extended family or community. This situation promotes intense familial interactions that result in unrealistic expectations regarding family members. Such isolation is one of the factors contributing to the high incidence of abuse among military families.

Some people argue that the family today is in terrible shape, like a rudderless ship in the dark. Idealizing past family arrangements and decrying change have become commonplace in the public media. Yet other people hail the changes that have occurred in families and approve the current diversity and options. Just as some families—both past and present—have engaged in behaviors destructive to individuals and to other social institutions, other families have provided healthy environments for individuals to grow and live. It is true that the sphere of activity of families is diminishing; however, although the structure, function, and processes of families have changed, the institution called "the family" survives. It is in fact the most tenacious unit in society.

CHANGING DEMOGRAPHICS OF AMERICAN FAMILIES

Major changes are taking place in American families today, with dramatic effects on family life and family health. Notable trends reported by the US Bureau of the Census (1989a,b,c,d; 1991a,b; 1992a,b,c,d) include increases in divorce, remarriage, age at first marriage, labor force participation of women, and delays and declines in childbearing. These developments have altered the structure, process, and function of American families in the span of just one generation. Today's families are smaller than 20 years ago, and they are more likely to be maintained by a single parent, to have multiple wage earners, to require child care assistance, and to contain stepchildren (Tables 1–1 and 1–2). Individual and family trajectories involve many more transitions today as people form, dissolve, and reform families.

TABLE 1–1

FAMILY DEMOGRAPHICS*

Type of Family	1970	1990	2000
Married with children (%)	49	36.9	34
Married without children (%)	37.1	41.7	42.8
Single-parent families (%)			
Female 88%	5.7	10.2	9.7
Male 12%	0.07	1.8	2.7
Same-sex households (%)	2	2	
Unmarried couples (cohabitation)	520,000	3 million	
People living alone (%)	20	30	
Births to single mothers (%)	11	27	

*Figures given as percentages of total number of households.
SOURCE: From *Current population reports*, Series P-20, No. 218, US Bureau of the Census, 1990.

TABLE 1–2

FAMILY COMPOSITION IN THE UNITED STATES, 1970–2000*

Type of Family	1970	1990	1995	2000
All families*	51.2	64.5	68.0	71.7
Total (%)	100.0	100.0	100.0	100.0
Married couple with children (%)	49.6	36.9	36.2	34.5
Married couple without children (%)	37.1	36.9	41.8	42.8
Female head with children (%)	5.7	10.2	10.0	9.7
Male head with children (%)	0.7	1.8	2.2	2.7
Other families (%)	6.9	9.4	9.8	10.3

*Figures given in millions.
SOURCE: From "New realities of the American Family," by D. A. Ahlburg & C. J. Vita, 1992, *Population Bulletin, 47*, p. 7. Copyright 1992 by the Population Referral Bureau, Washington, DC. Reprinted with permission.

Family Variation

In the past families were more homogeneous than they are today. The norm was a two-parent family living together with their biological children. Table 1–2 shows how families have changed from 1970 to 1990 and what we can expect in the year 2000. The percentage of families made up of married couples with children declined from 49% in 1970 to 37% in 1990 and is projected to decrease further to 35% in the year 2000. The percentage of couples without children will increase from 37% to 43% by the year 2000. All kinds of single-parent families have increased substantially. Births to single mothers (largely unmarried teens) have increased from 11% to 27% of all live births. Same-sex "households" stay steady at 2% of American families. It is apparent that married couples with children are decreasing, whereas married couples without children are increasing, single-parent families are increasing, and single fatherhood is becoming more common. Other family forms are also increasing, for example, families with foster children, skip-generation families (grandparents raising grandchildren), gay families, and so forth.

Marriages

The total number of marriages in the United States reached an all-time high in 1984 (2.4 million) and has leveled off since then. About two thirds of all marriages are first marriages and one third are remarriages (US Bureau of the Census, 1989a,b,c,d, 1991a,b, 1992a,b,c,d). Ninety percent of all people marry at some point in their lives, but the percentage of never-married women who eventually marry decreases with age. The median age for first marriage of women (24.1 years) and men (26.3 years) has moved up in recent years, approximating the figures at the turn of the century (US Bureau of the Census, 1992). One fourth of women who marry do so by 20 years of age and three fourths marry by 28 years of age. Thus, marriage for women is becoming a less age-concentrated event (US Bureau of the Census, 1989c).

Singleness

The proportion of men and women in their twenties and early thirties who have never married has grown substantially during the past two decades. The percentages of singles in these age groups have nearly tripled for both women and men, and are even higher for African-Americans and Hispanics (US Bureau of the Census, 1989d). The percentage of married persons declined from 72% to 61% between 1970 and 1991, while the percentage of unmarried persons rose to 39% (US Bureau of the Census, 1992b).

This vast rise in the number of single adults has occurred both because young adults are postponing marriage and because many are becoming single again through divorce. Also, elderly persons may find themselves single because of the death of their spouse, and there is an increasing divorce rate among older couples. Although singleness may be viewed as a temporary state (90% of people marry and of those who divorce, about 75% remarry), single people have needs for public and private sector services and these needs are unique. They include child care and economic equity for single parents, education and work opportunities for young adults, and housing and health care for the elderly, all of which are important issues for the well-being of the American people.

Interestingly, an increasing number of young adults are living with their parents today. Three out of 10 unmarried adults aged 25 to 29 years live in the home of their parents (US Bureau of the Census, 1992b,c), mainly due to the postponement of first marriage. This is creating a new kind of multigenerational family.

Divorces

The number of divorces has been increasing for years in the United States and is currently over 1.1 million per year. The prevalence of divorce varies within the population. Young adults most commonly experience divorce, the mean age at divorce being 34 years, and divorce rates are higher for African-Americans and Hispanics than for whites. In recent years, there has been an upward trend in divorce among couples over 60 years old, whose marriages survived many years before divorce. This despite the fact that divorce occurs most frequently after 7 years of marriage. The divorced state is generally temporary in nature, as about 75% of divorced persons remarry after a median interval of about 2 years, although 75% of these second marriages also end in divorce. If current divorce levels persist, approximately 50% to 60% of all recent marriages will end in divorce (Norton, 1992).

About two thirds of all divorces involve one or more children, so that, each year, more than 660,000 children experience the divorce of their parents. Most of these children are toddlers, preschoolers, or school-age children.

Remarriages and Stepparenting

An increasing number of children are living in stepparent or remarried families by the time they reach 16 years of age. One fourth of families (4.5 million) have at least one stepchild living in the household (US Bureau of the Census, 1989c,d). Most stepchildren live with biological mothers and stepfathers rather than stepmothers and biological fathers.

Skip-Generation Families

In the 1990s there has been an increase in what is termed the "skip-generation family": that is, children are being raised primarily by their grandparents for a number of reasons — mothers are working, parents are incapacitated by drugs, or the children are "throwaway" kids. In the most recent census, the number of children raised by their grandparents was 2.9 million, or 5% of all children under 18 years (US Bureau of the Census, 1989c,d). African-American children are more likely to live with grandparents than white children.

Single-Parent Families

Single-parent families are created through (1) divorce, (2) births out of wedlock, (3) spousal absenteeism, (4) death of a spouse, and (5) adoption (Hanson, Heims, Julian, & Sussman, 1995a–d). The proportion of single-parent households doubled from 1970 (12%) to 1992 (27%). Today, almost 4 out of every 10 children in the United States are either currently living with a single parent or have lived with one in the past (Bianchi, 1994). In addition to the 27% of children currently in single-parent households, another 11% are living with one biological parent and one stepparent (Saluter, 1991). While the increase in divorce fueled the growth in one-parent families in the 1960s and 1970s, delayed marriage and childbearing outside marriage contributed far more to the growth in mother-child families during the 1980s than did marital disruption. Eighty-six percent of single-parent households are headed by women. During the 1980s, however, father-child families increased more than mother-child families. By 1990, almost one in five single-parent families was maintained by a father, although only 3% of all children lived in this type of household (Bianchi, 1994). Projections are that half of the children born today will spend time living apart from one or both biological parents (Fig. 1–1).

Single parenting by unmarried mothers is much higher within the African-American community than the white community and racial differences in these percentages were

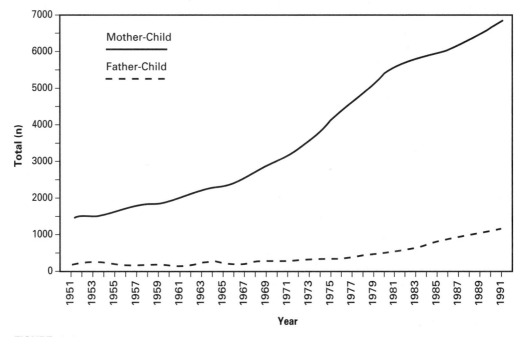

FIGURE 1–1
Growth in the number of mother-child and father-child families from 1951 to 1991. (From "The Changing Demographic and Socioeconomic Characteristics of Single-Parent Families," by S. M. Bianchi, *Marriage and Family Review*, 22: pp. 1–4, with permission.)

larger at the beginning of the 1990s than a generation earlier. While two thirds of white children currently live with both biological parents, only one quarter of African-American children do so (Bianchi, 1994). Far more African-American (54%) and Hispanic (30%) than white children (19%) live in single-parent households.

Compared with two-parent families, single-parent families are disadvantaged in terms of economic status, health, and housing conditions. The average income for families with two parents in 1990 was $41,260, while the income for single-father households was $25,211, and for single-mother households $13,092. The difference in income for single-father and single-mother households reflects the gap in men's and women's incomes; women earn two thirds of what men make. Many single-mother households are poor, and children living with never-married mothers are the most economically disadvantaged group of children (Bianchi, 1994). Of the 33 million Americans who are currently classified as poor, 13 million are children, and of these poor children 500,000 are homeless (Smith & Cutright, 1985).

Census figures afford a more detailed picture of mother-child households. There are 10 million single-mother households in the United States. Of these 58% are awarded child support (US Bureau of the Census, 1991a) and 32% are poor. The average child support payment is approximately $2995 per year and represents about 11% of the family income (US Bureau of the Census, 1989b; 1991a). Of women who are due payments, about half receive the full amount, the rest receive partial payment or nothing. The majority of absent fathers (55%) have visitation privileges and 7% have joint custody, while 38% have neither visitation nor custody rights. A volume recently published on single-parent families summarizes the latest theory, practice, and research on the various types of single-parent families (Hanson, Heims, Julian, & Sussman, 1995 a–d).

FUNCTIONS OF FAMILY

Traditional Functions

Throughout history, a number of functions have traditionally been performed by families. Six of these functions are summarized in the following discussion, not necessarily in the order of their importance. First, families have existed to *achieve economic survival*. Before the Industrial Revolution in Western Europe, all the members of most families worked on farms. Later, men were breadwinners, earning wages either through self-employment or working for others, while women were helpmates, homemakers, and nurturers of children. Until this century, families had many children for economic reasons: more children meant more wealth because they could work the land, and children also took care of their parents in old age. The children of earlier centuries did not experience what we think of as adolescence. Instead, they worked in the family business as mini-adults and stayed home until they married. The family was an economic unit to which all members contributed and from which everyone benefited.

Second, families existed *to reproduce the species*. Not many people elected to stay childless; they bore or adopted children. There was strong social pressure against sexual activity and childbearing outside of marriage. If unmarried women became pregnant, they were stigmatized and sent away to homes for unwed mothers.

Third, families *provided protection* from hostile forces. Family members protected those who could not protect themselves, such as the very young, the very old, and the handicapped. Family groups immigrated together to avoid hostile cultures and formed ethnic blankets (ghettoes) in an "us against you" world.

Fourth, *passing along the religious faith (culture)* was an important function for families. Families passed on religious stories, doctrines, traditions, and values. Significant family events such as births, baptisms, marriages, and death were ritualized, and faith was an integral part of daily family life.

A fifth function of families was *to educate (socialize) the young*. Boys worked with their fathers to learn trades or take over family farms, while girls worked with their mothers to learn homemaking and parenting. In young America children were largely taught by their parents. They learned to read from religious books like the *Bible* and *The Pilgrim's Progress*, an endeavor that produced faith and staved off ignorance, and they learned to use the gun to procure game for the table and to protect the family.

A sixth function of families was *to confer status*. In Europe, it was difficult to change status in society. If a person's father was a respected blacksmith, the son was expected to become one also. Similarly, if the father was the town drunk, the son had little chance to become something else. An untarnished family name was especially important in a non-mobile society. Many people immigrated to America to seek new opportunities (as well as riches) that their family names could not provide in the old country.

Families that performed all of these six functions were considered healthy or good. A "good family" was self-sufficient, did not ask for help from others, supported community institutions, was untainted by failure, starved before they went on welfare, and met the "good family" criteria of the community and church. That is, they looked good to the outside world. People paid little attention to what went on inside the family. Society was not concerned about good communication, emotional support, or trusting relationships. They were concerned about meeting visible family standards set by the community such as married parents, religious affiliation, affluence, home ownership, and community respect.

Contemporary Functions

In contemporary times, the functions of families have changed, and new ones have been added. First, the *economic* function of families has changed dramatically. Family members do not need each other to stay financially afloat as they did in the past. A woman does not need to stay married to a man for food, shelter, or respectability, nor need a man marry to have someone cook and clean for him. The spinster aunt has been replaced by the career woman. Now that over 50 percent of women with young children work outside the home, children are no longer economic assets but costly luxuries. Government programs such as Medicare, Social Security, Aid to Families with Dependent Children, and welfare help subsidize families economically, and some social reformers are even promoting a guaranteed income for all. Thus, families are no longer the basis of economic security.

The *reproductive function* of families has also changed in recent years. Sexual activity is more common among people of all ages and a whole complement of birth control measures are available, so that reproduction does not necessarily take place within the boundaries of the traditional family. For example, one third of live births in the United States today occur to women who are not married. Also, women who were infertile in the past have benefited from fertility drugs and other technology so that they can now bear children.

Third, the *protective functions* of families are no longer as important as they used to be. Social, welfare, and law enforcement agencies have largely taken over the protection of society. When families are not willing or able to protect their offspring, society takes over for them. For example, if parents are suspected of child abuse, the children are removed from the home and sent to foster parents. Also, because not all families protect their children against diseases, the society has recently mandated immunization for children.

Fourth, the responsibility for *passing on religious faith* has been largely relegated to churches and synagogues. Further, American culture has become more secular, and less religion is passed on to younger generations.

Fifth, the *education and socialization functions* of families have been largely transferred to public and private school systems. The majority of mothers and fathers work outside the home and place their children in day care and preschool until they are of school age. Further, the teaching that had traditionally taken place in the home has been eroded by television. Educators complain that too much responsibility has been placed in the hands of teachers and that families are delinquent in socialization.

Sixth, the family is no longer needed to *confer status*. If you are a Rockefeller or Kennedy your family name may be helpful, but for the majority of Americans, family heritage is not essential for success. Status today is gained through education, occupation, income, and address.

Several new functions have become prominent in families. The *relationship function* has become more important for contemporary families: People marry so they can love and be loved, instead of to meet basic needs; couples join in a search for intimacy, not protection; parents have children to connect to posterity rather than to be taken care of in their old age. In short, because the needs of basic sustenance have been met, this generation is able to focus on the quality of their relationships and families may define themselves on the basis of relationships, rather than by blood relationships or legal criteria. If our relational needs are not met in our families, we search elsewhere. If we are lonely or unhappy in our relationships, we seek alternatives through infidelity or divorce, through work, volunteerism, chemical dependency, or alienation. The focus on relationship has become paramount in contemporary families.

The *health function* of families has also become more evident in contemporary society. Researchers have recently noted the interaction between the health of individuals and the health of families. The family helps to keep its members well by passing along attitudes, beliefs, and habits that promote health and by caring for the ill. The family is thus the genesis of a lifetime of physical and mental health or lack thereof.

In sum, the functions that families serve have evolved and changed over time. Some have become more important and others less so. It is clear that not all traditional families were "good" families and not all contemporary families are having problems. Over the centuries our families have had their problems and strengths.

FAMILY HEALTH

What Is Family Health?

The World Health Organization (1992) has defined health as a state of complete physical, mental, and social well-being, and not merely the absence of disease and infirmity. This definition could apply to families as well as individuals; however, there is no consensus on what family health is and no precise definition of the term. Family health has been described as a state or process of the whole person in interaction with the environment, and the family represents a significant factor in the environment (Anderson & Tomlinson, 1992). Anderson and Tomlinson (1992) further said, ". . . the analysis of family health must include simultaneously both health and illness and the individual and the collective." There is growing evidence, for example, that when a family member is seriously ill, this has a powerful influence on family function and health, and that conversely families' behavior patterns can influence individual health (Campbell, 1986).

The term "family health" is often used interchangeably with the terms "family functioning," "healthy families," or "familial health." Some people define family health as the composite of individual family members' health, because it is impossible to characterize the physical health of a whole family at once. A "healthy" family is considered one that is functioning well in society, but this may or may not have much to do with physical health (Hanson, 1985). The term "unhealthy/dysfunctional family" is often used to refer to families who are mentally unhealthy, which may not have anything to do with physical health.

McEwan (1992) says that "family health" refers to the health status of the individuals within the family and that "familial health" is an evaluative description of the functions and structures of the family, with a dual focus on both the health of individual members and the health of the family as a whole.

Hanson (1985) defined family health as "a dynamic changing relative state of well-being, which includes the biological, psychological, spiritual, sociological, and cultural factors of the family system." This bio/psycho/socio/cultural/spiritual approach is useful for individual members as well as the family unit. An individual's health affects the entire family's functioning and, in turn, the family's functioning affects individuals' health. Thus, assessment of family health involves simultaneous assessment of individual family members and the family as a whole. Family nursing includes health promotion as well as treatment of chronic and acute illness.

Healthy Families

Various terms have been used to describe healthy families or family strengths. Otto (1963) developed criteria for assessing family strengths and emphasized the need to focus on positive family attributes instead of accentuating family weaknesses. Pratt (1976) introduced the idea of the energized family as one that encourages and supports persons to develop their capacities for full functioning and independent action. Curran (1983, 1985) looked not only at family stressors but at traits of healthy families; a list of these traits appears in Table 1 - 3.

TABLE 1–3

TRAITS OF HEALTHY FAMILIES

The healthy family—
    Communicates and listens
    Fosters table time and conversation
    Affirms and supports one another
    Teaches respect for others
    Develops a sense of trust
    Has a sense of play and humor
    Has a balance of interaction among members
    Shares leisure time
    Exhibits a sense of shared responsibility
    Teaches a sense of right and wrong
    Abounds in rituals and traditions
    Shares a religious core
    Respects the privacy of one another
    Values service to others
    Admits to and seeks help with problems

SOURCE: From *Traits of a Healthy Family*, by D. Curran, 1983, Minneapolis, MN: Winston Press. Copyright 1983 by Winston Press. Reprinted with permission.

FAMILY HEALTH PERSPECTIVES

Family social scientists have developed a number of views of family health care that are pertinent for family nursing. Four of these perspectives are presented below: the family health and illness cycle, levels of family care, when to assemble the family in health care, and the therapeutic triangle in health care (Doherty, 1985; Doherty & McCubbin, 1985; Doherty & Campbell, 1988).

The Family Health and Illness Cycle

The family health and illness cycle (Fig. 1–2) represents a series of temporal phases in the family's efforts to reduce the risks of illness, manage the initial onset of illness, and adapt to illness. The phases in the cycle represent different states of health and illness.

One phase of the cycle in which family nurses work is *family health promotion and risk reduction*. In this phase the emphasis is on environmental, social, psychological, and interpersonal factors that promote the family's health and reduce risk. These factors include family beliefs and activities that help individuals avoid behaviors that increase the likelihood of becoming ill, such as poor diet, lack of exercise, or smoking. Nurses can do a lot to promote family health and reduce risk.

Another part of the cycle that nurses get involved with is the phase of *family vulnerability and illness onset*, when life events and experiences render family members susceptible to illness or relapses of chronic illness. For example, nurses work with the family to reduce the stress associated with relapses or exacerbations of chronic disorders (e.g., diabetes, multiple sclerosis, or schizophrenia). Support groups represent one nursing strategy for dealing with family members who have chronic illness (e.g., a cancer support group for women).

A third part of the cycle pertinent to family nursing is *family illness appraisal*. This determines what meaning families give to the individual's symptoms and whether the

Family Health and Illness Cycle

Phase 1. Family health promotion and risk reduction

Phase 2. Family vulnerability and illness onset

Phase 3. Family illness appraisal

Phase 4. Family acute response

Phase 5. Family and health care system

Phase 6. Family adaption to illness

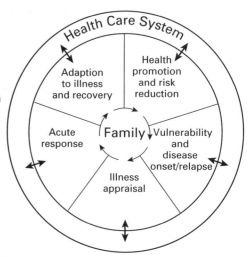

FIGURE 1–2

Family health and illness cycle. (From "Families and Health Care: An Emerging Arena of Theory, Research, and Clinical Intervention," by W. J. Doherty and H. I. McCubbin, 1985, *Family Relations*, 349, pp. 5–11, with permission.)

family is amenable to intervention. Nurses often intervene to help families cope with a difficult situation before it becomes critical. For example, they may lead groups for depressed adolescents to prevent them from committing suicide.

The *family's acute response* refers to the period immediately following a diagnosis of illness in a family member, and this is also an important area of intervention for family nurses. After an extraordinary event such as a heart attack or a diagnosis of cancer, families go through a crisis period and disorganization, and family nurses can intervene to help them cope with the crisis.

Next, there is *family adaptation to illness*, which refers to the role of the family in facilitating recovery or adaptation of individual members to illness. Families must adapt to the demands of a chronic condition; and a great deal of information has been accumulated on family coping and family compliance with medical regimens. Family nurses try to help families promote the recovery of ill members, while nurturing other family members and maintaining family functions. For example, the nurse might help the family find respite care for the family member who is the primary caregiver for an ill elderly relative, so that this caregiver does not burn out.

Finally, the *family and healthcare system* refers to the family's decision either to seek outside help for an illness or to handle it within the family. Family help-seeking behavior can take place in any phase of the family health and illness cycle, and the resources sought may include everything from traditioinal medical care to nontraditional modalities of health care.

Levels of Family Care

Doherty (1985), a family social scientist, proposes that health provider involvement when caring for families forms a continuum that can be divided into four levels. This continuum is also useful for family nursing.

At level 1, families are contacted only when necessary for practical or legal reasons. For example, a hospital intensive care nurse might contact the family to get a no resuscitation order signed. Nurses require little knowledge or skill in family nursing to handle this level of care.

At level 2, medical information and advice are given by generalist family nurses through regular contacts with families. The nurse may answer questions or advise families on managing care. For example, a clinic nurse might work with a family on diabetic foot care for an elderly patient.

At level 3, family nurses provide support and help families deal with feelings based on their knowledge of normal family development and the ways in which families react to stress. The family nurse encourages family members to discuss their reactions and supports them in their coping efforts. Care is individualized to the particular family. For example, the nurse may make a home visit to help family members cope with the situation when a newly discharged paraplegic patient goes home for the first time.

At level 4, systematic assessment of families and planning interventions, the nurse must understand family systems, be aware of the nurse's own family system, and understand the larger systems within which families and healthcare providers operate. More knowledge and skills are required for this level of care, and usually the nurse has graduate training. For example, a clinical nurse specialist in an inpatient acute setting may coordinate care for a trauma patient with multiple injuries, and this coordination will involve dealing with the family as well as other health care providers.

Level 5, the most complex level of care, requires advanced knowledge of family systems and patterns of dysfunctional interaction, and skill in working with dysfunctional

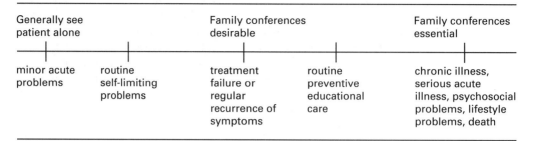

Generally see patient alone			Family conferences desirable			Family conferences essential
minor acute problems	routine self-limiting problems		treatment failure or regular recurrence of symptoms	routine preventive educational care		chronic illness, serious acute illness, psychosocial problems, lifestyle problems, death

FIGURE 1–3
When to assemble the family in health care.

families. The nurse who works at this level is a specialist in psychiatric mental health nursing and/or family therapy. The generalist nurse either refers a family to or consults with a psychiatric mental health nurse who is a specialist in this area. For example, the specialist nurse may be consulted about a difficult and complex family situation in which some members of the family want a dying family member resuscitated while other members do not. The situation would require holding a family conference, assessing the family functioning, and mediating the decision-making process.

When to Assemble the Family in Health Care

Doherty (1985) has also provided guidelines to help health providers know when to involve the family in the course of providing care. Figure 1–3 visualizes when to assemble the family in health care in terms of a two-part continuum. The upper half of the continuum ranges from seeing the individual patient alone to holding family conferences. The bottom half of the continuum shows the kind of health care problem being addressed; this ranges from minor acute problems (minor suturing) to serious acute illness (heart attack) and chronic illness. Such an organizational aid can assist nurses in making decisions about the degree of family involvement appropriate for any given situation and reassure nurses that "family nursing" can take place even when the whole family is not assembled.

The Therapeutic Triangle in Health Care

A third concept of importance to nurses in providing family care is the notion of the therapeutic triangle (Fig. 1–4). There are three main actors in the therapeutic triangle: the identified patient, the health care professional, and the family of the identified patient. The relationships exist primarily between the dyad in the triangle, while the third party in the triangle is in the background. Triangulated relationships are those in which a third party becomes involved in order to stabilize tensions that exist within the dyad. The third party distracts from the anxiety based in the dyad. As dyads change, so does the third party: with the patient-family dyad, the health care professional is the third party, but when the health care professional and identified patient make up the dyad, the family is the third party. For example, when there is difficulty in a nurse-patient relationship, the patient may engage the family to approach the nurse instead of directly confronting the nurse. Or the health care professional may provide a listening ear for a disgruntled patient complaining about the family's caregiving. Often health care providers find themselves positioned between family members. Detailed discussion of the therapeutic triangle is beyond the scope of this book, but others have described it in depth (see Broderick, 1983).

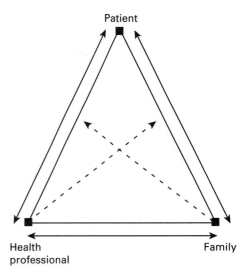

FIGURE 1–4
The therapeutic triangle in health care.

DEVELOPMENT OF FAMILY NURSING

Family nursing has existed since prehistoric times. It has usually been the primary responsibility of women to care for family members who fell ill and to seek remedies for their illness. Also, in their housekeeping, women have traditionally made efforts to provide a clean and safe environment for the maintenance of health and wellness (Bomar, 1989; Ham & Chamings, 1983; Whall, 1993).

In Colonial America, women continued the centuries-old tradition of nurturing and sustaining their families and caring for the ill. During the Revolutionary War women called "camp followers" nursed the wounded. During the Civil War (1861–1865), the nursing of wounded soldiers became more organized. Women formed Ladies' Aid Societies, which met regularly to sew, prepare food and medicines, and gather other items needed by the soldiers. Dorothea Dix was named the Superintendent of Women Nurses of the US Army and hundreds of women received a month's training to prepare them for nursing with military families.

In the late nineteenth century Florence Nightingale influenced both nursing of the sick and poor and the work of "health missionaries" through "health-at-home" teaching. She was convinced that cleanliness in the home could eradicate high infant mortality and morbidity and promoted both nurse-midwifery and home-based health services. Furthermore, she also encouraged family members of the fighting troops to come into the hospitals during the Crimean War and take care of their loved ones. In *Training Nurses for the Sick Poor*, published in 1876, Nightingale admonished nurses to do both sick nursing and health nursing in the home environment. She gave both home health nurses and maternal-child nurses the mandate to carry out nursing practice with the whole family (Nightingale, 1979).

During the industrial development of the United States in the nineteenth century, family members began to work outside the home. Immigrants in particular were in need of income, and many women went to work for the early hospitals. These nurses were involved in the beginning of the labor movement and were concerned with the health of workers and their families. Maternal-child nursing and family care were incorporated into basic nursing curricula of training schools being developed in the late nineteenth century.

Maternity nursing, nurse-midwifery, and community nursing have always focused on the quality of family health. Two pioneers in this area were Margaret Sanger, who fought for family planning, and Mary Breckenridge, who formed the famous Frontier Nursing Service (midwifery) to provide training to nurses to meet the health needs of mountain families.

During the Depression there were concerted efforts to expand public health nursing to work with families; however, during and after World War II, nursing became more focused on the individual, and care became centered in the hospital, where it remained until the 1960s, when nurses again began focusing on the family as the primary unit of care.

In recent decades, family studies in various disciplines have produced family assessment techniques, conceptual frameworks, theories, and other family research tools. This interdisciplinary work has now become known as "family social science." Many family nurses have become active in the National Council of Family Relations, and because of the influence of this organization and the large number of family publications they produce, family social science has had a large impact on family nursing in the United States. The influence of this field is reflected in the large number of nurses who have received advanced degrees in family social science.

Conceptual Models for Family Nursing

Nursing theorists began in the 1960s to systematize nursing practice and to articulate the philosophy and goals of nursing care. Initially, theorists were concerned only with individuals, though gradually individuals became viewed as part of larger social systems such as the family. In the 1970s only one theorist included the family in her system for nursing practice and other theorists' models did not speak specifically to families, though families could be the identified client (Orem, 1985; Roy, 1984; Neuman, 1989). During the 1980s nurses throughout the country began to focus on the family as a unit of care. Family nurses began to define the scope of their practice, explore family concepts, and decide how to teach this information to the next generation of nurses.

One conceptual framework for family nursing is depicted in Figure 1-5. This frame-

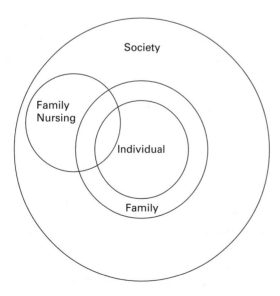

FIGURE 1-5
Family nursing conceptual framework.

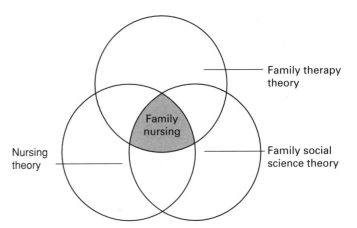

Family therapy
theory

Family
nursing

Nursing
theory

Family social
science theory

FIGURE 1-6
Family nursing practice.

work shows how family nursing intersects with the individual, the family, and the community. Figure 1-6 provides a framework for viewing family nursing practice based on the intersection of theories and strategies from nursing, family therapy, and family social science. Family nursing incorporates into practice many ideas from family therapy and family social science.

Wright and Leahey (1984) have proposed that nurses should receive generalist or basic preparation in family nursing during their undergraduate work, and that they should have advanced preparation in family nursing/family therapy at the graduate level or as continuing education. They suggest that there are a number of differences between the generalist family nurse and the specialist family nurse; these are summarized in Table 1-4. In brief, they consider that family assessment is an important skill for all levels of nurses and that advanced specialists in family nursing can take a much narrower, more intensive focus than generalists.

Interventions in Family Nursing

Gilliss, Roberts, Highley, and Martinson (1989, pp. 71-72) have identified 10 characteristic features of family nursing; all emphasize the complex relationships between family health and the health of individual members. These ten features are as follows:

1. Family care is concerned with the experience of the family over time. It considers both the history and the future of the family group.

2. Family nursing takes into consideration the community and cultural context of the group. The family is encouraged to receive and contribute to community resources.

3. Family nursing considers the relationships among family members and recognizes that individuals and the family group do not always achieve maximum health simultaneously.

4. Family nursing is directed at families whose members are both healthy and ill. The family's health is not indexed by the degree of individual health or illness.

5. Family nursing is often offered in settings to which individuals come with physiological or psychological problems. In addition to being competent in treating in-

TABLE 1–4

FAMILY NURSING: GENERALIST VERSUS SPECIALIST

Generalist	Specialist
1. Education The baccalaureate level with some focus on family assessment and family intervention skills. Minimal clinical supervision of family work.	**1. Education** The graduate level with heavy emphasis on family assessment and family therapy theory and skills. Extensive clinical supervision of family work.
2. Identity Perceives self as a generalist with adequate skills in family interviewing.	**2. Identity** Perceives self as a specialist in family nursing.
3. Context of Employment Family interviews from time to time, but represents less than 30% of work load. The major focus of intervention is on the individual within the family context.	**3. Context of Employment** Family assessment and intervention represent more than 70% of work load. The major focus is on the family as a unit.
4. Conceptualization of Human Needs/Problems The nurse uses systems and communication concepts to conceptualize needs and/or problems within families.	**4. Conceptualization of Human Needs/Problems** The nurse uses family social science, family therapy, and nursing concepts to conceptualize needs and/or problems within families.
5. Family Assessment Using a family assessment model, the nurse generally assess both normative and paranormative events in families.	**5. Family Assessment** Using a variety of family assessment models, the nurse generally assesses and intervenes in both normative and paranormative events in families.
6. Family Problems Families presenting problems with normative events (e.g., birth of a family member, retirement) and/or paranormative events (e.g., coping with chronic illness, divorce).	**6. Family Problems** Families predominantly presenting with paranormative events (e.g., adolescent runaways, miscarriage).
7. Family Intervention Nurses intervene with normative events in families by use of direct and straightforward interventions (e.g., psychoeducation).	**7. Family Intervention** Nurses intervene in both normative and paranormative events in families using various intervention models. Interventions may be direct but often include complex and indirect interventions. The nurse seeks supervision and/or consultation when appropriate.
8. Termination The nurse assesses, intervenes, and concludes with a therapeutic termination for families experiencing normative events. Following a thorough assessment, families experiencing paranormative events may be referred. The decision to refer depends upon the skill level of the nurse.	**8. Termination** The nurse assesses, intervenes, and concludes with a therapeutic termination for those families experiencing normative and/or paranormative events.

SOURCE: Adapted from *Nurses and Families, A Guide to Family Assessment and Intervention* (pp. 7–8), by L. M. Wright and M. Leahey, 1984, Philadelphia: F. A. Davis. Copyright 1984 by F. A. Davis.

dividual health problems, family nurses must recognize the reciprocity between individual and family health.

6. The family system is influenced by any change in its members; therefore, when caring for individuals in health and illness, the nurse should also attend to the family. Individual and family health are intertwined and both will be influenced by any nursing care given.

7. The family nurse tries to increase family interactions between the nurse and family and between family members; however, the absence of family members does not preclude the nurse from offering family care.

8. The family nurse recognizes that the person in a family who has the most symptoms may change over time, and thus the focus of the nurse's attention will change over time.

9. Family nursing focuses on the strengths of individual family members and the family group, and promotes their mutual support and growth where possible.

10. Family nurses must define with the family who constitutes the family and where nurses will place their therapeutic energies.

These distinctive characteristics of family nursing continually reappear in studies of family nursing and in family nursing practice, regardless of the theoretical model used.

Approaches to Family Nursing

There are several different approaches to family nursing. Wright and Leahey (1993) describe three: family nursing with the individual as focus; family nursing with the family as focus; and family systems nursing, in which the individual and family are both the focus. Friedemann (1993) describes individually focused family nursing, interpersonal family nursing, and family system nursing.

This chapter presents four different perspectives or approaches to family nursing: (1) the family as the context for individual development, (2) the family as a client, (3) the family as a system, and (4) the family as a component of the society. These four approaches have their roots in different specialties within nursing: maternal-child nursing, primary care nursing, psychiatric mental health nursing, and community health nursing (Hanson, 1987; Berkey & Hanson, 1991). The approach that nurses use is determined by many factors, including the health care setting, family circumstances, and the nurse's resources.

The first approach to family nursing focuses on the assessment and care of an individual client; in this approach, the *family is the context*. This is the traditional nursing approach, in which the individual is foreground and the family is background. The family is context for the individual in that it serves as either a resource or a stressor to the individual. This approach is also called "family-centered" or "family-focused" nursing. It is rooted in maternal-child nursing and underlies the philosophy of many maternity and pediatric health care settings. A nurse using this focus might ask an individual client: "How has your diagnosis of juvenile diabetes affected your family?" or "Will your nightly need for medication be a problem for your family?"

In the second approach to family nursing, all individual family members are assessed and the *family* is the client or the focus of care. In this approach, the family is in the foreground and individuals are in the background. However, the family is not necessarily the primary consideration. The family is considered the sum of its individual members, and the focus is on every individual member. All are assessed, and health care is provided for all. This approach to family care is rooted in medical primary care and, more recently, in care by family nurse practitioners. This approach is typically seen in health care settings in the community, where sooner or later family practice physicians or family nurse practitioners provide care to all family members. From this perspective, a nurse might say to a family member who has just become ill: "Tell me about what has been going on with your own health, and while you are here, tell me about how your sister is getting along with her juvenile diabetes."

The third approach to care focuses on the *family as a system*. The family is viewed as an interactional system in which the whole is more than the sum of its parts. The emphasis is on interactions between family members — for example, the interactions between parents, or between the parental dyad and the child (Fig. 1 – 7). The more children there are in a family, the more complex these interactions become. The interactions between family members are the target for nursing assessment and intervention; that is, the family is the client. Thus, this family approach focuses on the individual and the family simultaneously and views the family as a system. When something happens to one part of the system, the other parts of the system are also affected. So if one family member becomes ill, that affects all other members of the family. Thus the nurse might ask "What has changed between you and your spouse since your child was diagnosed with juvenile diabetes?" or "How has the diagnosis of juvenile diabetes affected the ways in which your family functions and you get along with each other?" This interactional model is rooted in psychiatric mental health nursing.

The fourth approach to care views the *family as a component of the society*. In this approach, the family is viewed as one of the many institutions in society, such as health, educational, religious, and economic institutions. The family is a basic or primary unit of society, as are all the other units. The family as a whole interacts with other institutions to receive, exchange, or give communication and services. Family social scientists have used this approach, and community health nursing, which focuses on the interface between families and community agencies, has drawn many of its tenets from this approach.

Variables Influencing Family Nursing

The evolution of family nursing has been influenced by the development of nursing theory, practice, education, and research; the family social sciences and health care sciences; national and state health care policies; changing health care behaviors and attitudes; and national and international political events. A detailed discussion of each of these is outside the scope of this text. However, Figure 1 – 8 gives a sample of the many variables that influence family health nursing and shows that the status of family nursing is dependent on what occurs in the wider society. For example, health practices and policies are changing today due to recognition that the costs of health care are escalating and increasing numbers of people are losing access to health care. The goal of health care reform is to make treatment available to all at an affordable cost. That will require a major shift in priorities, funding, and services, and a movement toward health promotion and family care in the community. This in turn will affect the evolution of family nursing.

Obstacles to Family Nursing Practice

While there is a vast amount of literature on the family, until the last decade there was little content on the family in nursing curricula. Further, many nurses still believe that family nursing is just common sense and does not need to be formally taught; and most undergraduate nursing students are more attracted to pathology than to wellness. Thus many practicing nurses have not been exposed to *family concepts* in their education and they use an individualist approach in their practice. Moreover, nursing has strong historical ties

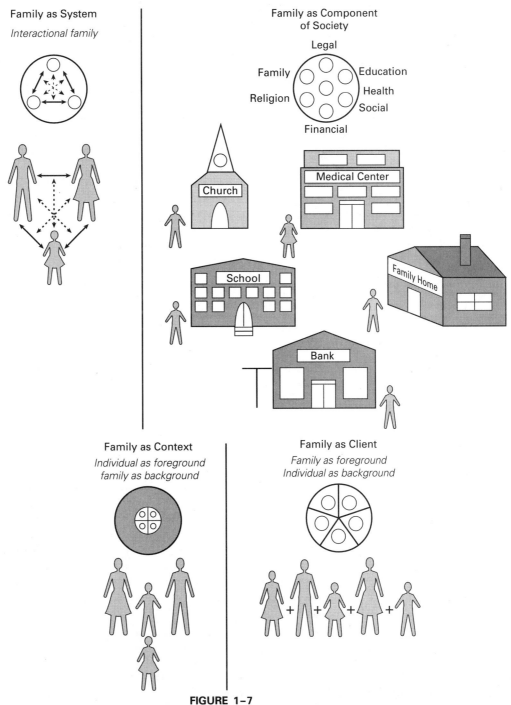

Family as System

Interactional family

Family as Component of Society

Legal

Family

Education

Religion

Health

Social

Financial

Church

Medical Center

School

Family Home

Bank

Family as Context

Individual as foreground family as background

Family as Client

Family as foreground Individual as background

FIGURE 1–7
Approaches to family nursing.

with the medical model of care, in which the focus is on the individual, not the family. Often families have been considered a nuisance in health care settings, an obstacle to providing care for the individual. At best, the family has been viewed as the context for care.

The charting system in health care has also been oriented to the individual. For example, the SOAP (subjective, objective, assessment, plan) format focuses on physical care of

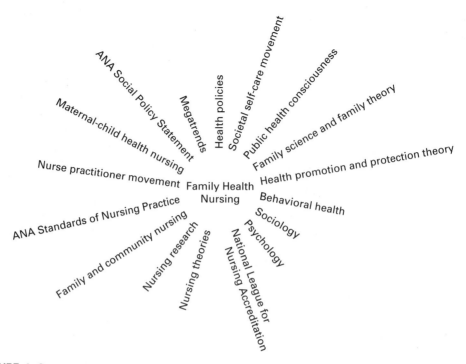

FIGURE 1–8
Variables influencing family health nursing. (From "Introduction to Family Health Nursing and Family Promotion," by P. J. Bomar, G. McNeely, and I. S. Palmer, 1989. In P. J. Bomar (Ed), *Nurses and Family Health Promotion: Concepts, Assessment, and Interventions.* Williams & Wilkins, Baltimore, with permission.)

the individual and does not lend itself easily to focusing on a whole family or several members of families. The medical and nursing diagnostic systems used in health care are similarly focused on individuals because they are disease centered. The International Classification of Diseases (ICD), the Diagnostic and Statistical Manual of Mental Disorders (DSM), and the North American Nursing Diagnosis Association (NANDA) have few diagnostic codes that take the whole family into consideration. Therefore nurses have few choices for family diagnoses that would make the family the focus for intervention. Another consideration is that most insurance carriers require that an individual patient be identified with a diagnosis drawn from the disease-centered diagnostic systems. Thus, even if the healthcare provider intervenes with an entire family, the provider must identify one person in the family as the patient and label that person with a physical or mental health disorder. Clearly, we need better family diagnostic codes that are accepted by insurers as legitimate reasons for reimbursement.

A further obstacle to the practice of family nursing is the lack of good comprehensive family assessment models, instruments, and strategies. Scholars and practitioners are now developing ideas and material in this area, and the chapter on family assessment and intervention (Chapter 7) presents three of the better-known assessment models. A final obstacle to family care is the traditional hours during which health care systems typically provide services, that is, during the day, when family members cannot accompany each other to seek care and become acquainted with the healthcare provider. Fortunately, urgent care settings and other outpatient settings are now incorporating evening and weekend hours in their schedules, making it possible for family members to come in together. Other obstacles to family-focused nursing practice are slowly shifting but nurses need to lobby for continued changes to make it easier to care for the family as a whole.

FAMILY NURSING ROLES

The roles of family nurses are evolving along with changes within the field. Figure 1–9 shows the many roles that family nurses can assume (Leavitt, 1982; Bomar, 1989; Friedman, 1992; Berkey & Hanson, 1991). These roles may vary in different health care settings, and some of these following roles are briefly described.

1. **Health Teacher** Family nurses teach the family about illness and wellness; for example, they might teach new parents how to care for their infant, give instructions about diabetes to a newly diagnosed adolescent and family members, and provide parenting education. Family nurses teach in all settings, both formally and informally.

2. **Coordinator/Collaborator/Liaison** The family nurse coordinates the care that families receive and collaborates with the family in planning this care. When a family member has been in an accident, the nurse plays a key role in helping the family gain access to inpatient care, outpatient care, home health care, social services, or rehabilitation. The nurse often serves as the liaison among these various services.

3. **Deliverer and Supervisor of Care/Technical Expert** The family nurse either delivers or supervises the care that families receive in various settings. For example, the nurse may go into the family home every day to consult with the family and help take care of a child on a respirator. This requires expertise, knowledge, and skill on the part of the family nurse.

4. **Family Advocate** Family nurses advocate for the families with whom they work. The nurse empowers family members to speak for themselves or speaks out for the family. A nurse might advocate for family safety by supporting legislation requiring air bags for motor vehicles.

5. **Consultant** Family nurses often serve as consultants to families, and sometimes they consult with agencies to facilitate family-centered care. A clinical nurse specialist in a hospital may help a family find the appropriate long-term care setting

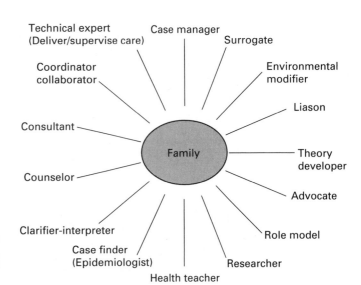

FIGURE 1–9
Family nursing roles. (Data from Leavitt [1982], Bomar [1989], Friedman [1992], and Hanson [1991].)

for their sick grandmother. The nurse thus comes into the family system, by request, for a short period of time and with a specific purpose.

6. **Counselor**   The family nurse plays a therapeutic role in helping individuals and families solve problems or change behavior. When a family member is diagnosed with schizophrenia, the family may require help in coping with this long-term chronic condition.

7. **Case Finder/Epidemiologist**   The family nurse gets involved in case finding and becomes a tracker of disease. When a family member is diagnosed with a sexually transmitted disease, the nurse tries to discover the source of the disease and helps to get sexual contacts in for treatment. The nurse may also screen the whole family and make referrals for treatment.

8. **Environmental Modifier**   The family nurse consults with families and other health care professionals to modify the environment. When a paraplegic is about to be discharged from the hospital, the nurse helps the family modify the home environment so that the patient can move around in a wheelchair and engage in self-care.

9. **Clarifier/Interpreter**   The family nurse clarifies and interprets information for families in all settings. If a child develops a complex disease like leukemia, the nurse clarifies and interprets information about the child's diagnosis, treatment, and prognosis for parents and other family members.

10. **Surrogate**   The family nurse sometimes serves as a surrogate, or stand-in for another person. For example, the nurse may stand in temporarily as a loving mother to an adolescent who is giving birth to a child by herself in the labor and delivery room.

11. **Researcher**   The family nurse identifies practice problems and tries to find the best solutions to the problems through the process of scientific investigation. A family nurse might collaborate with another nurse to find a better way to help families cope with elders living at home who have trouble with bladder control.

12. **Role Model**   The family nurse continually serves as a role model for other people. Family nurses working in schools serve as role models for parents and children alike.

13. **Case Manager**   As case manager, the nurse coordinates the collaboration between a family and the health care system. The case manager is formally empowered to be in charge of a case. A family nurse working with seniors in the community may be assigned to be the case manager for a patient with Alzheimer's disease.

STATE OF THE ART AND SCIENCE OF FAMILY NURSING PRACTICE

Family Nursing Practice

Family nursing practice is still in the process of being defined and developed. According to Friedman (1992), family nursing can be practiced at three levels: (1) the individual or most basic level, where the family is seen as the context for the individual; (2) the interpersonal level, where the family is seen to consist of dyads, triads, and larger units; and (3) the highest or system level, where the family is viewed as a system with its own structural and functional components, interacting with systems in the environment and with its own subsystems. Family nurses who practice on a higher level also include the lower level(s) in their practice (Friedemann, 1993).

The focus at the *individual level* is the physical health and personal well-being of family members; interpersonal change and system change are by-products. At the *interpersonal level*, family nurses have as their main goal the mutual understanding and support of family members. Personal change is anticipated and the interaction between personal and interpersonal factors is taken into consideration in the nursing care plan. System change is anticipated so that harmful situations can be avoided. For nurses who practice at the *system level*, the goal is change in the family system as a whole and increased harmony between the family system and its subsystems, as well as between the family and the environment. Changes at all levels are carefully predicted, monitored, and corrected if the need arises.

Friedemann (1993) says that family nursing can and should be practiced at all three levels by all nurses. Nurse generalists are equipped to care for families functioning relatively well at both the individual and the interpersonal levels. Nursing of families with dysfunctions and nursing at the level of the family system require advanced knowledge and skills in family theory and practice.

Nursing practice at the systems level focuses on family health and strengths and requires knowledge of the complex interaction of a multitude of family factors at all system levels. The reciprocal relationships between health problems and family functioning are well known to clinicians and are well documented. Health problems influence family perceptions and behaviors; likewise, family perceptions and behaviors influence health. Wright and Leahey (1993) call this level of nursing "family systems nursing." The nurse focuses on the whole family as the unit of care, simultaneously concentrating on both the individual and the family. It is not "either/or," but rather, "both/and." Family systems nursing integrates theories of nursing, systems, cybernetics, and family therapy. Wright and Leahey suggest that in the future, nurses will be more involved with families in all types of healthcare settings. Families will be invited in more for interviews, and more interventions will take place at a systems level.

In a recent survey of family nurses (Kirschling et al., 1994), 201 nurses were asked to describe their success in family-centered nursing interventions. Five types of successful outcomes were identified as a result of family nursing interventions:

1. Families were able to identify a problem and seek help; for example, they called the nurse when a family member was experiencing great stress.

2. Families and family members behaved differently as a result of family nursing interventions; for example, an asthmatic child's family member stopped smoking in order to provide the child a smoke-free environment.

3. Family members felt more satisfied with their ability to solve their own problems as a result of nursing interventions.

4. As a result of nurses' interventions, family members knew more about the terms used in health care, about family process, and about each others' beliefs and views; for example, as a result of the nurse teaching them to care for their high-risk infant at home.

5. The family and individuals continued to develop in spite of illness because family nurses assisted families to allow children to lead normal rather than protected lives, even when they had a chronic illness such as diabetes.

These family nurses involved families and family members in assessment and interventions and provided support, education, and opportunities to explore feelings.

Family Nursing Research

Families have been neglected in nursing research, which has focused on the individual (see Chapter 2). Recently, however, nursing has awakened to the fact that family dynamics and health and illness are related, though research on the family and mental health is further advanced than research on the family and physical health (Campbell, 1986).

Studies of the family's impact on physical health have generally taken the perspective of social epidemiology. For example, studies have shown that poor diabetic control and hypertension are associated with unresolved marital conflicts. Further, marital status has been found to be an important factor in mortality and morbidity from cardiovascular disease. Recent studies have shown that patients often respond more to their family's response to illness than to the disease itself.

Murphy (1986), Feetham (1990), Moriarty (1990), and Gilliss and Davis (1993) have summarized the family nursing research to date and some of the methodological problems in this type of research. Wright and Leahey (1993) note that family assessment techniques must be further developed, and the reciprocal relationships between family functioning and the course and treatment of illness need more study. They conclude that the efficacy of family treatment will become more obvious when family interventions are both used and studied more.

Family Nursing Education

Family nursing education has come of age in the United States and Canada. Hanson and Heims (1992) looked at the status of family nursing education in all schools of nursing in the United States. Wright and Bell (1989) modeled a Canadian study after the American study. Both studies found that:

1. More general family content is included in undergraduate and graduate nursing curricula than in the past. However, family content and clinical experience need to be more family-specific, and family content also needs to be integrated into other courses.

2. An eclectic approach to family assessment is taught. Nurses need to learn models and assessment strategies so as to become more systematic and thorough in family assessment.

3. Clinical practicums in a variety of settings still focus on individuals rather than families. Clinical experiences that focus on family relationships and interactions need to be developed.

4. Students are supervised primarily through case discussion and process recordings. Audio- and videotapes are now frequently used to review case material, but there is a need for more direct and live supervision, for example, through the use of one-way mirrors.

5. Those faculty responsible for family nursing often lack advanced knowledge, experience, and skills. More faculty need to do graduate work in family nursing and in the family social sciences, therapy, sociology, and psychology.

6. Schools are better at teaching family assessment than family intervention strategies, reflecting the fact that family nursing interventions are still in an early stage of development. More emphasis and resources should be focused on developing interventions with families.

7. Faculty who teach family nursing have varied backgrounds; many are maternal-child, community, or psychiatric mental health nurses. People who are trained in the family and expert in this area need to be teaching the family content.

Education, for family nurses, begins during undergraduate education and may continue through postdoctoral training. There is still a question of whether family nursing education prepares the nurse for generalist or specialist practice. The ANA (1995) says that nurse generalists take a comprehensive approach to health care and can meet the diverse health concerns of individuals, families, and communities, whereas nurse specialists are expert in providing care to specific clusters of people or problems. Gilliss says that "a nurse who views the family in context may be a generalist in family nursing and a specialist in another field of practice. Conversely, those nurses who practice family nursing are specialists in family care and generalists in other areas of practice" (1993, p. 36). Gilliss has proposed a schema to conceptualize the levels of preparation for family nursing (Fig. 1–10).

LEVELS OF PREPARATION FOR FAMILY NURSING

At the baccalaureate level, students should be prepared to work with the family as context and the family as a component of society. This is consistent with the generalist orientation of undergraduate nursing education. Family content is usually found in undergraduate nursing courses that deal with children's, women's, or community health. However, family content is needed in other courses as well.

Masters level preparation is required for advanced practice in which nurses work with the family as a client or the family as a system. This preparation consists of courses on family theory, nursing interventions with families, advanced practice, and clinical supervision. At one northwest school of nursing, all master's students (nurse practitioner and clinical nurse specialists) are required to take these courses.

Doctoral study usually focuses on family theory development and research. The National Institute of Nursing Research is now funding institutional and individual National Research Service Awards (NRSAS) to support pre- and postdoctoral students in family nursing research.

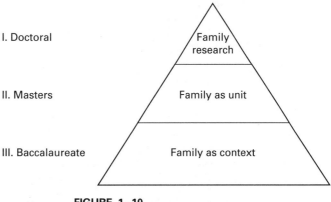

FIGURE 1–10
Levels of preparation for family nursing.

SUMMARY   The purpose of this chapter was to provide a broad overview of family nursing. First, family nursing was defined and the reasons for learning about the family were discussed. Next, the history of families in America and the history of family nursing were summarized. The roles of family nurses and the contemporary state of the art, practice, research, and education pertaining to family nursing were introduced. All of these are evolving as families and society change and grow.

STUDY QUESTIONS

1. Define family.
2. Define family health.
3. List five traits that are common in healthy families.
4. Define family health care nursing.
5. Which of the following statements are true about family nursing practice?
   a. Family care is concerned with the experience of the family over time.
   b. Family nursing is directed at families whose members are both healthy and ill.
   c. The family nurse is responsible, along with the family itself, for defining who is the family.
   d. If family nursing practice is successful, the family members will simultaneously achieve maximum health.
6. Describe the difference between family as a client and family as a system.
7. Name and describe three of the many roles that nurses can assume with families.
8. The primary mode of supervising students studying family nursing is through:

   a. Audio tapes of interactions between students and families
   b. Video tapes of interactions between students and families
   c. Process recordings developed by the student
   d. Direct supervision of student and family interactions

9. Which of the following nursing specialties has historically focused on the quality of family health?
   a. Maternity nursing
   b. Pediatric nursing
   c. Public health nursing
   d. All of the above
10. Family health care nursing is a specialty that started near the end of the twentieth century. True or False; explain your answer.
11. Discuss three traditional functions performed by families over history and that still exist today. What are two functions that have become more meaningful in modern times?

REFERENCES

Ahlburg, D. A., & DeVita, C. J. (1992, August). New realities of the American family. *Population Bulletin, 47,* 1–44.

Altergott, K. (Ed.). (1993). *One world, many families.* Minneapolis, MN: National Council on Family Relations.

American Nurses' Association. (1995). *Nursing: A social policy statement.* Kansas City, MO.

Anderson, K. H., & Tomlinson, P. S. (1992). The family health system as an emerging paradigmatic view for nursing. *Image: Journal of Nursing Scholarship, 24,* 57–63.

Bell, J. M., Watson, W. L., & Wright, L. M. (Eds.). (1990). *The cutting edge of family nursing.* Calgary, Alberta: University of Calgary, Faculty of Nursing.

Berkey. K. M., & Hanson, S. M. H. (1991). *Pocket guide to family assessment and intervention.* St. Louis, MO: Mosby Year Book.

Bianchi, S. M. (1994). The changing demographic and socioeconomic characteristics of single-parent families. *Marriage and Family Review, 20,* 71–98.

Bomar, P. J. (Ed.). (1989). *Nurses and family health promotion: Concepts, assessment, and interventions.* Baltimore: Williams & Wilkins.

Bomar, P. J. (Ed.). (1995). *Nurses and family health promotion: Concepts assessment, and interventions* (2nd ed.). Philadelphia: W. B. Saunders.

Broderick, C. B. (1983). *The therapeutic triangle.* Beverly Hills, CA: Sage Publications.

Burgess, E. W., & Locke, H. J. (1953). *The family: From institution to companionship.* New York: American Book.

Campbell, T. (1986). *Family's impact on health: A critical review and annotated bibliography* (DHHS Publication No. ADM 861461). Washington, DC: US Government Printing Office.

Curran, D. (1983). *Traits of a healthy family*. Minneapolis, MN: Winston Press.

Curran, D. (1985). *Stress and the healthy family*. Minneapolis, MN: Winston Press.

Danielson, C. B., Hamel-Bisselli, B., & Winstead-Fry, P. (Eds.). (1993). *Families, health and illness: Perspectives on coping and intervention*. St. Louis, MO: Mosby.

Department of Family Nursing, Oregon Health Sciences University. (1985). *Department of Family Nursing: Philosophy, conceptual framework, objectives and definitions*. Unpublished manuscript. Portland: Oregon Health Sciences University School of Nursing.

Doherty, W. (1985). Family intervention in health care. *Family Relations, 34,* 129–137.

Doherty, W., & Campbell, T. (1988). *Families and health*. Newbury Park, CA: Sage Publications.

Doherty, W. J., & McCubbin, H. I. (1985). Families and health care: An emerging arena of theory, research and clinical intervention. *Family Relations, 34,* 5–11.

Feetham, S. L. (1990). Conceptual and methodological issues in research of families. In J. M. Bell, W. L. Watson, & L. M. Wright (Eds.), *The cutting edge of family nursing* (pp. 35–50). Calgary, Alberta: University of Calgary.

Feetham, S. L., Meister, S. B., Bell, J. M., & Gilliss, C. L. (Eds.). (1993). *The nursing of families: Theory/research/education/practice*. Newbury Park, CA: Sage Publications.

Ford, D. Y. (1994). An exploration of perceptions of alternative family structures among university students. *Family Relations, 43,* 68–73.

Friedemann, M. L. (1993). The concept of family nursing. In G. D. Wegner & R. J. Alexander (Eds.), *Readings in family nursing* (pp 13–22). Philadelphia: J. B. Lippincott.

Friedman, M. M. (1992). *Family nursing: Theory and practice* (3rd ed.). Norwalk, CT: Appleton & Lange.

Gilliss, C. (1989). Family research in nursing. In C. L. Gilliss, B. L. Highley, B. M. Roberts, & I. M. Martinson (Eds.), *Toward a science of family nursing* (pp. 37–63). Menlo Park, CA: Addison-Wesley.

Gilliss, C. L. (1990). Forward. In J. M. Bell, W. L. Watson, & L. M. Wright (Eds.), *The cutting edge of family nursing* (pp. iii–v). Calgary, Alberta: University of Calgary, Faculty of Nursing.

Gilliss, C. L. (1993). Family nursing research, theory and practice. In G. D. Wegner & R. J. Alexander (Eds.), *Readings in family nursing* (pp. 34–42). Philadelphia: J. B. Lippincott.

Gilliss, C. L., & Davis, L. L. (1993). Does family intervention make a difference? An integrative review and meta-analysis. In S. L. Feetham, S. B. Meister, J. M. Bell, & C. L. Gilliss (Eds.), *The nursing of families: Theory/research/education/practice* (pp. 259–265). Newbury Park, CA: Sage Publications.

Gilliss, C. L., Roberts, B. M., Highley, B. L., & Martinson, I. M. (1989). What is family nursing? In C. L. Gilliss, B. L. Highley, B. M. Roberts, & I. M. Martinson (Eds.), *Toward a science of family nursing* (pp. 64–73). Menlo Park, CA: Addison Wesley.

Ham, L. M., & Chamings, P. A. (1983). Family nursing: Historical perspectives. In I. Clements & F. B. Roberts (Eds.), *Family health care: A theoretical approach to nursing care* (Vol. 1), (pp. 88–109). San Francisco: McGraw-Hill.

Hanson, S. M. H. (1985). *Defining family health*. Paper presented at the Annual Conference of the Oregon Council of Family Relations, 1984, Portland, OR.

Hanson, S. M. H. (1986). Healthy single parent families. *Family Relations, 35,* 125–132.

Hanson, S. M. H. (1987). Family nursing and chronic illness. In M. Leahey & L. Wright (Eds.), *Families and chronic illness* (pp. 2–32). Springhouse, PA: Springhouse.

Hanson, S. M. H., & Heims, M. L. (1992). Family nursing curricula in U. S. schools of nursing. *Journal of Nursing Education, 31,* 305–308.

Hanson, S. M. H., Heims, M. L., Julian, D. J., & Sussman, M. B. (Eds.). (1995a). *Single parent families: Diversity, myths and realities*. New York: Haworth.

Hanson, S. M. H., Heims, M. L., Julian D. J., & Sussman, M. B. (1995b). Single parent families: Present and future perspectives. In S. M. H. Hanson, M. L. Heims, D. J. Julian, & M. B. Sussman (Eds.), *Single parent families: Diversity, myths and realities*. New York: Haworth.

Hanson, S. M. H., Heims, M. L., Julian, D. J., & Sussman, M. B. (Eds.). (1995c). Single parent families: Diversity, myths and realities. *Marriage and Family Review, 22,* 550.

Hanson, S. M. H., Heims, M. L., Julian D. J., & Sussman, M. B. (Eds). (1995d). Single parent families: Present and future perspectives. *Marriage and Family Review, 22,* 1–26.

Hanson, S. M. H., & Kaakinen, J. (1996). Family assessment. In M. Stanhope & J. Lancaster (Eds.), *Community health nursing: Process and practice for promoting health*. St. Louis: C.V. Mosby.

Kirschling, J. M., Gilliss, C. L., Krentz, L., Camburn, C. D., Clough, R. S., Duncan, M. T., Hendricks, J., Howard, J. K. H., Roberts, C., Smith-Young, J., Tice, K. S., & Young, T. (1994). "Success" in family nursing: Experts describe phenomena. *Nursing and Health Care, 15,* 186–189.

Kissman, K., & Allen, J. A. (1993). *Single-parent families*. Newbury Park, CA: Sage Publications.

Leavitt, M. B. (1982). *Families at risk: Prevention in nursing practice*. Boston: Little, Brown.

Loveland-Cherry, C. J. (1989). Family health promotion and health protection. In P. J. Bomar (Ed.), *Nurses and family health promotion: Concepts, assessment and interventions* (pp. 13–25). Baltimore: Williams & Wilkins.

McCubbin, M. A., & McCubbin, H. I. (1993). Families coping with illness: The resiliency model of family stress, adjustment, and adaptation. In C. B. Danielson, B. Hamel-Bissell, & P. Winstead-Fry (Eds.), *Families, health and illness: Perspectives on coping and intervention* (pp. 21 - 65). St. Louis, MO: Mosby.

McEwan, P. J. M. (1992). The social approach to family health studies. *Social Science and Medicine, 8,* 487 - 493.

Mischke, K., & Hanson, S. M. H. (1995). Family health assessment and intervention. In P. J. Bomar (Ed.), *Nurses and family health promotion: Concepts, assessment, and interventions* (2nd ed.). Philadelphia: W. B. Saunders.

Mischke-Berkey, K., Warner, P., & Hanson, S. M. H. (1989). Family health assessment and intervention. In P. J. Bomar (Ed.). *Nurses and family health promotion: Concepts, assessment and interventions* (pp. 115 - 154). Baltimore: Williams & Wilkins.

Moriarty, H. J. (1990). Key issues in the family research process: Strategies for nurse researchers. *Advances in Nursing Science, 12,* 1 - 14.

Murphy, S. (1986). Family study and nursing research. *Image: Journal of Nursing Scholarship, 18,* 170 - 174.

Neuman, B. (1989). *The Neuman Systems Model. Application to nursing education and practice* (2nd ed.). Norwalk, CT: Appleton & Lange.

Nightingale, F. (1979). *Cassandra.* Westbury, NY: The Feminist Press.

Norton, A. J., & Miller, L. F. (1992). Marriage, divorce, and remarriage in the 1990s. *Family Relations, 35(6),* 9 - 17.

Olson, D. H., & Hanson, M. K. (Eds.). (1990). *2001: Preparing families for the future.* Minneapolis, MN: National Council on Family Relations.

Orem, D. (1985). *Nursing: Concepts of practice* (3rd ed.). New York: McGraw-Hill.

Otto, H. (1963). Criteria for assessing family strengths. *Family Process, 2,* 329 - 338.

Pearson, A., & Vaughan, B. (1986). *Nursing models for practice.* Rockville, MD: Aspen.

Pender, M. H. (1987). *Health promotion in nursing practice* (2nd ed.). Norwalk, CT: Appleton-Century-Crofts.

Pender, N., Barkauskas, V., Hayman, L., Rice, V., & Anderson, E. (1992). Health promotion and disease prevention: Toward excellence in nursing practice and education. *Nursing Outlook, 40,* 106 - 109.

Pratt, L. (1976). *Family structure and effective health behavior: The energized family.* Boston: Houghton Mifflin.

Price, S., & Elliott, B. (Eds.). (1993). *Vision 2010: Families and health care.* Minneapolis, MN: National Council on Family Relations.

Ross, B., & Cobb, K. L. (1990). *Family nursing: A nursing process approach.* Redwood City, CA: Addison-Wesley.

Roy, C. (1984). *Introduction to nursing. An adaptation model* (2nd ed.). Englewood Cliffs, NJ: Prentice-Hall.

Saluter, A. F. (1991). Marital status and living arrangements: March 1990. US Bureau of the Census. *Current Population Reports.* Series P-20, No. 458.

Smith, H. L., & Cutright, P. (1985). Components of change in the number of female family heads ages 15 to 44, update and reanalysis: United States, 1940 to 1983. *Social Science Research, 14,* 226 - 250.

Stanhope, M., & Lancaster, J. (1992). *Community health nursing: Process and practice for promoting health* (3rd ed.). St. Louis, MO: Mosby.

Stinnett, N., Chesser B., & DeFrain, J. (Eds.). (1979). *Building family strengths: Blue prints for action.* Lincoln, NE: University of Nebraska Press.

Sussman, M. B., & Steinmetz, S. K. (1987). *Handbook of marriage and the family.* New York: Plenum Press.

US Bureau of the Census. (1989a). Current population reports, Series P-25, No. 1018. *Projections of the population of the United States, by age, sex, and race: 1988 to 2080.* Washington, DC: US Government Printing Office.

US Bureau of the Census, (1989b). Current population reports, Series P-60, No. 163. *Poverty in the United States: 1987, and earlier report.* Washington, DC: US Government Printing Office.

US Bureau of the Census. (1989c). Current population reports, Series P-23, No. 162. *Studies in marriage and the family.* Washington, DC: US Government Printing Office.

US Bureau of the Census. (1989d). Current population reports, Series P-20, No. 445. *Marital status and living arrangements: March, 1989.* Washington, DC: US Government Printing Office.

US Bureau of the Census. (1991a). Current population reports, Series P-60, No. 173*, Child support and alimony: 1989.* Washington, DC: US Government Printing Office.

US Bureau of the Census. (1991b). Current population reports, Series P-20, No. 461. *Marital status and living arrangements: March 1991.* Washington, DC: US Government Printing Office.

US Bureau of the Census. (1992a). Current population reports, Series P-20, No. 458. *Household and family characteristics: 1991.* Washington, DC: US Government Printing Office.

US Bureau of the Census. (1992b). Current population reports, Series P-23, No. 180. *Marriage, divorce, and remarriage in the 1990s.* Washington, DC: US Government Printing Office.

US Bureau of the Census. (1992c). Current population reports, Series P-20, No. 468. *Marital status and living arrangements: March 1992.* Washington, DC: US Government Printing Office.

US Bureau of the Census. (1992d). Current population reports, Series P-23, No. 181. *Households, families and children: A 30-year perspective.* Washington, DC: US Government Printing Office.

Wegner, G. B., & Alexander, R. J. (Eds.). (1993). *Readings in family nursing.* Philadelphia: J. B. Lippincott.

Whall, A. L. (1993). The family as the unit of care in nursing: A historical review. In G. D. Wegner & R. J. Alexander (Eds.), *Readings in family nursing* (pp. 3 – 12). Philadelphia: J. B. Lippincott.

Whall, A. L., & Fawcett, J. (Eds.). (1991). *Family theory development in nursing: State of the science and art.* Philadelphia: F.A. Davis.

World Health Organization. (1992). *Basic documents.* Geneva: World Health Organization.

Wright. L. M., & Bell, J. M. (1989). A survey of family nursing education in Canadian universities. *The Canadian Journal of Nursing Research, 21,* 59 – 74.

Wright, L. M., & Leahey, M. (1984). *Nurses and families: A guide to family assessment and intervention.* Philadelphia: F.A. Davis.

Wright, L. M., & Leahey, M. (1993). Trends in nursing of families. In G. D. Wegner & R. J. Alexander (Eds.), *Readings in family nursing* (pp. 23 – 33). Philadelphia: J. B. Lippincott.

Wright, L. M., & Leahey, M. (1994). *Nurses and families: A guide to family assessment and intervention* (2nd ed.). Philadelphia: F.A. Davis.

BIBLIOGRAPHY

Boss, P. G., Doherty, W. J., LaRossa, R., Schrumm, W. R., & Steinmetz, S. K. (Eds.). (1993). *Sourcebook of family theories and methods: A contextual approach.* New York: Plenum.

Bozett, F. W., & Hanson, S. M. H. (1991). *Fatherhood and families in cultural context.* New York: Springer.

Carpenito, L. (1993). *Nursing diagnosis: Application to clinical practice.* (5th ed.). Philadelphia: Lippincott.

Clemen-Stone, S., Eigsti, D., & McGuire, S. (1991). *Comprehensive family community health nursing.* (3rd ed.). St. Louis: Mosby.

Danielson, C. B., Hamel-Bissell, B., & Winstead-Fry, P. (1993). *Families, health and illness: Perspectives on coping and intervention.* St. Louis: C.V. Mosby.

Grotevant, H. D. (1989). The role of theory in guiding family assessment. *Journal of Family Psychology*, 3, 104 – 117.

Nettle, C., Pavelich, J., Jones, N., Beltz, C., Laboon, P., & Pifer, P. (1993). Family as client: Using Gordon's health pattern typology. *Journal of Community Health Nursing*, 10, 53 – 61.

Shaw, G. C. (1993). (Ed). *Nursing process in clinical practice.* Springhouse, PA: Springhouse Corp.

von Bertalanffy, L. (1968). *General systems theory: Foundations, development, applications.* New York: George Braziller.

von Bertalanffy, L. (1972). The history and status of general systems theory. In G. Klir (Ed.), *Trends in general systems theory.* New York: John Wiley & Sons.

Whall, A. L. (1986). *Family therapy theory for nursing: Four approaches.* Norwalk, CT: Appleton-Century-Crofts.

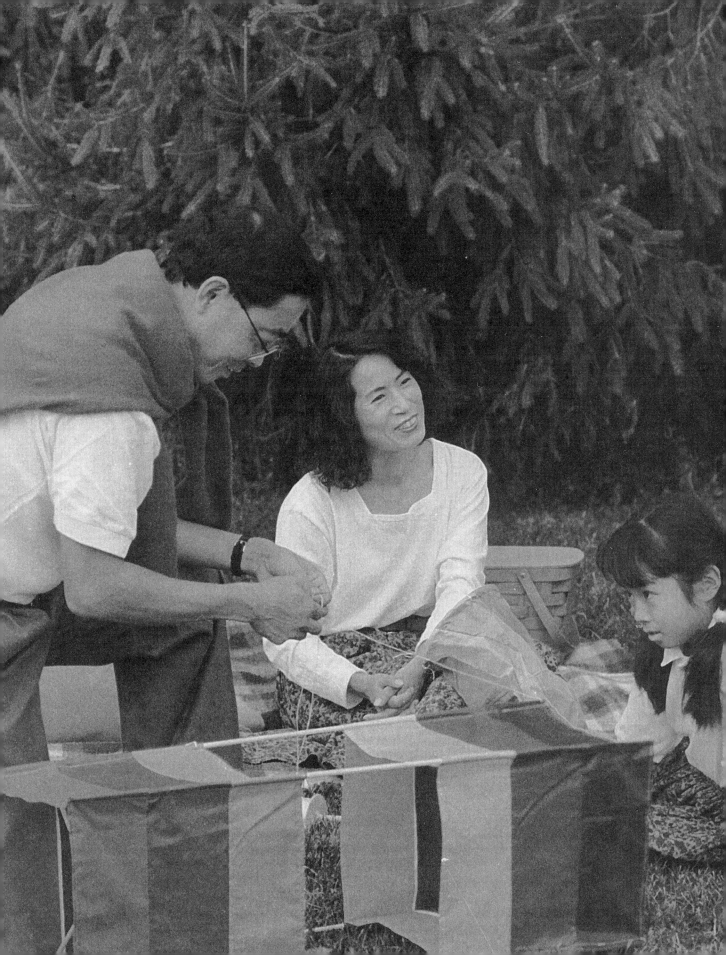

Theoretical and Research Foundations of Family Nursing

The introduction you received in the first chapter provided some answers to important questions about why one should study family nursing. This chapter, which covers family nursing theory and family nursing research, will help to answer more of those questions. It will also challenge you to think clearly and methodically. Many nursing students find theory classes difficult. This is understandable because nursing students typically want to be *doing* nursing rather than just *learning* about it. This chapter will help you understand the importance of theory and research to the development of family nursing.

If you are the typical nursing student your previous course work provided an introduction to nursing theory. You learned about the need to carefully identify and examine concepts and think critically about their relevance to the practice of nursing. You will rely on previous learning, especially course work related to theory in nursing and nursing research, to master the important information in this chapter.

After exploring the importance of non-nursing theory to the development of nursing, students will be introduced to developmental theory, adaptation theory, structural-functional theory, and systems theory, all of which are illustrated with examples of how each assists our understanding of the family. Differences between conceptual models and theories of nursing are identified, and conceptual overviews of many theorists are described, including those of King, Neuman, Orem, Rogers, and Roy.

As baccalaureate students you are expected to become familiar with nursing research, to incorporate research developments into the practice of nursing, and to employ the research process in your professional activities. The second part of this chapter reviews the research process and provides examples of nursing research with families.

CHAPTER 2

Theoretical and Research Foundations of Family Nursing

Sheryl Thalman Boyd, RN, PhD, FAAN

OUTLINE

FAMILY NURSING THEORY: AN OVERVIEW
    The Development of Family Nursing Theory
    Use of Theoretical and Conceptual Frameworks in Family Nursing

FAMILY NURSING RESEARCH: AN OVERVIEW
    Historical Perspective
    Design and Measurement Issues
    Ethical Considerations
    Analysis of Family Nursing Research

OBJECTIVES

Upon completion of this chapter, the reader will be able to:

1. Discuss the development of family nursing theory and research.
2. Describe the integration of theory, practice, and research in family health care nursing.
3. Identify four theoretical frameworks that are used by family health care nurses to guide clinical practice.
4. Discuss the distinction between family-related nursing research and family nursing research.
5. Summarize sampling issues related to family nursing research.
6. Describe three measurement issues in family nursing research.
7. Identify two data analysis issues that are pertinent to family nursing research.

With the emergence of family nursing as a recognized area of practice, the theoretical and research foundations of family nursing have become better delineated, and knowledge in this area of nursing is expanding. This chapter reviews the development of family nursing theory and research, and the development of the broader area of family science. Throughout the discussion, the relationships between family theory, practice, and research are emphasized, and the interdependence of all three is stressed.

Theory and research flow from practice, practice is guided by theory, and research influences both practice applications and theory development; all three elements thus have direct and indirect effects on one another. For example, a family nurse clinician might be frustrated by a father's lack of involvement with his infant during the postpartum hospitalization period and wonder whether the father would be more involved if the hospital staff made more efforts to help him. In this instance, the nurse has posed a question that can be examined through research. It would be possible to set up a study to determine whether teaching the father would affect his involvement in child care activities and his involvement in the spousal relationship. When the nurse identifies research problems, the same conceptual and theoretical framework that guides practice may serve as a framework for development of the research design. In the previous example, a family nurse who uses a systems framework would be interested in the relationships between the members of the family system as well as how the family system interacts with the hospital. Findings of the study might then improve understanding of these relationships and in turn affect nursing practice with childbearing families. In some instances family nurse clinicians can find answers to questions through research that has been completed previously. Research in a practice discipline is designed to influence the practice of clinicians, though some research must go through many steps before it is ready for use in practice. It is through this integration of theory, practice, and research that nursing ultimately contributes to family health.

FAMILY NURSING THEORY: AN OVERVIEW

The Development of Family Nursing Theory

The definition of family provides the foundation for family nursing theory. Over the past two decades, the definition of family has changed extensively. The family was once thought of as two parents who were bound by marriage, with one or more offspring. Less conservative definitions began to emerge in the 1970s and 1980s. For example, in 1985, Boyd defined family as "a social system composed of two or more individuals who have a strong emotional involvement and live within a common household" (p. 164). Today, the family is defined by family members and is not limited by walls or by individual relationships. Although it is not crucial to have full agreement on the definition of family, to ensure that their work is interpreted on the basis of a common understanding, researchers and theorists need to be specific about their definitions of family. Chapter 1 provides an in-depth discussion on the definition of family.

Reviewing the published nursing literature beginning with the writings of Florence Nightingale, Whall and Fawcett (1991) found that nursing has consistently had an interest in family members and acknowledged the importance of family in relation to health. In their efforts to provide a theoretical framework for nursing practice, early nursing theorists tended to be overly general and their theories were cumbersome in application to specific nursing situations. For the most part, these theories were oriented toward individual health care and were difficult to adapt to family assessment and intervention. However, some of these theories have been revised to place greater emphasis on the family (Andrews & Roy, 1986; Chin, 1985; King, 1983; Neuman, 1983, 1989; Orem, 1983a, b; Reed, 1989; Rogers, 1983; Roy, 1983, 1984; Whall & Fawcett, 1991).

Family nursing has also drawn heavily on theory and research in other social sciences, including anthropology, sociology, and psychology. Theoretical frameworks from other disciplines have guided the evolution of family nursing science. In particular, systems theory, developmental theory, symbolic interactionism, and social exchange theory have provided useful frameworks for nurses studying family phenomena. Family science, or the interdisciplinary study of families, is now recognized as a separate discipline:

> Family science is the discipline devoted to the study of the unique realm of the family. Its primary concentration focuses on the inner workings of family behavior and centers on family processes such as emotion in families, love boundaries, rituals, paradigms, rules, routines, decision making, and management of resources. When the family is studied from a family-science perspective, researchers, practitioners, and clinicians treat information from other related disciplines (i.e., sociology, psychology, anthropology) as vital background information. The foreground emphasis, however, is on the family system and its intimate workings (Burr, Day, & Bahr, 1993 pp. 17–18).

A major difference in theory developed by other disciplines and theory in family nursing is that nurses are interested in the relationships between family environment, family health, family structure and function, and the actions of nurses in promoting wellness and optimal health. That is, family study by nurses focuses on the interactions between nursing actions and family health. Nurses who study the family try to determine how nursing actions will influence the family's health or the health of family members, and how the health of the family influences the nursing interventions selected for use with that family.

Use of Theoretical and Conceptual Frameworks in Family Nursing

There is no one theory that is right for everyone. Nor is there just one theory consistently relevant for nursing practice. Some theories are more relevant to family nursing practice than others. In practice, however, nurses are likely to take an eclectic approach, using portions of more than one theory when these are relevant to specific aspects of practice and integrating concepts from several theoretical frameworks.

The most frequently used frameworks for family nursing clinical practice are systems theory, developmental theory, communication theory, and the structural-functional theory. Throughout the clinical specialty chapters of this text, authors have presented these and other theories in greater depth as they uniquely relate to specific areas of family nursing practice, research, and education.

Systems Theory

Systems theory is used by many nurses to guide practice in their area of family nursing. The major principles of systems theory are: (1) Each system has its own characteristics, and the whole is greater than the sum of the parts, rather than just the sum of the characteristics of individual parts of the system. (2) All parts of the system are dependent on one another, even though each part has its own role within the system. (3) There are mechanisms for exchange of information with the system (subsystems) and within the broader environment (suprasystem). Subsystems within the family system include parent-child dyads, spousal dyads, triads of siblings, and so forth. Examples of suprasystems that are relevant to families include schools and the health care system. Systems theory as related to various facets of family nursing is covered in more depth in later chapters. Chapters 10 and 12 provide excellent overviews of systems theory as related to the areas of childbearing and medical-surgical nursing. In addition, Chapter 12 discusses the Resiliency Model of Family Stress, Adjustment, and Adaptation, which is based upon systems theory and emphasizes the family's response to stressful life events such as illness. This chapter also furnishes an overview of family stress theory. In Chapter 14, Gerontological Family Nursing, the author presents two systems-based models of family nursing: the Resiliency Model and the Family Life Cycle Model, which incorporates concepts from systems theory as well as family developmental theory.

Developmental Theory

Developmental theory was originally used to explain individual growth and development but it has been adapted to examine different stages in the development of the family. Duvall's (1979) Family Life Cycle Model is the most widely used developmental approach and the one on which most other developmental approaches are based. Duvall identified eight chronological stages through which the family passes, each of which includes predictable tasks that the family must master prior to proceeding to the next stage:

1. Beginning family
2. Childbearing family
3. Family with preschool children
4. Family with teenagers
5. Launching center family
6. Family with middle-aged parents
7. Family with old age and retirement

Terkelsen (1980), another developmental theorist, also divides the family life span into different stages with different tasks. Terkelson, however, views the family as a social system and places greater emphasis on relationships and interactions among family members. Thus, Terkelson takes into consideration socioeconomic status and events such as divorce and considers the effects of these on the progression of developmental stages. Unfortunately, although developmental theories provide criteria for assessing a family's current stage and its ability to accomplish the tasks of this stage, these theories offer little help in developing intervention strategies (Boyd, 1985).

In Chapter 10, Martell and Imle provide an overview of Duvall's theory applied to the childbearing family, as well as a developmental model based on transition concepts. In Chapter 11, Gedally-Duff and Heims have incorporated developmental theory and symbolic interaction theory as components of an interactional model they describe to guide family child health nursing.

Structural-Functional Model

The structural-functional family nursing model emphasizes the organization or structure of the family and how this structure facilitates the family functioning (Friedman, 1992). It characterizes the family as a social system and examines the relationships between family members as they relate to carrying out family functions. Friedman (1992) defines the five basic family functions as: (1) affective function — the maintenance of personalities of family members; (2) socialization and social placement function — socializing the child to be a productive member of society; (3) reproductive function; (4) economic function; and (5) health care function. A limitation of the structural-functional model is that it tends to be situational and circumscribed to a specific time frame. Chapters 10, 12, and 14 provide more in-depth discussions of theoretical models that emphasize family structure and function.

Communication Theory

Communication theory emphasizes the sending and receiving of both verbal and nonverbal messages. According to this theory, communication that has a high level of clarity and congruence between the sender and the receiver promotes positive behavior within the family; communication that lacks clarity is apt to lead to problematic family behaviors or relationships. In Chapter 13, Shepard and Moriarity use communications theory as a guide for family mental health nursing.

The models and theories discussed previously provide various frameworks for family nursing practice and research. No one specific theory best suits this specialty. What is important is that a conceptual and theoretical framework provides a rationale and guide for decision making in a range of practice situations. Selection of a model that corresponds with the nurse's practice philosophy is essential.

FAMILY NURSING RESEARCH: AN OVERVIEW

Nursing research involves investigation of actual and potential health problems that may be affected by the actions of nurses; family nursing research is a relatively new area in nursing endeavors. As nurses have recognized the need in their practice to provide health care for the whole family, research with an emphasis on family health care and family relationships has emerged. It is beyond the scope of this text to provide a general overview of nursing research, but we will examine research concerning family nursing practice. Emphasis is placed on the unique aspects of nursing research when the focus is on the family.

Historical Perspective

Family nursing research includes examination of the family's impact on the health of individual family members, as well as the impact of the health of family members on the family unit. The goal of the research is to add to the body of knowledge that guides nursing practice and to improve the health care that family members and the family receive. As families are increasingly recognized as the context, if not the focus, of nursing interventions, family research has evolved as an important part of nursing science. The emergence of family nursing research has brought with it complex research issues related to the design and measurement of relationships between individuals.

There is controversy, moreover, about which studies can actually be considered family research. The more conservative view is that family research includes only studies that examine the relationships between family members when all family members are present and participating in the study. This definition suggests that collecting data from family members independently may preclude the possibility of examining exchanges among family members (Fisher, 1982). However, research in which the family is the unit of measurement is extremely expensive and time-consuming.

A less conservative view is that research that examines family members' perceptions or observes family members independently is also an important part of the science of family nursing. Feetham (1991) calls research that collects data from individuals "family-related research" and research that studies the family, "family research." She says that both types of research are "of equal importance, and both can contribute to knowledge about families" (p. 56).

In a review of family research conducted in the 1980s, Berardo (1990) identified three major themes. First, economic variables affect the family's health and welfare. Second, the fact that increasing numbers of women work outside the home influences roles within the family and the division of labor between spouses. Third, the research shows a "recognition and acceptance of the diversity of American families and their lifestyles" (p. 817). Today, these three themes remain significant in family nursing research as families continue to face major challenges in developing economic independence and healthy home environments.

Design and Measurement Issues

In any study, the research questions guide decisions regarding design and methodology. Some design and measurement issues, however, are particularly relevant to research with families, including sources of data, family nursing interventions, and measurement of family data.

Articulation of the conceptual and theoretical framework and definition of family, as well as other significant concepts within the framework, provides the basis for designing the research study. It is essential to make the definition of the family explicit and to ensure that this definition is congruent with the conceptual or theoretical model upon which the study is based. For example, to define family as only those family members who live together may not be consistent with a theoretical framework that focuses on intergenerational families. An explicit definition of family gives others a clear understanding of how the research has been conceptualized and facilitates replication of the research.

Having decided upon the conceptual framework and clearly defined the significant concepts in the research, the research team has a foundation for making other decisions, including decisions about (1) the design of the study, (2) the family members who will be included as subjects in the study, (3) if an experimental design is to be used, the intervention(s) to be implemented, and with which family members, (4) the setting for interventions and data collection, (5) the methods to be used for data collection, and (6) data analysis procedures. Thus, once the conceptual framework is articulated, design and methodology decisions are guided by this framework. For example, when examining data from a systems perspective, the researcher is interested in the interactions of family members within the family system. If a developmental framework is used, the researcher may be more likely to use a longitudinal design that examines development of the family or individual family members over time.

Sources of Data

Decisions about the sources of data are influenced by the nature of the research. Which family members to include in the study, what setting to use for data collection, and whether to collect data simultaneously or separately from family members are all decisions based on the researcher's intent. When children are involved in the family unit, decisions must be made about age-appropriate measures and how best to involve the children in family unit analysis. Just as in practice, the nurse conducting research needs to have alternative plans, since some options may be eliminated by the family's structure, the availability of family members, or individual family members' decisions about whether to participate in the study. As the number of family members required for the study increases, so will the difficulty of recruiting families to the study. For example, in the author's research examining parent-child interaction, it was found that when couples were recruited together during the postpartum hospitalization period, they were more likely to choose to participate. When the mother was approached alone, she often played the role of gatekeeper, declining participation while often stating that she knew her partner would not want to participate. However, when the father was included, he frequently expressed gratification and expressed his frustration with his limited opportunities to be involved in the health care of his wife and baby.

Another factor affecting family research is the mobility of the contemporary family. Whenever the data collection process includes more than one data collection point, research protocols must incorporate strategies for locating families that move while the study is in process. This is an important consideration since the results of the study may be affected if procedures for tracking families have not been incorporated into the study. One common strategy is to give the subject a postcard pre-addressed to the researcher at the first data collection point and to ask the subject to mail it if the family moves; another strategy involves obtaining the name, permanent address, and telephone number of a family member or friend who can be contacted if future tracking is necessary.

Just as it may be difficult for the practicing nurse to find a time when both parents are available to provide patient education, the nurse researcher often finds it very complex and time-consuming to schedule time with family members. It may be necessary to schedule appointments with the family in the evening hours, on weekends, or at other times when family members are available. In addition, as the sensitivity of the research questions increases, subjects are more likely to decline involvement. For example, families having marital problems may opt out of a study measuring marital satisfaction, though it may be these very subjects who are of interest to the family nurse researcher and who may benefit from a family intervention aimed at improving communication between spouses. Families tend to be more amenable to participating in research when they understand the rationale for the study and how it may benefit them or the future health care of others.

Another incentive for families to participate in a study is the opportunity to learn more about themselves. Learning about one another can occur during group measurement or when sharing the results of a study with participants. Recruitment procedures should include educating the family members about the potential benefits and risk of the study. Although a study may be designed in such a way as to reduce or eliminate stress or negative outcomes of the research for individual family members, outlining a process for managing any consequences of family members' increased understanding of the family is a necessary part of the research process. Exploring relationships can sometimes be painful, and family members may need help in dealing with the emotions elicited through the research process. All family members need to be offered an opportunity to discuss thoughts or feelings that result from their participation in the study.

The rationale for sample selection is especially relevant because informed consent requires researchers to provide complete information to potential research subjects, including a "full explanation of the project, a description of the risks involved, if any, a disclosure of alternative procedures that might be used, and an offer to answer any and all questions concerning the project" (Gelles, 1978, p 420). Subjects must also be informed that they can withdraw from the study at any time. Such information can be a source of apprehension, which may cause some potential subjects to decline to participate. Thus, accurate information about the number of eligible subjects, the number approached to participate, and the number who actually participate is essential. The major reasons for nonparticipation are also important in understanding who the study actually represents and the generalizability of the study. Finally, it is important that families in the control group are similar to those families in the intervention group.

Family Nursing Intervention

The majority of studies in family nursing research have been descriptive and correlational (Moriarity, 1990). However, more and more studies are examining interventions within family systems. Attention must be given to the process of the research intervention as well as the outcomes of the intervention, including who receives the intervention, who delivers the intervention, and where the intervention takes place.

It is essential to know who will be the recipient of the intervention. Will it be one member of the family? Selected family members? The whole family? For example, in a study testing an intervention to decrease smoking in pregnant women, the researcher must decide whether to intervene only with the mother-to-be or to include other family members in the intervention. Another consideration is whether the intervention will be delivered to the family as a group or to individual family members. These decisions are influenced by such factors as the time and cost of interventions. For instance, funding may be available to invite the father-to-be into the clinic as part of a smoking-cessation intervention, or funding may only permit sending home a brochure discussing the importance of not using tobacco.

Research that involves contacts between researchers and subjects requires that researchers be able to communicate with the study population. For example, a research project in which the author is currently involved uses paraprofessionals to provide the parent education portion of the intervention. This approach is effective with the study population since the intervention regarding parenting skills comes from members of the community, to whom the subjects can relate more easily and who are thus not seen as outsiders or authority figures. Another concern in family nursing research involving ethnic groups or people of color is whether the persons contacting subjects will be more effective if they are of the same group or race. The effectiveness of such strategies needs to be studied further to assess their impact.

Another consideration pertaining to family research is the setting in which the intervention will take place, and the design and methods of the study influence this decision. The advantages and disadvantages of various settings will need to be explored. For example, if the nursing intervention needs to be provided in a setting in which the family can be observed, and the researcher believes that their behavior would be most natural in a homelike setting, the ideal setting would be the home. Subjects are sometimes more willing to participate in a study when there is no additional burden of going out of their home. Research in the home is expensive, however, and cost may be an issue for the investigators; thus, the researcher may need to create a room that resembles a home setting where subjects may be more comfortable sharing intimate information. If the study includes videotaping or sophisticated computer coding, this also may necessitate data collection in a laboratory setting.

Measurement of Family Data

Selection of instruments that are sensitive to family data is critical. An instrument may provide information only about individual family members or it may provide insight into how the family functions as a whole. From a systems perspective, the family whole is more than simply a sum of its parts. Thus comparison of individual data within a family is one method of trying to get at this whole, while observation of family members interacting or responding to an interview as a whole is another. Stein and Riessman's (1980) "Impact on Family" scale is an example of a tool that seeks data on how the family copes with the chronic illness of a child. When only one family member completes the scale, the researcher has only one perspective. When two or more family members complete the scale, comparison of different members' perspectives provides more in-depth information.

Whether data are collected from individuals or the group of family members, the researcher needs to be aware of the complexity of family issues. For example, when examining the partner relationship, the researcher needs to carefully consider the implications of measuring only one individual's perception. Data from only one family member, that is, individual data, may not take into consideration the perceptions or actions of any other family members (Fisher, Kokes, Ransom, Phillips, & Rudd, 1985). When data is collected from more than one family member individually and is then combined for analysis, Fisher et al. (1985) refer to this research as being relational. The researcher is responsible for determining the manner in which the scores will be combined from the individual data.

Another method for examining the marital relationship is to observe a couple together; even more data would result from observation of the entire family as a group. Fisher and colleagues refer to this type of data collection as "transactional," because the data are derived from observation of the functioning of the family unit.

In using observation techniques, the extent to which behavior of family members changes in observed situations needs to be considered, so as to minimize the effects of the observational technique. In family studies where individual family members are asked to respond to the same questionnaire, another issue arises. It is essential that each family member answer the questionnaire independently, and data collection procedures need to establish privacy whenever possible. Having a researcher or research assistant present during self-report data collection is ideal. When this is not possible, for example with mailed questionnaires, subjects should be asked to respond independently and not to discuss their answers until after their questionnaires have been completed and returned. In interview situations, it is critical to decide who should be present. Answers to questions may vary depending on the whether the subject is alone or other family members are present.

Just as subjects may be sensitive to issues raised in family research, so may researchers. Members of the research team who are involved in data collection are especially prone to having their own concerns emerge as a result of working on issues with families. A process for helping the research team resolve such issues is particularly important in family research. If the researcher is unaware of or does not come to terms with feelings and issues that arise in the research process, these feelings may affect the researcher's behavior with subjects. Debriefing the research team, as well as the subjects, helps to overcome the problems that may arise during the study of families.

As family assessment tools become more sophisticated, they are being used more in practice as well as in research. When appropriate, the family nurse clinician can serve a dual role as the data collector and as the individual who provides the nursing intervention or, in other words, as researcher and clinician.

The ongoing debate in nursing science regarding quantitative and qualitative research methods also exists within the area of family nursing research. Qualitative methods have gained greater acceptance within nursing science in the past decade and are being conducted more frequently. Until recently, the primary method of examining the family was quantitative and based on self-report questionnaires, structured interviews, and surveys. A critique of quantitative methods for measuring the family unit asserts that family nursing practice is more sophisticated and further advanced than the quantitative instruments available (Moriarty, 1990). Qualitative approaches, including unstructured interviews with families and participant observation, have been found more useful than quantitative approaches in measuring the family's subjective experiences and provide information on the family's motivations and behaviors (Moriarty, 1990).

Ethical Considerations

The ethical considerations that are inherent in all research are particularly relevant in research with the family. The researcher must balance the desire to gain information that is private and generally emotional against the need to protect the family's right to confidentiality and to respect the hospitality offered by the family. The nature of qualitative research often means that the researcher does not know where an interview may be leading or what may be the outcome of an observation session. Thus, it is important to establish boundaries that will provide research subjects with the opportunity to discontinue at any time. Although informed consent establishes guidelines for this, it is critical that the researcher remain aware of the family's potential vulnerability.

Analysis of Family Nursing Research

Data analysis in family research offers another set of issues to consider. The conceptual framework and definition of the family guide the investigator in analysis of the data. In addition, "your plan for data analysis is derived from your question, your design, your method of data collection, and the level of measurement of your data" (Brink & Wood, 1994, p. 212). Data analysis is simplified when data are collected from only one family member; however, having only one individual's perspective limits the generalizability of the study and does not adequately examine the dynamic and relational aspects of the family unit.

When more than one family member completes a data collection instrument, the researcher must decide whether to examine the data as individual data or select a method of combining the data to create "family responses." For example, the researcher can combine the scores of two or more family members and use the average of their scores as the family response. Careful consideration of the meaning of both individual scores and combined scores is necessary in family research. Uphold and Strickland (1989) provide an excellent review of the advantages and disadvantages of several strategies for combining scores from more than one individual family member.

Family studies usually involve not only the study of more than one individual, but also the study of more than one variable. Consequently, data analysis can be very complex. Generally it involves multivariate techniques since the complexities of marriage and family phenomena are best approached with these techniques (Miller, 1986). At times the researcher may analyze the same data using several different techniques. When similar results are obtained using different techniques of data analysis, the specific data analysis technique becomes less significant and the researcher is often more confident of the findings. However, as Feetham (1991) warns, the data analysis technique should not be chosen arbitrarily, but rather, "technique[s] must be linked conceptually to the study and be appropriate for the data" (p. 45).

SUMMARY

The clinical skills of the practicing nurse include those same skills that can be effectively used in the research process (Gillis, 1983). That is to say, assessment of the patient and family requires the same observation and critical analysis that is needed in gathering research data. For example, preparing to teach parents about the care of their newborn first involves assessing the parents' knowledge regarding infant care. The nurse uses listening skills to assess this and plan his or her intervention. Unfortunately, nursing research often has not taken advantage of those skills of the practicing nurse that could contribute to research. Similarly, practicing nurses have not taken advantage of critical information gathered by researchers. For example, evidence concerning the influence of the relationship between the family and patient is more than 20 years old, yet little progress has been made in systematically organizing and using this information (Gillis, 1989).

It is important that, as a practice discipline, nursing integrate theory, practice, and research. As questions arise in practice and nurses examine the nature of their practice, scientific inquiry can challenge the models upon which practice is based and ultimately advance both theory and practice. Today, hospitals are persistent in their use of quality assurance mechanisms to evaluate the care provided in their institution. The emphasis on such measures provides nurses with the opportunity to develop evaluation techniques and more sophisticated outcome measures. Partnerships between nurse clinicians and researchers will strengthen the development of nursing science. Every research project benefits when the perspective and skills of practicing nurses are brought together with the skills of researchers; conversely, collaboration between researchers and practitioners facilitates the use of new knowledge in the practice arena.

STUDY QUESTIONS

1. In discussing the integration of theory, practice, and research in family healthcare nursing, which of the following statements would apply?
   a. Family nursing practice will guide the development of family nursing research and theory.
   b. Theory related to family nursing will provide a framework for family nursing practice.
   c. Family nursing research will influence the development of theory relevant to family nursing.
   d. All of the above.

2. State why it is important for family nurse researchers to clearly define family.

3. Identify three social science disciplines that have influenced the development of family nursing science.

4. Which of the following statements are true?
   a. A characteristic of systems theory is that each subsystem is independent of all others.
   b. Developmental theory is based on chronological stages through which the family passes.
   c. An advantage of the structural-functional model is that it characterizes a family over time.
   d. Communication theory emphasizes the sending and receiving of both verbal and nonverbal messages.

5. List three major themes of family research over the past decade.

6. Once the research question is formulated, it is important to articulate the _____, as it will provide a basis upon which design and methodology decisions can be made.

7. Identify three factors in collecting data from family members that add to the complexity of doing research within families.

8. A family may be more willing to participate in a research study if:
   a. The health care setting requires that they participate

b. The researcher is seen as someone authoritarian and outside their own community.
c. The research is carried out in their family home.
d. All of the above.

9. Discuss how the researcher would deal with both research subjects and the research team when investigating a sensitive research topic.

10. Describe how family nurse clinicians can be involved in family nursing research.

REFERENCES

Andrews, H. A., & Roy, C. (1986). *Essentials of the Roy Adaptation Model.* Norwalk, CT: Appleton-Century-Crofts.

Berardo, F. M. (1990). Trends and directions in family research in the 1980s. *Journal of Marriage and the Family*, *52*, 809–817.

Boyd, S. T. (1985). Conceptual basis for nursing intervention with families. In J. E. Hall & B. R. Weaver (Eds.), *Distributive nursing practice: A systems approach to community health* (pp. 163–177). Philadelphia, J. B. Lippincott.

Brink, P. J., & Wood, M. J. (1994). *Basic steps in planning nursing research: From question to proposal.* Boston: Jones & Bartlett.

Burr, W. R., Day, R. D., & Bahr, K. S. (1993). *Family science.* Pacific Grove, CA: Brooks/Cole.

Chin, S. (1985). Can self-care theory be applied to families? In J. P. Riehl-Sisca (Ed.), *The science and art of self-care* (pp. 56–62). Norwalk, CT: Appleton-Century-Crofts.

Duvall, E. M. (1979). *Marriage and family development* (5th ed.). Philadelphia: J. B. Lippincott.

Feetham, S. L. (1991). Conceptual and methodological issues in research of families. In A. L. Whall & J. Fawcett (Eds.), *Family theory development in nursing: State of the science and art* (pp. 55–68). Philadelphia: F. A. Davis.

Fisher, L. (1982). Transactional theories but individual assessment: A frequent discrepancy in family research. *Family Process, 21*, 313–320.

Fisher, L., Kokes, R. F., Ransom, D. C., Phillips, S. L., & Rudd, P. (1985). Alternative strategies for creating "relational" family data. *Family Process, 24*, 213–224.

Gelles, R. J. (1978). Methods for studying sensitive family topics. *American Journal of Orthopsychiatry, 48*, 408–424.

Gilliss, C. L. (1983). The family as a unit of analysis: Strategies for the nurse researcher. *Advances in Nursing Science, 5*, 50–59.

Gilliss, C. L. (1989). Family research in nursing. In C. L. Gilliss, B. L. Highley, B. M. Roberts, & I. M. Martinson (Eds.), *Toward a science of family nursing.* Menlo Park, CA: Addison-Wesley.

Hanson, S. M. H., Kaakinen, J., & Friedman, M. M. (in press). Theoretical approaches to family nursing. In M. M. Friedman (Ed.), *Family nursing: Theory and practice* (5th ed.). Norwalk, CT: Appleton & Lange.

Hill, R. (1980). Status of research on families. In J. A. Calhoun, E. H. Grotberg, & W. R. Rackley (Eds.), *The status of children, youth, and families, 1979* (pp. 191–251) (DHHS Publication No. (OHDS) 80-30274). Washington, DC: US Department of Health and Human Services.

King, I. M. (1983). King's theory of nursing. In I. W. Clements and F. B. Roberts (Eds.), *Family health: A theoretical approach to nursing care* (pp 177–188). New York: Wiley.

Miller, B. C. (1986). *Family research methods.* Newbury Park, CA: Sage Publications.

Moriarty, H. (1990) Key issues in the family research process: Strategies for nurse researchers. *Advances in Nursing Science, 12*, 1–14.

Murphy, S. (1986). Family study and nursing research. *Image: Journal of Nursing Scholarship, 18*, 170–174.

Neuman, B. (1983). Family intervention using the Betty Neuman Health-Care Systems Model. In I. W. Clements and F. B. Roberts (Eds.), *Family Health: A theoretical approach to nursing care* (pp. 239–254). New York: Wiley.

Neuman, B. (1989). *The Neumann Systems Model. Application to nursing education and practice* (2nd ed.). Norwalk, CT: Appleton & Lange.

Orem, D. E. (1983a). The family coping with a medical illness. Analysis and applications of Orem's theory. In I. W. Clements and F. B. Roberts (Eds.), *Health: A theoretical approach to nursing care* (pp. 385–386). New York: Wiley.

Orem, D. E. (1983b). The family experiencing emotional crisis. Analysis and application of Orem's self-care deficit theory. In I. W. Clements and F. B. Roberts (Eds.), *Health: A theoretical approach to nursing care* (pp. 367–368). New York: Wiley.

Reed, K. S. (1989). Family theory related to the Neuman's System Model. In B. Neuman (Ed.), *The Neuman Systems Model: Application to nursing education and practice* (2nd ed.) (pp. 385–395). Norwalk, CT: Appleton & Lange.

Rogers, M. E. (1983). Science of unitary human beings: A paradigm for nursing. In I. W. Clements & F. B. Roberts, *Health: A theoretical approach to nursing care* (pp. 219–228). New York: Wiley.

Roy, C. (1983). Roy Adaptation Model: In I. W. Clements and F. B. Roberts (Eds.), *Health: A theoretical approach to nursing care* (pp. 255–278). New York: Wiley.

Roy, C. (1984). *Introduction to nursing: An adaptation model* (2nd ed.). Englewood Cliffs, NJ: Prentice Hall.

Stein, R., & Riessman, C. (1980). The development of an impact-on-family scale: Preliminary findings. *Medical Care, 18,* 465–472.

Terkelsen, K. G. (1980). Toward a theory of the family life cycle. In E.A. Carter & M. McGoldrick (Eds.), *The family life cycle: A framework for family therapy.* New York: Gardener Press.

Uphold, C. R., & Strickland, O. L. (1989). Issues related to the unit of analysis in family nursing research. *Western Journal of Nursing Research, 11,* 405–417.

Whall, A. L., & Fawcett, J. (1991). *Family theory development in nursing: State of the science and art.* Philadelphia: F.A. Davis.

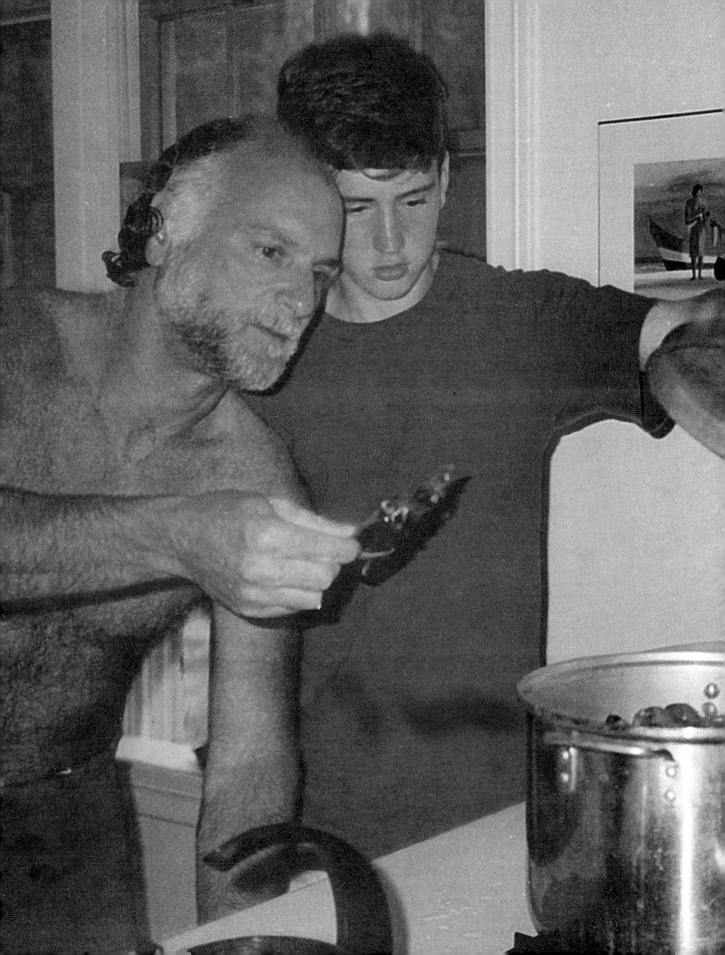

Family Structure, Function, and Process

This chapter is designed to answer questions like: What makes families "work"? How do they do what they do? Why are some families healthy and nurturing and others unhealthy and dysfunctional? What goes on in families that affects the overall health of individual family members and the health of the entire family unit?

As you are well aware, your own family of origin is different from that of your grandparents. Although you and your grandparents share a common genetic code, it is unlikely that the structure of your current family is the same as theirs when they were the same age. The social acceptability of alternative lifestyles has increased in recent years and new family types have proliferated. As you read, keep in mind that different family structures are constantly emerging. Because these new types of families may be your clients, it is essential that you have the knowledge to work with them.

Family structure refers to the individuals who comprise the family and the connections between household members. Structure also refers to relationships between the family and other social systems. In this chapter, structure is defined as an ordered set of relationships among the parts of the family and you will find a cogent discussion of family composition, types of families, family size, and the importance of the family's social network.

The chapter proceeds to explore the purpose or function the family serves in relation to individual family members, to the family as a whole, to other social systems, and to society. As you learn how family structure affects family function and, conversely, how family function influences structure, you will be challenged to sort out the cause-and-effect relationships between family structure and function.

Finally, family process, or the ongoing interaction among family members, is examined. In this section you will learn about the roles of family members and how they are enacted. Role strain as a potential major stressor to family systems is examined. Communication, power, marital satisfaction, and coping strategies complete the discussion of family process.

CHAPTER 3

Family Structure, Function, and Process

Naomi R. Ballard, RN, MA, MS, CNRN

OBJECTIVES   *Upon completion of this chapter, the reader will be able to:*

1. Identify the major limitation underlying the analysis of family structure, function, and process.
2. Describe four types of family structure present in American society in the late twentieth century.
3. Analyze the relationship between family structure and health status.
4. Identify four functional prerequisites of the family system.
5. Identify two functions of the American family in the late twentieth century.
6. Analyze the relationship between family function and health status.
7. Describe eight familial roles.
8. Identify five sources of role strains and five mechanisms to alleviate the strains.
9. Differentiate between effective and ineffective familial communication.
10. Analyze the relationship between familial power and decision making.
11. Identify the characteristics of a healthy family system.
12. Analyze the nursing implications of alterations in family structure, function, and process.

Does the family have a future? This question has preoccupied lay people, social scientists, and health professionals for at least four decades (Bane, 1976; Otto, 1970; Spanier, 1989). The demographic and social changes that the family is undergoing are viewed by many as indicators of the family's instability, if not its impending demise. These arguments, however, are based on ideas about what a traditional family is supposed to be but, in reality, never was. Coontz's (1988, 1992) historical analyses of the American family document an ongoing evolution in **family structure, function** and **processes**. Change is the norm, not the exception. This is true both of the family as an institution in society and of individual family units, which undergo dynamic changes throughout their life cycle. Change enables the family to continue to play a viable role in society.

The family is, or should be, the primary unit of health care. The structure, function, and process of the family influence, and are influenced by, the health status of the individuals in the family and the health of the family unit. For example, the breadth of a family's social network determines when and how a child gets chicken pox, and a child with a contagious disease limits parents' ability to meet their social responsibilities. Family health care requires a multidisciplinary knowledge base. This foundation enables the nurse to assess the family's health status, ascertain the effect of the family on individuals' health status, predict the impact of alterations in individual health status on the family, and work with the family in the development and implementation of an action plan to improve health.

The nurse also needs to understand the role of the family as a social institution. The family is linked to almost every other institution within society; consequently, understanding of family change requires understanding the historical, social, cultural, economic, political, and psychological context in which it occurs. This facilitates understanding the effect of change on the health of the individual, the family, and society.

Any analysis of family structure, function, and process is limited by the knowledge on which it is based. Despite the predominance of nontraditional families in American society today, little is known about them. The traditional nuclear family remains the standard by which individual families are evaluated (Ganong, Coleman, & Mapes, 1990; Spanier, 1992). Indeed, most of our knowledge about the American family is derived from research on nuclear families. Blumstein and Schwartz's study of American couples (1983) is a notable exception.

This chapter analyzes changes in family structure, function, and process that have implications for the delivery of family health care. The discussion of family structure focuses on the decline of the nuclear family and the emergence of other family types in American society in the late twentieth century. The function of the family in relation to society and to the maintenance of the family system is analyzed. In the discussion of family processes, changes in the delineation and enactment of familial roles are examined, and the effects of communication, power, and decision making on the enactment of these roles are explored.

FAMILY STRUCTURE

The most clear-cut change that has occurred in the American family during the past few decades has been in its structure. Family structure is the ordered set of relationships among the parts of the family and between the family and other social systems. In determining family structure, the nurse needs to identify the individuals that make up the family, the relationships between them, and the relationships between the family and other social systems. A family's patterns of organization tend to be relatively stable over time. However, they are modified — gradually throughout the family life cycle, or radically by divorce or death. In a rapidly changing society, several types of family structure may coexist. Each family type has its strengths and weaknesses, which directly or indirectly affect the health of the individuals in the family and the family unit.

Composition of the Family

When does a set of individuals compose a family? Traditionally, the family was organized around the biological function of reproduction; therefore, the family was composed of a husband, a wife, and their biological children. Throughout American history, this has been the most common type of family (Bane, 1976; Degler, 1980; Coontz, 1988, 1992). However, during the past two decades, the reproductive function has become increasingly separated from the traditional family unit (Robertson, 1991), and defining a family has become more difficult. The criteria most often used to define a family are structure and function (Winch, 1977). When the family is defined according to its structure, the positions that the individuals in the family assume and the relationships between them are emphasized. The US Bureau of the Census uses this kind of criterion in its definition of a *household*, a concept that overlaps that of *family*. When a functional criterion is used to define family, the individuals making up the family must engage in activities that are considered familial; for example, childrearing. A third option, which ignores both the structural and functional criteria, is that the family is whatever the set of individuals making up the family say it is. In reality, the definition of a family may be less important to the individuals who compose a family than to the scholars who study families. Basically, individuals organize themselves into families to meet cultural prescriptions and basic human needs. As cultural prescriptions and needs change, families change.

Types of Families

The traditional family, composed of a husband and wife, married for the first time, and their biological children, is no longer the predominant type of family in American society. The US Bureau of the Census (1993) currently uses five variables to describe various types of households, or families: marital status, gender of sexual partners, presence of children, parentage of children, and age of children. For example, a remarried or blended family contains a man and woman, at least one of whom has been married before. They may or may not have children living in the household. If they do, the children may be his, hers, or theirs. The children may be under or over 18 years of age. Another type of family may be composed of two unmarried men or women who have no children.

Married Couples

Households headed by married couples are undergoing marked change in their structure. The number of households without children is rising as a result of the increased length of the postparental stage of the family life cycle. Further, in approximately one third of the households headed by married couples, one or both of the spouses has been married previously (Spanier & Furstenberg, 1987). Remarried families, stepfamilies, or blended families differ from traditional families both in their interactions with children and in their larger social network.

Single-Parent Families

The single-parent family is one in which the head of the household has never been married or is not currently married. Single-parent families make up 23% of all households with children under 18 years of age (US Bureau of the Census, 1993). This high percentage is due to the high divorce rate, the increase in births to adolescents, and the limited availability of mates in some portions of the population. Single parenthood is particularly common among African-Americans (Jayakody, Chatters, & Taylor, 1993). Fifty-four percent of African-American children under 18 years of age reside in households headed by their mothers. This is related, in part, to the lack of African-American men in the marriage market. The high mortality rate for African-American men, their high level of incarceration, and limited opportunities in the labor market reduce marital options for African-American women (Fossett & Kiecolet, 1993). Thirty percent of Hispanic children and 18.1% of white children reside in households headed by their mothers. The single-parent structure alters the relationship between men and women (Guttentag & Secord, 1983) and between parents and children (Dawson, 1991; Thomson, McLanahan, & Curtin, 1992). It is also correlated with high rates of poverty and has ominous implications both for children and for the future of American society.

Cohabiting Couples

An alternative for sexual partners who do not wish to marry or who, because of legal proscription, cannot marry is cohabitation. Since 1970, the number of unmarried heterosexual couples living together has increased markedly (Cherlin, 1992). By 1986, 6% of all unmarried adults in the United States were cohabiting (Glick, 1988). Cohabitation has not resulted in a decrease in the marriage rate: 9 out of 10 Americans eventually marry. However, cohabitation has altered the timing of marriage. Today, many young adults postpone marriage until their mid or late twenties or even their thirties. Cohabitation thus seems to be a part of the courtship process, not an alternative to marriage. However, cohabitation prior to marriage is associated with a higher divorce rate; moreover, divorced people are more likely to cohabit.

Little is known about the cohabitation patterns of homosexual couples. Since 1950, date on unmarried and unrelated adults of the same sex, 25 years of age and older, who share a household have been included in the census. The data are limited, however, because these householders may or may not be sexual partners. Nevertheless, the number of cohabiting homosexual couples is consistently half as numerous as the number of unmarried heterosexual couples (Glick, 1988). Currently, marriage is not a legal alternative for homosexual couples.

Family Size

The size of households has decreased during the past few decades. This is related to a decline in the birth rate and the mortality rate (Santi, 1987; Teachman, Polonko, & Scanzoni, 1987). The decline in the birth rate has reduced the proportion of large families, and the decline in the mortality rate has increased the proportion of postparental families. In addition, more individuals are choosing to live alone. In 1990, approximately 22 million households were composed of one person (US Bureau of the Census, 1993). The only trend that seems to be offsetting this decline in household size is the tendency for adult children to return temporarily to their parents' home.

Marital Dissolution

The change that has had greatest impact on family structure is the increase in the rate of divorce. The divorce rate rose from the middle of the nineteenth century until the 1980s (Cherlin, 1992). In the 1980s, the rate began to decline slightly, but is has remained higher than in the 1960s. By 1974, more marriages ended in divorce than in death. From 1960 to 1980, the rise in the divorce rate was greater than would have been predicted by the trend line. What accounted for this? Divorces tend to increase after wars and decrease in times of economic difficulty; the end of the Vietnam War and the burgeoning economy probably contributed to the high divorce rate from 1960 to 1980. In addition, the options available for women outside of marriage improved. Certainly, people were not disenchanted with marriage, because the majority remarried. However, their expectations for marriage may have exceeded reality.

At the current divorce rate, about half of all marriages will end in separation or divorce. This means that two fifths of all children will experience disruption in their parents' marriage by age 16 years. The majority of them will live in a single-parent household headed by their mother for at least 5 years before their mother remarries or they reach the age of 18 years. The social and economic consequences of divorce for women and children have been well documented (Weitzman, 1985). The long-term impact of high rates of marital dissolution on adult children and society is just beginning to become apparent (Amato & Keith, 1991).

Social Network

People outside the home who engage in activities of an affective or material nature with the members of the household constitute the family's social network. The presence of a strong social network improves the health status and life satisfaction of the family members. For an individual, the best single predictor of the size and richness of the social network is education; that is, better-educated individuals are more likely to have a substantial social network. This in turn benefits the family. Familial social networks change with changes in marital status, the family's developmental level, and the family's geographic location; for example, an individual's social network declines markedly after divorce or separation. Even remarried or blended families have a smaller social network than traditional families. The reason for this is unclear. Indeed, because of contacts with ex-spouses and their families, remarried or blended families might be expected to have a larger social network.

Families operate on a continuum from a closed to an open system in their interactions with the outside world (Kantor & Lehr, 1975). A closed family system, functioning in isolation from other social systems and social institutions, is impossible to sustain. However, a few families — for example, cult members and survivalists — try to achieve total isolation from the larger society. More commonly, families who operate as somewhat closed systems maintain only essential contacts with the outside world. Their primary interactions with the outside world are through their work. They send their children to school, but they do not become involved in school activities. Their drapes remain pulled, their doors closed. They have no visitors and may have only a nodding acquaintance with their neighbors. They may not even have a radio or television. Under ordinary circumstances the closed family may be able to maintain homeostasis, but it may be poorly equipped to deal with change or with the stress of an illness. At the opposite extreme, open families have many interchanges with the outside world. They are involved in multiple activities both inside and outside the family. Visitors are encouraged, drapes are open, lights are on, and doors may be unlocked. Indeed, the open family system's boundaries may become blurred, leaving them vulnerable to breakdown of the family structure. Most families lie somewhat between these extremes. They have clearly defined boundaries but enough flexibility to capitalize on their contacts with the outside world.

The family's social network provides both instrumental and expressive support. This is particularly true of the extended family, which, contrary to popular belief, remains the major source of social support for American families. Intergenerational interaction is the norm, not the exception (Stull & Borgatta, 1987). This source of support is especially important for the frail elderly and for single parents. The majority of elderly persons live within a short travel time of at least one child. Even those who live 3000 miles away from their children usually maintain contact. Most elderly people who need either material or affective support are able to depend on family members to provide it. In addition, families seem to go out of their way to help single parents. This is particularly true of African-Americans; an extensive system of kin networks has been documented in African-American communities. Nevertheless, the extent of aid to African-American single parents may be overstated. Despite the presence of extensive networks, only a quarter of African-American never-married mothers receive financial assistance and less than one fifth receive help with child care (Jayakody, Chatters, & Taylor, 1993). Unlike single-parent families, married families have the advantage of being able to seek support from both families of origin. To determine the usefulness of a family's social network, data on the type of support provided, the proximity of the network, the interactions within the network, and the affinity of the kin need to be evaluated.

Nursing Implications

Every family experiences strain in dealing both with daily hassles and with crises. Households headed by married couples usually have more resources to draw on in dealing with day-to-day strains. Single-parent families, especially those headed by women, are particularly vulnerable because they have fewer resources of time, energy, and money with which to cope. Cohabiting families, both heterosexual and homosexual, have to cope with this additional stressors of social censure and legal restraints, which limit the coping strategies they can invoke.

Nurses, as citizens and as health professionals, need to play an active role in enacting social policies to reduce the strains for families. For example, more available child care would reduce the burden of many families. In addition, families today are being asked to assume more responsibility for health care. They are expected to care for acutely and chronically ill family members who were once cared for by health professionals. This portends disaster for families already strained to the limit. Until social policies reduce the burden on families, nurses, through counseling and education, need to help families develop more adaptive interaction patterns and more effective coping strategies (see Bomar, 1989; Wright & Leahey, 1984, 1987; and Leahey & Wright, 1987a, b for a discussion of specific interventions).

FUNCTION OF THE FAMILY

Family function is the purpose that the family serves in relation to the individual, the family, other social systems, and society. However, family function is very difficult to describe. One quickly gets caught in circular reasoning: family function is a consequence of family structure, but the structure exists to fulfill one or more functions. In everyday life, the function of the family is questioned only when a social need — for example, social control — is not being met.

For example, recently the family's function as instrument of social control has been questioned. Several social trends, including the increase in violence in our society, the increase in substance abuse, and the increase in teenage pregnancies, have been attributed to the family's ineffectiveness in transmitting family values. Unfortunately, this is a simplistic explanation for very complex problems because it ignores the interaction of the family and other social institutions. The complexity of these relationships makes describing the function of the family difficult.

To ascertain the effect of the family on the individual's and family's health, the function of the family must be analyzed at two levels. At the microlevel, the effects of the family unit on the growth and development of its members and maintenance of the family system are analyzed. On the macrolevel, the effect of the family as a social institution is examined.

The Family as a Social System

Functional Prerequisites

In order for the family to meet society's needs, the family unit has to maintain its integrity as a social system. In order to survive as a social system, the family must meet certain prerequisites: adaptation, goal attainment, integration, and pattern maintenance/tension management (Parsons, 1951).

Adaptation

Adaptation refers to the necessity to accommodate to the family's external and internal environments. The external environment includes the physical environment, other social systems with which the family interacts, and the predominant culture. The internal environment is composed of the family members as biological organisms and as personalities. In order to adapt, the family must carry out a range of tasks (Bell & Vogel, 1960), and the family must have the resources, skills, and motivation to perform these tasks. For example, one of the basic needs of family members is to obtain food. One or more family members must assume responsibility for growing food or for making the money to buy food; further, someone has to obtain and cook food that is compatible with the family members' biological needs and their cultural prescriptions, the family members have to be motivated to eat the food, and someone has to clean up afterwards. Failure to perform these tasks puts individual family members in physical jeopardy and leads to the breakdown of the family as a social system.

Goal Attainment

The family as a social system needs to identify its goals and the means to attain them. This is not always conscious. Sometimes goals can be inferred from the actions of the family members. At other times, the actions of family members seem incongruent with identified goals. For example, many parents state that spending quality time with their children is a top priority. However, when caught in a bind between the demands of their job and their family, they may attend to their jobs first. In identifying and attaining goals, the family member who has most influence in decision making may vary from situation to situation; however, over time, the leadership structure of the family is fairly stable.

Integration

Integration is the means by which a family acquires the cohesion, solidarity, and identity that enable the family to maintain close relationships over time. Overt and covert expressions of affection promote family cohesion, as do family rituals and celebrations. Symbols of family solidarity include photograph albums, heirlooms, and favorite jokes. Family ties operate to prevent the disintegration of the family system and to motivate family members to abide by the family's norms.

Pattern Maintenance and Tension Management

Like integration, pattern maintenance and tension management have to do primarily with the internal state of the family. In their interactions with each other, family members develop expectations about how each should behave. In order for a family to survive, it must agree, to a certain extent, on the values that regulate family activities. There may or may not be conscious, but they must be flexible enough to allow some deviation. For example, a family who expects everyone to show up for a 6:00 PM dinner needs to make allowances when a family member is delayed by a traffic jam. Furthermore, the family's expectations have to be modified as the family develops. For example, the constraints placed upon a child's travel outside of the home are reduced as the child ages.

Role of the Family in Society

Before the Industrial Revolution, the family played a much larger role in society than it does today. It was the primary source of economic production, education, and health care. Later, other institutions — for example, schools and hospitals — assumed many of the functions that were once the responsibility of the family. Today, the economic and reproductive functions of the family are undergoing change. Significant functions of the family include the socialization of children and the stabilization of adult personalities (Parsons & Bales, 1955). Through these two functions, the family has a major effect on the health of its members.

Economic Function

In the early period of American history, the household was the major source of commodity production (Coontz, 1988). Economic relationships within the household reflected familial relationships, and the family worked under the leadership of a household head. Usually the head of the household was a man; however, a woman who, because of the death of her husband or father, assumed the position as family head exerted more power than before or since. With the emergence of capitalism in the early nineteenth century, the patriarchal household served as a source of workers. The household head, who received the wage for the family, contributed family members as workers for fledgling industries. This left a gap at home, and eventually married women returned home to resume their domestic duties. Thus, young women, unmarried women, and men constituted the labor pool and the division between work and home — between men's work and women's work — increased. This trend continued until World War II, when many married women moved back into the labor force. After the war, many women returned to their homes, but many elected to remain in the labor force. With the shift in recent years from an industrial to a service economy, the number of women in the labor force has once more increased. This reflects not only the need for their services but also the inability of many men to earn a family wage in the evolving economy. Young men, in particular, are experiencing a worsening of their economic position, while older men are leaving the labor force in record numbers. In economic terms, families today are no longer a source of commodity production. Instead, their economic function is to consume goods and services to keep the economy viable.

Reproduction

In the past the primary function of the family in society was the regulation of reproduction. Families today, however, have much less control over reproduction than in the past (Robertson, 1991) and seem unable or unwilling to control reproduction by family members. In the United States, more than a million adolescents become pregnant each year; approximately half of these pregnancies result in live births (Kalmuss, Namerow, & Baeur, 1992). This essentially means that children are having children. Because only about 5% of teenagers choose adoption, teenage mothers and their babies are either integrated into their families of origin or left to fend for themselves. Adolescent childbearing may increase as religious and legal threats to abortion increase. For centuries, the state, religion, and the family have fought over the right to control reproduction. Twenty years ago, in the *Roe v. Wade* decision, the US Supreme Court ruled that during the first trimester of pregnancy, the decision to have an abortion should be left solely to a woman and her physician (Leslie & Korman, 1985). However, the *Roe v. Wade* decision has been constantly challenged. Many argue that it negates the rights of the unborn child and the father. The ethical dilemmas embedded in the abortion controversy are mirrored by those introduced by technological advances in reproduction. Artificial insemination by husband or donor, in vitro fertilization, and artificial embryonation, in which a woman other than the wife donates an egg for fertilization, further remove the family from control of the reproductive process. In some cases, fertilization has moved out of the bedroom into the laboratory – out of the body and into the petri dish. Gestation may occur in the biological mother, even if she is 60 years of age, or in a surrogate. Religious, legal, and technological challenges to the family's control over reproduction will increase in the years ahead.

Socialization of Children

An important function of the family in American society is the socialization of children. Through this process, children acquire the social and psychological skills to take their place in the adult world. On the parents' part, this seems to involve a combination of social support and social control (Peterson & Rollins, 1987). Traditional American families composed of a man, a woman, and their biological children seem to be more effective than nontraditional families in the socialization of children. In 1988, 61% of children under 18 years of age lived with both biological parents. Those children had fewer health and behavioral problems than children reared in nontraditional families (Dawson, 1991). Nock (1988) suggest that the hierarchy of the nuclear family, with its formal authority structure, seems to be more effective in preparing children for adult roles (Nock, 1988). In other words, the attitudes and values learned in dealing with authority figures in the family are internalized, and consequently the child reared in a traditional family is more likely to achieve at school or work, because achievement in these settings also requires functioning in a hierarchial environment.

According to Nock (1988), children in nontraditional families are less likely to internalize the attitudes and values needed for success. The generational boundaries in single-parent families are not as clearly defined as in traditional families, and single parents tend to be more lax disciplinarians. Indeed, a working single parent of school-age children is probably too tired to do otherwise. In most cases, support from noncustodial spouses is minimal. Children from single-parent homes have less success in school, lower earnings, and lower occupational prestige than children from intact, two-parent families (Nock, 1988). They also have a higher rate of divorce and out-of-wedlock births. Of course, the effects of nontraditional family structure on the socialization process need to be considered in the context of economic deprivation and psychological stress. For instance, the presence of a second adult in the home, for example, a grandmother, helps offset the deleterious effects of being reared by a single parent (Demo, 1992; Thomson, McLanahan, & Curtin, 1992).

Remarried or blended families also seem to experience more problems with childrearing than do traditional families. The role of a stepparent is not clearly defined and, frequently, has many negative connotations. Stepparents show less warmth and communicate less well with stepchildren than biological parents (Thomson, McLanahan, & Curtin, 1992). They participate in fewer child-related activities, and this does not seem to change over time. The lack of engagement of stepparents may contribute to the development of more behavioral problems in children; however, it does not seem to affect the achievement of children. Most likely, remarried or blended families have a hierarchial structure similar to that of traditional families.

Stabilization of Adult Personalities

Another function of the American family is the stabilization of adult personalities. Married men and women have better physical and mental health than never-married, separated, divorced, or widowed persons (Barnett, Marshall, & Pleck, 1992; Gove, 1973; Verbrugge, 1979, 1983; Hahn, 1993). Older persons who have never married have a higher rate of mental disorders than married individuals of similar age. Widows are five times more likely than married persons to be institutionalized in long-term care facilities; separated or divorced persons are ten times more likely (Stull & Borgatta, 1987). Married persons have much lower age-standardized death rates. Unmarried persons have death rates above average from cirrhosis of the liver, pneumonia, motor vehicle accidents, suicide, and homicide. However, the cause of the inverse relationship between marriage and poor health of both men and women is unclear.

Are healthier people more likely to get married and stay married? Or does the psychological stress from the loss of a marriage increase one's susceptibility to illness? Marriage seems to have a buffering effect on the health status of both men and women, but the effect seems stronger for men. The marital role, both as spouse and as father, may be more central to men's physical and mental health than to women's (Barnett, Marshall, & Pleck, 1992). In a satisfactory marriage, both men and women receive psychological support from each other, which may improve their immunological response. In addition, married men and women are more likely to engage in health-enhancing activities (Hahn, 1993). This is particularly true of married men, who tend to rely upon their wives for many health-enhancing activities—for example, the provision of a balanced diet. Married women have a higher family income, are more likely to own a home, and are more likely to have health insurance than single women. Because socioeconomic status is positively related to health status, it may be a confounding variable for women in the relationship between marriage and health.

What effect does individual happiness have on the relationship between marriage and health? Traditionally, personal happiness has been positively correlated with marriage. However, in the past two decades, the difference in happiness between married and never-married persons has decreased (Lee, Seccombe, & Shehan, 1991). Among the never-married, both men and women demonstrate an increase in personal happiness. Among the married, women, particularly young women, report a decrease in personal happiness.

The change is most pronounced among employed mothers who are trying to balance multiple, demanding roles. However, married people still tend to be happier than unmarried people. Finally, the greater economic, psychological, and social support available to married people serves to stabilize their personalities and, consequently, to enhance their health (Lee, Seccombe, & Shehan, 1991).

Nursing Implications

Nursing interventions to promote family functioning vary with the degree of strain faced by the family. A family that is unable to meet the functional prerequisites of a social system — adaptation, goal attainment, integration, and pattern maintenance — is in danger of disintegrating. Family therapy by a nurse in advanced practice or by another health professional is needed (Bulechek & McCloskey, 1992). Most families can benefit from health teaching or counseling on health promotion, including instruction on safety, nutrition, exercise, stress management, sleep, hygiene, childrearing, and sexuality (Bomar, 1989). However, health teaching is unlikely to enhance the family's protective health function unless it is tailored to the learning needs of the family and the cultural context. Nurses may also strengthen the family's social support network by offering themselves as therapeutic agents and by identifying other support services. This is particularly important during times of family transition, for example, at the onset of chronic illness.

FAMILY PROCESS

Family process is the ongoing interaction between family members through which they accomplish their instrumental and expressive tasks. In part, this is what makes families unique. Families with the same structure and function may interact very differently. Family process, at least in the short term, seems to have a greater effect on the family's health than family structure and function, and, in turn, to be more affected by alterations in health status. It certainly has the most implications for nursing action. For example, for the chronically ill, an important determinant of successful rehabilitation is the ability to assume familial roles. This often requires a great deal of adaptation from all family members, and the familial power structure may or may not enhance this process. Moreover, the success or failure of the adaptation process in turn has an impact on the family structure and marital satisfaction.

Roles

Role Delineation

Within the nuclear family, each position within the family, for example, husband or wife, has a number of roles attached to it. Each role is composed of a set of expectations about what one *should* do. Nye (1976) identified eight roles attached to the position of spouse:

- Provider
- Housekeeping
- Child care
- Socialization
- Sex
- Therapeutic role

■ Recreation
■ Kinship

Traditionally, the provider role was assigned to the husband and the housekeeper and child care roles to the wife. However, the traditional assignment of these roles has been replaced by the members of the family negotiating their roles. For example, a newly married couple has to decide who writes the thank-you notes after the wedding. According to old etiquette books, this is the bride's responsibility. Today, however, many couples decide that the bride writes thank-you notes to her kin, and the groom to his. The husband and wife do not make these decisions in isolation; they are influenced by the culture in which they live. For the nuclear family, many culturally prescribed behavioral expectations exist. When norms are not met, social sanctions may occur; for example, the groom's grandmother may express her displeasure at what she perceives as a lack of social grace. At other times, legal sanctions are incurred—for example, when parents go on vacation and leave their children alone without arranging appropriate care. Nontraditional families, in which roles are not traditionally prescribed, may actually have more freedom in the negotiation process; too often, however, they are subjected to social sanctions for even existing.

Role Enactment

The Provider Role   The behaviors of family members in their various roles are not necessarily congruent with their expectations. The enactment of the provider role has undergone change in recent decades. The proportion of households in which men were the sole breadwinner had declined to 15% by 1988 (Wilkie, 1991). This decline is related to growth in multiple-earner families, a decrease in the proportion of families with a man living in the house, an increase in the number of families with no wage earners, and growth in the number of families solely supported by women. In industrialized nations, the participation of women in the labor force has increased dramatically (Kalleberg & Rosenfeld, 1990). At the same time, work conditions have become increasingly stressful for both men and women. Therefore, work obligations outside of the home increasingly impinge on the ability of family members to meet their familial role obligations.

Housekeeping and Child Care   Women experience a great deal of role strain in balancing the provider role with other familial roles. That is because women continue to be responsible for most of the family housekeeping and child care (Kalleberg & Rosenfeld, 1990; Ward, 1993). When a wife is employed, the husband spends only a small amount of additional time on housework. Women with children spend the most time on housework. Although husbands' roles in child care are increasing, their focus still tends to be on playing with the children, rather than meeting their basic needs. The portion of time women spend fulfilling housekeeper and child care roles may be related, in part, to the family income. Women with higher incomes spend less time on housekeeping and child care; they pay others to do it for them. Many women, however, earn less because of their familial responsibilities and they have more familial responsibilities because they earn less. Thus, they are caught in a vicious circle.

Socialization   In relation to socialization of the children, role expectations tend to be more egalitarian. The involvement of both parents is necessary for the development of healthy children because the father-child relationship is qualitatively different from the mother-child relationship. However, the wife still assumes the larger share of responsibility for the socialization of children. Men take more responsibility for the socialization of boys than of girls (Harris & Morgan, 1991).

After separation or divorce, the majority of children have little or no contact with nonresident fathers (Seltzer, 1991). Fathers may limit contact with children for whom they do not have custody in order to protect themselves from loss or to avoid conflict. Fathers who visit and pay child support are more likely to be involved in childrearing decisions; however, less than half of nonresident fathers pay child support. When children are born outside of marriage, the fathers are even less likely to be involved.

Sexual Roles The sexual and therapeutic familial roles also require a more egalitarian relationship between the adult partners, because in a satisfactory relationship, each needs to play an active role in meeting the sexual and therapeutic needs of the other. The main predictor of an egalitarian sexual relationship seems to be socioeconomic status and, more specifically, education. More highly educated women tend to be more assertive; more highly educated men tend to be more sensitive and emotionally expressive (Francoeur, 1987). More highly educated men and women are also more accepting of alternative sexual behaviors and tend to rate their sexual intimacy more positively. Women and men in the lower socioeconomic classes are more likely to experience early sexual intercourse and to follow more traditional sexual practices.

Two opposing trends that affect sexual relationships seem to be becoming more important in American society. One is the increase in the number of different ethnic groups who hold traditional sexual values. The other is the decrease in the sex ratio. Guttentag and Secord (1983) argue that the sex ratio is correlated with sexual attitudes, values, and behaviors. Thus, the clear surplus of females in American society may contribute to an environment in which adultery is considered acceptable or normal, marriage is viewed as temporary, sexual liberation is encouraged, and women are encouraged to work outside the home (Francoeur, 1987). The relative impact of these two opposing trends is yet to be determined.

The Therapeutic Role The therapeutic role involves helping each other with intra- and extrafamilial problems. This includes a willingness to share one's own concerns, a willingness to listen to others, active involvement in problem solving, and emotional support. It embodies what small-group theorists call the expressive role. However, families cannot depend on one member to assume the expressive role and another the instrumental or more directive role. In order to survive as a family, all members have to assume both roles at one time or another. One study of family roles found that over 60% of husbands and wives believed they had a duty to enact the therapeutic role (Nye, 1976). Sixty-three percent of the men and 80% of the women in the study enacted the role. Over three fifths disapproved of a husband or wife who refused to help a spouse with a problem. The husbands and wives in the study also thought that a family member who reacted with criticism to the person confiding a problem, who disclosed the problem to a third party, or who imposed solutions on the confider deserved verbal sanctions.

The therapeutic role includes supporting family members in activities that promote health and prevent disease. Individuals are more likely to engage in health-promoting activities, such as exercise, when they are accompanied by a significant other. When individuals become sick, they turn to members of their family for validation of their symptoms. For example, one woman knew it was time to seek medical help when her husband found her with all the doors and windows open despite freezing temperatures outside and said, "You're screwed up." This verified her own perceptions. She was eventually diagnosed with hyperthyroidism. In addition to supporting each other in seeking health care, family members also play a therapeutic role in helping the sick person decide on treatment options. They frequently assist in the administration and evaluation of long-term treatments. Family support is a major determinant in rehabilitation.

The Recreation Role Most recreation is engaged in with other family members (Hawks, 1991). However, the recreational role is not as culturally prescribed as many other familial roles. Families do not assign recreational responsibilities to a particular member. They do not care who does the planning, as long as it gets done. The quantity and types of recreation engaged in vary with the stages of the family life cycle. Also, families with higher incomes have more formal, organized, and expensive activities; families from a lower socioeconomic status tend to rely on more inexpensive activities such as visiting relatives (Hawks, 1991). Recreation is also affected by the wife's participation in the labor force. When the woman works outside the home, social activities outside the family decrease, but intrafamily activities and commercial recreation are not as greatly affected (Carlson, 1976). The major complaint about recreation is the lack of time available for it (McCown, Delamarter, Schroeder, & Liegler, 1989). Perceived satisfaction with leisure time is positively associated with marital sociability, marital satisfaction, marital stability, and marital intimacy (Hawks, 1991). The family's involvement in leisure time activities promotes integration of the family system. However, recreation is often the first role to be dropped when the family is under stress.

The Kinship Role Enactment of the kinship role involves maintaining contact with the extended family and friends. According to Marks and McLanahan (1993, p. 482), "Women continue to function as 'kinkeepers.'" Women maintain a higher level of interaction with the extended family than men; they give and receive more family help; and they tend to rely on parents, children, or siblings for support. Fathers in traditional families are more likely than men in nontraditional families to give instrumental social support to their parents and children, including child care, transportation, and repairs to home or car. Single fathers and single mothers are more likely than other families to receive support from parents. On the other hand, mothers with a cohabiting partner are less likely to receive social support from parents. Cohabiting homosexual couples rely more heavily on networks of friends. Middle-aged and elderly parents receive help from their children. A high level of exchange occurs between middle-aged and elderly parents and daughters, even when the daughter is not a caregiver (Walker & Pratt, 1991). Therefore, the kinship role is important throughout the family life cycle and in all types of families.

Role Competence

The competent performance of familial roles is a determinant of marital success. Blood and Wolfe (1960) hypothesized that power in marriage is related to the comparative resources that the husband and wife bring to the marriage, and it has been pointed out that competent performance of familial roles is one of the primary resources that a person brings to marriage (Bahr, 1976). It constitutes a reward to one's partner. The more rewards, for example — money, love, and status, one receives from a spouse, the more likely one is to comply when differences in opinion arise. Furthermore, the more rewards one receives from a spouse, the more likely one is to be satisfied in the marriage. If the exchange is inequitable, one or both spouses may seek other alternatives.

Role Strain

Lack of competence in role performance may be a result of role strain, that is, difficulty in the delineation and enactment of familial roles. Heiss (1981) identified five sources of difficulties in this process:

1. Inability to define the situation
2. Lack of role knowledge
3. Lack of role consensus

4. Role conflict
5. Role overload

All of these problems place strain on the family system; but solutions to the problems differ greatly.

Inability to Define the Situation   With changes in family structure and in gender roles, family members increasingly encounter situations in which the guidelines for action are unclear. For example, nowadays a couple who has just begun dating has to decide who opens the car door, whereas in the 1950s, the man automatically opened the door. Single parents, stepparents, nonresident fathers, and cohabiting partners deal daily with situations for which there are no norms. What right does a stepparent have to discipline the new spouse's child? Is a nonresident father expected to teach his child about AIDS? What name or names go on the mailbox of cohabiting partners? Whether or not the issues are substantive, they present daily challenges to the people involved. One method of dealing with the difficulty is withdrawing from the situation, an alternative that many nonresident fathers choose. A second way of handling the problem is to redefine the situation. For instance, a newly blended family might decide to operate in the same way as a traditional nuclear family. Finally, family members might resort to trial and error. The cohabiting couple might put only one name on the mailbox. If this presents problems, the option to change their strategy exists. If there are no guidelines, or conflicting guidelines, and a solution cannot be found, family members suffer role strain.

Lack of Role Knowledge   A second source of role strain is inability to choose a role, either because the people involved do not know a role appropriate to the situation or they know several and have no basis for choosing between them. For example, in American society, many people are not taught how to be parents. They may not know how to keep their children from running over the neighbor's dog with their bicycles. Anticipatory socialization in the care of chronically ill family members is also inadequate. Whether the individual is learning how to be a parent or a caregiver, "on the job" training may be required. Information may be acquired by observation of peers; reflexive role-taking, in which individuals deduce what others expect them to do in the situation; or explicit instruction. In the case of parents and caregivers, opportunities to observe peers may be limited and other family members may not have the knowledge to help; therefore, other means of obtaining the information need to be explored. These might include classes in child care, self-help groups, and instruction from health professionals. If individuals are unable to figure out their roles in a situation, this may limit their problem-solving abilities.

Lack of Role Consensus   The third source of role strain is a lack of role consensus. Family members may be unable to agree on the expectations attached to a role. The role that currently seems to be the source of most dissension in families is the housekeeping role. This is a major problem for dual-career couples. A man who has been socialized into the traditional male role is not often inclined to increase the amount of time he spends on household activities. If he does participate actively, and his wife has been socialized into the traditional housekeeping role, his performance may not meet the wife's standards. Their lack of agreement is associated with decreased marital satisfaction. Negotiation is required to reach a working consensus. Persuasion, manipulation, and coercion are also sometimes used, but over the long term they are less likely to be effective.

Role Conflict   A fourth source of role strain is role conflict. This occurs when the expectations of different familial roles or within one familial role are incompatible. For example, the therapeutic role might involve being a caregiver to an elderly parent. The expectations attached to this role may be incompatible with those of the provider, housekeeper, and child care roles. Does one go to the child's baseball game or to the doctor with the elderly parent? Most often, individuals have to set priorities. The caregiver and provider roles generally are maintained, and other familial roles may suffer. The first role to be limited is the recreational role. The caregiver may withdraw from activities that, in the short term, seem superfluous but, in the long term, are sources of much-needed energy.

Role Overload   A source of role strain that is closely related to role conflict is role overload. In role overload, individuals lack the resources, time, and energy to meet the demands of all the roles they are involved in. The first option considered is usually withdrawal from one of the roles. An alternative might be to add roles that are energy-producing — for example, the role of bridge-player, artist, or tennis player. An individual who experiences role overload might also consider delegating some responsibilities to others. This requires skill in negotiation.

Communication

The negotiation of familial roles requires effective communication. In healthy families, communication occurs among autonomous individuals in an environment that is relatively free of unresolved conflicts. Healthy communication is characterized by clear but flexible rules, clarity in the verbalization of feelings and thoughts, freedom to express a wide variety of feelings, and receptivity to and acknowledgment of the other person's communication (Hoffer, 1989; Lewis, Beavers, Gossett, & Phillips, 1976; Lewis, 1989). The psychological defense mechanisms of projection, denial, blaming, and scapegoating are infrequent.

Communication difficulties are probably the most common problem in families who seek help to improve their interactions. Miscommunication may occur because of differences in the cultural or developmental makeup of family members (Varenne, 1992). Communication difficulties may also be related to the different communication styles of men and women. Hawkins, Weisberg, and Ray (1984) found that women tended to prefer a communication style that conveys interest in, respect for, and validation of the internal realities of self and other; but many believed that their husband's communication style prohibited this openness. Husbands preferred to explore various facets of an issue, but they believed that their wives tended to avoid or gloss over the issues. These findings, however, may reflect differences in familial power, rather than gender. More study is needed to ascertain whether differences exist between men's and women's communication styles.

Power

Power is one of the most important, albeit controversial factors in family processes. According to Szinovacz (1987, p. 652), power is:

> . . . the net ability or capability of actors (A) to produce or cause (intended) outcomes or effects, particularly on the behavior of others (O) or on others' outcomes.

The exercise of power is a dynamic and multidimensional process. Its antecedents include the structural context and the characteristics of the individuals or groups involved.

Gillespie (1984) argues that the class/caste system operating in American society always gives the power to the man of the family. She says (p. 208), ". . . women are *structurally* deprived of equal opportunities to develop their capacities, resources, and competence in competition with males." Gillespie cites three sources of men's marital power: (1) the socialization process; (2) the marriage contract, which, in many states, legally favors men; and (3) economic resources. Married women have less sense of control over their lives than unmarried women. If income is constant, marriage decreases a woman's sense of control (Ross, 1991).

Blood and Wolfe (1960) studied individual and family characteristics that determined power in the decision-making process. Individual characteristics that contributed to their power included economic resources, education, and organizational participation. A family characteristic that tends to give power to the husband is suburbanization. This may reflect the economic power of a husband who is able to provide a home in the suburbs; the isolation of the wife from her family or origin; or, simply, the isolation of the suburban family from others, which allows the stronger individual to assume power. Another important family characteristic affecting power is race; African-American families are more egalitarian than white families. This probably reflects the African-American man's lack of access to sources of power.

Decision Making

Since the traditional norms governing familial interactions have become outmoded, decision making has become increasingly important in identifying and attaining family goals. Family decision making is not an individual effort, but a joint effort. Each decision has at least five features (Scanzoni & Szinovacz, 1980, p. 54):

1. *Who* raises the matter
2. *What* is said
3. *Supporting actions* to what is being said
4. *Importance* of what is being said to party saying it
5. *Response* of the other party

For example, a 2-year-old boy who refused to eat his spinach until after he had dessert involved the mother in a decision-making process. She had to decide whether the real issue was spinach, dessert, or control. If she defined the issue as the child's dislike of spinach, she could choose to omit it, substitute carrots, or coerce him into eating it. Instead, she defined the issue as control. Rather than withholding dessert until he had eaten his spinach, she decided that she did not want to get into a power struggle over the issue. She chose to let the child decide. Subsequently, he ate both his spinach and his dessert. This example emphasizes the importance of looking at the decision-making process. If one looked only at the outcome, one might conclude that the child controlled the situation. By looking at the process, one sees that the mother made the decision to give the child control.

Communication and power are basic to decision making. Members of the family may have their own spheres of power. The father may choose the car; the mother, the house; the child, the toy. Or the allocation and exercise of power may vary from situation to situation. In a healthy family, the balance of power resides in the parent coalition. Their relationship may be complementary, in that each person does the opposite or reciprocal of the other; or it may be symmetrical, that is, based on similarities rather than differences. Symmetrical participation in decision making is more likely to be satisfactory.

Communication style is a strong predictor of decision-making outcomes (Godwin & Scanzoni, 1989). Certain interactional strategies disrupt, such as the expression of negative emotions (Forgatch, 1989), and tend to lead to conflict; while others, such as reciprocity, enhance problem solving. Consensus or, at the very least, continuation of negotiations is the preferred outcome.

Marital Satisfaction

Even with the leveling off of divorce rates in the United States, marital satisfaction has continued to decline (Glenn & Weaver, 1988; Glenn, 1991). This may be related to higher expectations of marriage or to the breakdown of consensual norms. Although research findings are contradictory, a curvilinear relationship seems to exist between marriage and the life cycle (Suitor, 1991; Vannoy & Philliber, 1992). Marital satisfaction is relatively high among newly married and older couples. The presence of children in the home reduces marital satisfaction, particularly for husbands (Vannoy & Philliber, 1992). The increased marital satisfaction of older couples may reflect the fact that they experience less role strain because they carry out traditional familial roles. Overall, wives with nontraditional orientations seem to experience more dissatisfaction with marriage, while wives of husbands with nontraditional orientations experience more satisfaction.

The quality of marital interaction is related to the spouses' involvements and responsibilities both within and outside the household (McHale & Crouter, 1992; Ward, 1993). Satisfaction with the division of household labor has become increasingly important (Suitor, 1991). Newly married and aging wives, who are more satisfied with marriage than other wives, have fewer child care and housekeeping responsibilities. Yet Ward (1993) found that the number of hours spent on household tasks were not related to marital satisfaction. Instead, the marital happiness of wives was associated with the perceived fairness of household labor. Employment of the wife, in and of itself, does not seem to affect marital satisfaction. Husbands of employed wives do not appear to experience less marital satisfaction than others (Vannoy & Philliber, 1992). Instead, the relative occupational attainment of the spouses seems to be significant. Couples are less satisfied when the wife's occupational attainment is higher than the husband's.

Time constraints are an underlying factor in the relationship between marital satisfaction and child care, household labor, and employment (Zuo, 1992). Marital interaction promotes marital happiness and marital happiness promotes marital interaction. This holds true for both men and women throughout the life cycle. When there is less time for interaction, there is less marital happiness.

Coping Strategies

According to Lazarus and Folkman (1984, p. 141) coping consists of:

> . . . constantly changing cognitive and behavioral efforts to manage specific external and/or internal demands that are appraised as taxing or exceeding the resources of the person.

Each family has its own repertoire of coping strategies, which may or may not be adequate in times of stress. Although coping strategies are almost as numerous as individuals, they may be classified in three broad categories (Pearlin & Schooler, 1982): (1) responses that change the stressful event, (2) responses that control the meaning of the stressful event, and (3) responses that control the stress itself. The family's structure, function, and process; the family's resources of time, energy, money, knowledge, and skills; and the family's past experiences with crisis all influence family coping; but even functional families may experience difficulty coping when stressful events pile up. By definition, ineffective coping does not reduce or control stress (Measley, Richardson, & Dimico. 1989), but coping outcomes are difficult to evaluate in the short term. The long-term results of various coping strategies must be analyzed. For example, dysfunctional grieving may appear functional during the first few weeks after a loss. Others may comment that the mourner is "taking it well." Years later, however, another loss may evoke a disproportionate grief response, reflecting the fact that the mourner did not effectively grieve in the earlier situation.

Nursing Implications

The goal of nursing is to promote a healthy family system. According to Lewis et al. (1976, p. 202), the following are characteristics of a healthy family system:

1. An affiliative rather than an oppositional attitude about human encounters
2. A respect for one's own subjective world view and that of others
3. Openness in communication versus distancing, obscuring, and confusion mechanisms
4. A firm parental coalition without evidence of competing parent-child coalitions
5. An understanding of varied and complex human motivations versus a simplistic, linear, or controlling orientation
6. Spontaneity versus rigid, stereotyped interactions
7. High levels of initiative rather than passivity
8. The encouragement of unique versus bland human characteristics

In coping with the stress of an illness, particularly a chronic illness, the family experiences alterations in role performance and in power. Incompetent role performance results in dependency; dependency, in turn, results in a loss of power for the individual. In order to help the family adapt to the changes, the nurse needs to facilitate communication, enhance decision making, and promote coping. (See Bomar, 1989; Wright & Leahey, 1984, 1987; and Leahey & Wright, 1987a, b for specific interventions.)

SUMMARY   An understanding of family structure, function, and process provides a foundation for nursing practice and enables the nurse to provide care that is tailored to the individual family. Because information on nontraditional families is still limited, the nurse needs to maintain an open, inquiring mind. The nurse's role is to promote the health of individual family members and of the family. Because the interactions between the two are reciprocal, neither can be ignored.

STUDY QUESTIONS

1. Analyses of family structure, function, and process are limited because the majority of family studies focus on:
   a. Extended, multigenerational families
   b. Nontraditional family structures
   c. Poor, black, single-parent families
   d. White, middle-class, two-parent families

2. Which of the following family types is most likely to have the fewest resources to cope with stress?
   a. Blended families
   b. Cohabiting families
   c. Extended families
   d. Single-parent families

3. Married men are healthier than single men because they:
   a. Are less readily sanctioned
   b. Engage in more healthy activities
   c. Experience fewer stressors
   d. Tend to be much happier

4. Which of the following is a functional prerequisite for the family system?
   a. Adaption
   b. Determination
   c. Recreation
   d. Socialization

5. Which of the following familial roles has undergone the most change in the last two decades?
   a. Housekeeper
   b. Provider
   c. Recreational
   d. Therapeutic

6. What is the most common source of role strain in young married women with children under 6 years of age?
   a. Definition of the situation
   b. Lack of role consensus
   c. Lack of role knowledge
   d. Role overload

7. The woman is most likely to influence the outcome of familial decision-making when she is:
   a. Educated
   b. Rich
   c. Pregnant
   d. White

8. In a healthy family, power:
   a. Is equally divided among family members
   b. Is the purview of the husband
   c. Resides in the parental coalition
   d. Is an outmoded notion

9. A healthy family system is characterized by
   a. Absence of disease
   b. Parent-child coalitions
   c. Open communication
   d. Stereotyped interactions

REFERENCES

Amato, P. R., & Keith, B. (1991). Parental divorce and adult well-being: A meta-analysis. *Journal of Marriage and the Family, 53,* 43–58.

Bahr, S. J. (1976). Role competence, role norms, and marital control. In F. I. Nye (Ed.), *Role structure and analysis of the family* (pp. 179–189). Beverly Hills: Sage Publications.

Bane, M. J. (1976). *Here to stay: American families in the twentieth century.* New York: Basic Books.

Barnett, R. C., Marshall, N. L., & Pleck, J. H. (1992). Men's multiple roles and their relationship to men's psychological distress. *Journal of Marriage and the Family, 54,* 358–367.

Bell, N. W., & Vogel, E. F. (Eds.). (1960). *A modern introduction to the family.* Glencoe, IL: Free Press.

Blood, R. O., Jr., & Wolfe, D. M. (1960). *Husbands and wives: The dynamics of married living.* New York: Free Press.

Bomar, P. J. (Ed.). (1989). *Nurses and family health promotion: Concepts, assessment, and intervention.* Baltimore: Williams & Wilkins.

Bulechek, G. M., & McCloskey, J. C. (Eds.) (1992). *Nursing interventions: Essential nursing treatments* (2nd ed.). Philadelphia: Saunders.

Carlson, J. (1976). The recreational role. In F. I. Nye (Ed.), *Role structure and analysis of the family* (pp. 131–147). Beverly Hills: Sage Publications.

Cherlin, A. J. (1992). *Marriage, divorce, and remarriage* (rev. ed.). Cambridge, MA: Harvard University Press.

Coontz, S. (1988). *The social origins of private life: A history of American families 1600–1900.* New York: Verso.

Coontz, S. (1992). *The way we never were: American families and the nostalgia trap.* New York: Basic Books.

Dawson, D. A. (1991). Family structure and children's health and well-being: Data from the 1988 National Health Interview Survey on Child Health. *Journal of Marriage and the Family, 53,* 573–584.

Degler, C. N. (1980). *At odds: Women and the family in America from the revolution to the present.* New York: Oxford University Press.

Demo, D. H. (1992). Parent-child relations: Assessing recent changes. *Journal of Marriage and the Family, 54,* 104–117.

Forgatch, M. S. (1989). Patterns and outcome in family problem solving: The disrupting effect of negative emotion. *Journal of Marriage and the Family, 51,* 115–124.

Fossett, M. A., & Kiecolt, K. J. (1993). Mate availability and family structure among African Americans in U.S. metropolitan area. *Journal of Marriage and the Family, 55,* 288–302.

Francouer, R. T. (1987). Human sexuality. In M. B. Sussman & S. K. Steinmetz (Eds.), *Handbook of marriage and the family* (pp. 509–534). New York: Plenum Press.

Ganong, L. H., Coleman, M., & Mapes, D. (1990). A meta-analytic view of family structure stereotypes. *Journal of Marriage and the Family, 52,* 287–290.

Gillespie, D. (1984). Who has the power? The marital struggle. In B. N. Adams & J. L. Campbell (Eds.), *Framing the family: Contemporary portraits* (pp. 206–228). Prospect Heights, IL: Waveland Press.

Glenn, N. D. (1991). The recent trend in marital success in the United States. *Journal of Marriage and the Family, 53,* 261–270.

Glenn, N. D., & Weaver, C. N. (1988). The changing relationship of marital status to reported happiness. *Journal of Marriage and the Family, 50,* 317–324.

Glick, P. C. (1988). Fifty years of family demography: A record of social change. *Journal of Marriage and the Family, 50,* 861–873.

Gove, W. R. (1973). Sex, marital status, and mortality. *American Journal of Sociology, 79,* 45–67.

Guttentag, M, & Secord, P. G. (1983). *Too many women? The sex role question.* Beverly Hills: Sage Publications.

Hahn, B. A. (1993). Marital status and women's health: The effect of economic marital acquisitions. *Journal of Marriage and the Family, 55,* 495–504.

Harris, K. M., & Morgan, S. P. (1961). Fathers, sons, and daughters: Differential paternal involvement in parenting. *Journal of Marriage and the Family, 53,* 531–544.

Hawkins, J. L., Weisberg, C., & Ray, D. W. (1984). Spouse differences in communication style: Preference, perception, behavior. In B. N. Adams & J. L. Campbell (Eds.), *Framing the family: Contemporary portraits* (pp. 229–240). Prospect Heights, IL: Waveland Press.

Hawks, S. R. (1991). Recreation in the family. In S. J. Bahr (Ed.), *Family research: A sixty-year review, 1930–1990* (Vol. 1) (pp. 387–433). New York: Lexington Books.

Hoffer, J. (1989). Family communication. In P. J. Bomar (Ed.), *Nurses and family health promotion: Concepts, assessment, and interventions* (pp. 78–89). Baltimore: Williams & Wilkins.

Jayakody, R., Chatters, L. M., & Taylor, R. J. (1993). Family support to single and married African American mothers: The provision of financial, emotional, and child care assistance. *Journal of Marriage and the Family, 55,* 261–276.

Kalleberg, A. L., & Rosenfeld, R. A. (1990). Work in the family and in the labor-market: A cross-national, reciprocal analysis. *Journal of Marriage and the Family, 52,* 331–346.

Kantor, D., & Lehr, W. (1975). *Inside the family: Toward a theory of family process.* San Francisco: Jossey-Bass.

Lazarus, R. S., & Folkman, S. (1984). *Stress, appraisal, and coping.* New York: Springer.

Leahey, M., & Wright, L. M. (Eds.). (1987a). *Families and life-threatening illness.* Springhouse, PA: Springhouse.

Leahey, M., & Wright, L. M. (Eds.). (1987b). *Families and psychosocial problems.* Springhouse, PA: Springhouse.

Lee, G. R., Seccombe, K., & Shehan, C. L. (1991). Marital status and personal happiness. *Journal of Marriage and the Family, 53,* 839–844.

Leslie, G. R., & Korman, S. K. (1985). *The family in social context* (6th ed.). New York: Oxford University Press.

Lewis, J. M. (1989). *The birth of the family: An empirical inquiry.* New York: Brunner/Mazel.

Lewis, J. M., Beavers, W. R., Gossett, J. T., & Phillips, V. A. (1976). *No single thread. Psychological health in family systems.* New York: Brunner/Mazel.

McCown, D. E., Delamarter, P., Schroeder, & Liegler. (1992). Family recreation and exercise. In P. J. Bomar (Ed.), *Nurses and family health promotion: Concepts, assessment, and interventions* (pp. 216–236). Baltimore: Williams & Wiklins.

McHale, S. M., & Crouter, A. C. (1992). You can't always get what you want: Incongruence between sex-role attitudes and family work roles and its implications for marriage. *Journal of Marriage and the Family, 54,* 537–547.

Measley, A. R., Richardson, H., & Dimico, G. (1989). Family stress management. In P. J. Bomar (Ed.), *Nurses and family health promotion: Concepts, assessment, and interventions* (pp. 179–196). Baltimore: Williams & Wilkins.

Nock, S. L. (1988). The family and hierarchy. *Journal of Marriage and the Family, 50,* 957–966.

Nye, F. I. (1976). Role structure and analysis of the family. Beverly Hills: Sage Publications.

Otto, H. A. (Ed.). (1970). *The family in search of a future: Alternate models for moderns.* New York: Appleton-Century-Crofts.

Parsons, T. (1951). *The social system.* New York: Free Press.

Parsons, T., & Bales, R. F. (Eds.). (1955). *Family, socialization, and the interaction process.* Glencoe, IL: Free Press.

Pearlin, L. I., & Schooler, C. (1982). The structure of coping. In H. I. McCubbin, A. E. Cauble, & J. M. Patterson (Eds.)., *Family stress, coping, and social support.* Springfield, IL: Charles C. Thomas.

Robertson, A. F. (1991). *Beyond the family: The social organization of human reproduction.* Berkeley: University of California Press.

Ross, C. E. (1991). Marriage and the sense of control. *Journal of Marriage and the Family, 53,* 831–838.

Santi, L. L. (1987). Change in the structure and size of American households: 1970 to 1985. *Journal of Marriage and the Family, 49,* 833–837.

Scanzoni, J., & Szinovacz, M. (1980). *Family decision-making: A developmental sex role model.* Beverly Hills: Sage Publications.

Seltzer, J. (1991). Relationships between fathers and children who live apart: The father's role after separation. *Journal of Marriage and the Family, 53,* 79–101.

Spanier, G. B., & Furstenberg, F. F., Jr. (1987). Remarriage and reconstituted families. In M. B. Sussman & S. K. Steinmetz (Eds.), *Handbook of marriage and the family* (pp. 419–434). New York: Plenum Press.

Stull, D. E., & Borgatta, E. F. (1987). Family structure and proximity of family members. In T. H. Brubaker (Ed.). *Aging, health, and family: Long-term care* (pp. 247 – 261). Newbury Park, CA: Sage Publications.

Suitor, J. J. (1991). Marital quality and satisfaction with the division of household labor across the family life cycle. *Journal of Marriage and the Family, 53,* 221 – 230.

Szinovacz, M. E. (1987). Family power. In M. B. Sussman & S. K. Steinmetz (Eds.), *Handbook of marriage and the family* (pp. 651 – 693). New York: Plenum Press.

Teachman, J. D., Polonko, K. A., & Scanzoni, J. (1987). Demography of the family. In M. B. Sussman & S. K. Steinmetz (Eds.), *Handbook of marriage and the family* (pp. 3 – 36). New York: Plenum Press.

Thomson, E., McLanahan, S. S., & Curtin, R. B. (1992). Family structure, gender, and parental socialization. *Journal of Marriage and the Family, 54,* 368 – 378.

Vannoy, D., & Philliber, W. W. (1992). Wife's employment and quality of marriage. *Journal of Marriage and the Family, 54,* 387 – 398.

Varenne, H. (1992). *Ambiguous harmony: Family talk in America.* Norwood, NJ: Ablex Publishing.

Verbrugge, L. M. (1979). Marital status and health. *Journal of Marriage and the Family, 41,* 267 – 285.

Verbrugge, L. M. (1983). Multiple roles and physical health of women and men. *Journal of Health and Social Behavior, 24,* 16 – 30.

Walker, A. J., & Pratt, C. C. (1991). Daughters' help to mothers: Intergenerational aid versus caregiving. *Journal of Marriage and the Family, 53,* 3 – 12.

Ward, R. A. (1993). Marital happiness and household equity in later life. *Journal of Marriage and the Family, 55,* 427 – 438.

Weitzman, L. J. (1985). *The divorce revolution: The unexpected social and economic consequences for women and children in America.* New York: Free Press.

Wilkie, J. R. (1991). The decline in men's labor force participation and income and the changing structure of family economic support. *Journal of Marriage and the Family, 53,* 11 – 122.

Winch, R. F. (1977). *Familial organization: A quest for determinants.* New York: Free Press.

Wright, L. M., & Leahey, M. (1984). *Nurses and families: A guide to family assessment and intervention.* Philadelphia: F.A. Davis.

Wright, L. M., & Leahey, M. (Eds.). (1987). *Families and chronic illness.* Springhouse, PA: Springhouse.

US Bureau of the Census (1993). 1990 census of population and housing: United States summary. CD90-3C-1. Washington, DC: US Department of Commerce, Data User Services Division.

Zuo, J. (1992). The reciprocal relationship between marital interaction and marital happiness: A three-wave study. *Journal of Marriage and the Family, 54,* 870 – 878.

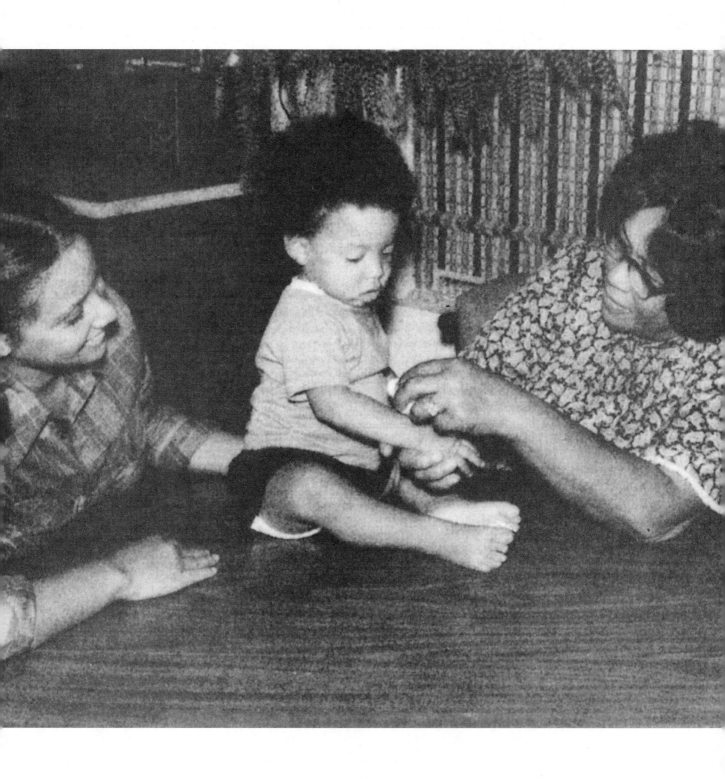

Sociocultural Influences on Family Health

Every student who reads this text comes from a unique sociocultural background, with specific variations determined by social class and the predominant cultural group of the student. Look around your classroom. What sort of cultural and ethnic variations do you see? What influence do you think those variations might have on study habits, food choices, or family relationships? On health habits?

The influence of culture is pervasive; it shapes choices about what we eat, drink, wear, how we are entertained, how we determine health, illness, what we study in school, as well as a myriad of other aspects of our daily lives. This chapter sorts out some of the complex sociocultural influences on family health. Sociocultural influences refer to both the family's social class background and the family's cultural heritage. These influences shape family behaviors, including health behaviors.

This chapter begins by defining key concepts of cultural heritage and ethnicity, social class, and family health. The discussion continues by examining the growth in cultural diversity and the disparity between social classes in the United States, identifying how the health status of socially disadvantaged and minority populations differs from that of the dominant culture. These observations raise important questions for nursing students regarding social justice and the role of the family nurse as client advocate.

The chapter moves on to examine the extent to which health beliefs and practices, family values, patterns of communication, family power, family roles, and family coping styles influence health care. This is followed by an exploration of social class structure in the United States and poverty as a decisive factor in family health. The interaction of culture and social class and its impact on family health are then discussed. Finally, implications for family nursing practice are suggested.

CHAPTER 4

Sociocultural Influences on Family Health

Marilyn M. Friedman, RN, PhD ■
Eleanor G. Ferguson-Marshalleck, RN, MPH

OUTLINE

KEY CONCEPTS
  Cultural Heritage and Ethnicity
  Socioeconomic Status or Social Class
  Family Health

CULTURAL DIVERSITY AND DISPARITIES BETWEEN SOCIAL CLASSES IN THE UNITED STATES
  Growth in Cultural Diversity in the United States
  Growth in the Disparity Between Social Classes in the United States
  Health Status of Socially Disadvantaged and Culturally Diverse Populations

THE INFLUENCE OF CULTURE ON FAMILY HEALTH
  Health Beliefs and Practices
  Family Values
  Family Roles, Power, and Communication Patterns
  Family Coping

THE INFLUENCE OF SOCIAL CLASS ON FAMILY HEALTH
  America's Social Class Structure
  Poverty in Families
  Who Are the Poor?
  Social Class Effects

THE EFFECTS OF THE INTERACTION OF CULTURE AND SOCIAL CLASS ON FAMILY HEALTH

IMPLICATIONS FOR FAMILY NURSING PRACTICE

OBJECTIVES   *Upon completion of this chapter, the reader will be able to:*

1. Identify two prime molders of family values, family behaviors, and family structure and functions.
2. Discuss the growth in cultural diversity and the increasing disparity between social classes in the United States.
3. Define culture and discuss its relationship to health beliefs and practices, family health, and family coping behaviors.
4. Differentiate among the terms culture, ethnicity, social class, acculturation, and ethclass.
5. Describe the social class structure of the United States.
6. Explain cultural (ethnic) differences in family and family members' health status.
7. Analyze the differences in family health status and health-related behaviors of families from different social classes.
8. Discuss the separate influences of culture and social class and the influence of the interaction of these two variables on family health.
9. Discuss the importance of incorporating a cultural assessment in the care of families.
10. Describe some nursing intervention strategies that can be used to enchance ethnic and social class sensitivity and competency in the care of culturally and socially diverse families.

Sociocultural influences on family health include both the family's socioeconomic or social class background and the family's cultural heritage. A family's cultural legacy plays a central role in influencing the family's value system, family functions, and family behavior. The influence of culture is pervasive; it permeates and circumscribes individual, familial, and social actions (Friedman, 1992).

The family's socioeconomic or social class status also plays a primary role in shaping family behavior, and particularly family lifestyle. Families are subjected to very different experiences — both stress-producing and growth-promoting — which exert great influence on family behavior and lifestyle. Family lifestyles vary as a result of these different exposures. Basic to the discussion of sociocultural influences are the key concepts of cultural heritage or ethnicity, socioeconomic status, and family health. Family health is viewed here as an outcome not only of sociocultural influence, but also of family developmental stage, historical factors, and the family's own idiosyncratic family culture.

This chapter focuses on culture and social class, two prime molders of family behavior and values. The chapter begins with basic definitions of the chapter's key concepts, followed by a description of the influence of culture on family health. The growing significance of culture is emphasized in a discussion of the growth in cultural diversity in the United States. The influence of social class on family health is then presented, with demographic data illustrating the widening gap between the affluent and poor in the United States today. How social class affects family health in each of the three primary social classes is explored, with special attention given to the poor and the concepts of poverty and homelessness. The interaction between culture and social class and its impact on family health are also discussed. Lastly, implications for family nursing practice are suggested.

KEY CONCEPTS

Cultural Heritage and Ethnicity

All families are bearers of the culture of the society they live in (Ablon & Ames, 1989) and the culture they identify with. In this sense, many families are multicultural — they are part of both the dominant culture or society and part of their particular subculture. The term **culture** refers to

> those sets of shared world views and adaptive behaviors derived from simultaneous membership in a variety of contexts, such as ecological setting (rural, urban, suburban), religious background, nationality and ethnicity, social class, gender-related experiences, minority status, occupation, political leanings, migratory patterns, and stage of acculturation; or values derived from belonging to the same generation, partaking of a single historical moment, or particular ideologies (Falicov, 1988, p. 336).

Patterned lifeways, values, ideals, beliefs, and practices are embedded in this definition. Patterns of learned behaviors, values, and beliefs are transmitted from one generation to the next by the family. **Ethnicity**, a major component of culture, is defined as a group's sense of "peoplehood" based on a combination of race, religion, ancestral history, and nationality; "it involves a many-layered sense of group identification — of shared values and understandings, that fulfill a deep psychological need for identity and historical continuity" (McGoldrick, 1993, p. 337).

Socioeconomic Status or Social Class

The terms "socioeconomic status," "social status," and "social class" (which are often used interchangeably in the sociological literature) are used to refer to large groups of persons who have relatively similar incomes, amounts of wealth, life conditions, life chances, and lifestyles (Ropers, 1991). Socioeconomic status is a major component within the chapter's broad definition of culture. Because this variable is so crucial in understanding families, it is addressed explicitly. Social class has a pervasive effect on family and family members' lives, especially within complex, heterogeneous societies such as the United States. A family's social class affects the family's lifestyle (where and how the family lives), family members' health status and longevity, their educational and occupational opportunities, and a multitude of other life conditions. Differences in social class are associated with differences in power, privilege, and prestige—resources vital to life conditions (Erickson & Gecas, 1991).

A person's social class status often is determined by the family's social class; and the family's social class, in turn, is determined by the spouses' (in traditional families, primarily the husband/fathers) occupational prestige, level of education, income, employment status, or a combination of these.

Family Health

The term "family health" refers to the health of both individual family members and the family as a whole. Because the health of individual family members affects the health of the whole family system and vice versa, it is difficult to separate the family and its health status from that of its members and their personal health status. Therefore, this chapter focuses on sociocultural influences on both individual family members' health and the family unit's or system's health.

CULTURAL DIVERSITY AND DISPARITIES BETWEEN SOCIAL CLASSES IN THE UNITED STATES

Growth in Cultural Diversity in the United States

Since the 1960s and 1970s, there has been a steady growth in racial and ethnic diversity (also referred to as cultural diversity) in the United States. Currently, more than one resident in four is nonwhite or of Hispanic origin (US Bureau of the Census, 1992b). The white majority is shrinking and aging, while the African-American, Hispanic, Asian-American, and Native American populations are young and growing (US Bureau of the Census, 1992b). If the present rate of births and immigration to the United States continues, the Asian-American presence will increase by 22% by the turn of the twenty-first century, Hispanic Americans will increase by 21%, African-Americans by 12%, and Americans of European descent by only 2% (Henry, 1990).

Dramatic changes have taken place in the American population over the past decade, as depicted in Tables 4–1 and 4–2. Table 4–2 summarizes the changes in the growth patterns of selected racial and ethnic minorities between 1980 and 1990. Although the sizes of the groups vary, the number of racial and ethnic groups profiled attests to the increasingly diverse nature of the population in the United States.

Ethnic minorities—African-Americans, Hispanics, Native Americans, and Asian-Americans—make up a far larger proportion of the United States population than they did in

TABLE 4–1

MAJOR RACIAL AND ETHNIC DIVISIONS OF THE UNITED STATES POPULATION, 1980 AND 1990

	1980(n)*	1990(n)*	1980(%)	1990(%)
RACE				
Anglo-American	188.4	199.7	83.2	80.3
African-American	26.5	30.0	11.7	12.1
American Indian, Eskimo, Aleut	1.4	2.0	0.6	0.8
Asian and Pacific Islander	3.5	7.3	1.5	2.9
Other	6.8	9.8	3.0	3.9
HISPANIC ORIGIN†				
Hispanic origin (of any race)	14.6	22.4	6.4	9.0
Not of Hispanic origin (all other ethnicities)	211.9	226.4	93.6	91.0
Total	226.5	248.7	100.0	100.0

*Data are reported in millions and rounded off to the closest 100,000.

†It should be noted that persons of Hispanic origin may be of any race; hence, there is a separate category for persons of Hispanic origin.

SOURCE: Data are abstracted from the US Bureau of the Census, *1980 Census of Population. General Population Characteristics* (1983, Tables 38 and 39) and *1990 Census of the Population. General Population Characteristics* (1992b, Table 3)

the past. From 1980 to 1990, the Hispanic population grew proportionally by 53%, that is, from 14.6 million (6.4%) to 22.4 million (9.0%); the Asian and Pacific Islander population grew proportionally by 108%, that is, from 3.5 million (1.5%) to 7.3 million (2.9%); and the Alaskan Indian, Eskimo, and Aleut Native American populations grew by 38%, that is, from 1.4 million to 2 million (0.8%).

The growth of the Hispanic population has been due to both legal and illegal immigration and to the high fertility rate among Hispanic families (Friedman, 1992b). In contrast, the rapid growth of the Asian population has been due primarily to immigration.

Representing 12% of the American population, African-Americans remain the largest minority group within the United States. However, this population showed a more modest growth from 1980 to 1990, increasing in size from 26.5 million (11.7%) in 1980 to 30 million (12.1%) in 1990 (US Bureau of the Census, 1992b). Low immigration, a high infant mortality rate, and shorter life spans are factors in the slower rate of increase in the number of African-Americans (National Center for Health Statistics, 1992; US Bureau of the Census, 1992a). Although the actual number of non-Hispanic whites increased in 1990, they declined in percentage of the total United States population, from 79.6% to 75.6% (US Bureau of the Census, 1992b). United States population growth today is clearly a function primarily of growth in racial and ethnic minority populations.

Growth in the Disparity Between Social Classes in the United States

Recent increases in income inequality in the United States and the implications for working-class and poor families have been widely addressed in the sociological and public health literature (Braun, 1991; Gilbert & Kahl, 1987; Ropers, 1991; Winnick, 1991). In the 1980s and early 1990s, the rich have continued to become richer and the poor poorer (Peterson, 1993; Braun, 1991; Ropers, 1991; United Press International, 1990), a change charac-

TABLE 4–2

CHANGE IN UNITED STATES POPULATION BY RACE AND ETHNICITY FOR SELECTED RACIAL AND ETHNIC GROUPS, 1980 AND 1990

Racial/Ethnic Group	1980(n)*	1990(n)*	Increase(%)
African-American	26.5	30.0	13.2
American Indian	1.4	1.9	37.7
Asian			
Chinese	0.8	1.6	104.1
Filipino	0.8	1.4	81.6
Japanese	0.7	0.8	20.9
Asian Indian	0.4	0.8	125.3
Korean	0.4	0.8	125.3
Vietnamese	0.3	0.6	134.8
Pacific Islander			
Hawaiian	0.17	0.2	26.5
Samoan	0.04	0.06	50.1
Guamanian	0.02	0.05	53.4
Hispanic origin			
Mexican	8.7	13.5	54.4
Puerto Rican	2.0	2.7	35.4
Cuban	0.8	1.0	30.0
Other Hispanic	3.0	5.1	66.7

*Data reported in millions. Most data are rounded off to the closest 100,000.
SOURCE: From US Bureau of the Census, *1980 Census of Population. General Population Characteristics* (1983, Tables 38 and 39) and *1990 Census of the Population* (1992b, Table 3).

terized by the sociologist Winnick (1991) as a shift toward two societies, separate and unequal. The shift in the distribution of income and wealth and the consequent growing gap between rich and poor began in the early 1970s but accelerated during the Reagan administration because of the reduction of all social programs serving the poor. The escalating national debt, sluggish economic growth, rising unemployment rate, and declining wages have only exacerbated the problems of America's poor families. The increase in income inequality has adversely affected access to education and employment, particularly for lower- and working-class families. This widening income gap means that the middle class is shrinking while both ends of the income continuum are expanding (i.e., there are increased proportions of rich and poor).

Health Status of Socially Disadvantaged and Culturally Diverse Populations

The health status of individuals in the United States differs dramatically between different cultural groups and social classes. There are several reasons for this: family and personal lifestyle differences; differing access to health care resources, including both services and health insurance; and differing exposure to environmental hazards. Unequal distribution of preventive and basic health care resources results in morbidity and mortality rates that vary significantly between white people and nonwhite people and between different socioeconomic classes. Major indicators of health status clearly demonstrate that the health status of minority Americans is substantially poorer than that of white Americans (Nickens, 1991; US Department of Health and Human Services, 1985). The same is true in terms of social class differences: health status is poorer among poor Americans. One glaring indication of this is the difference in infant mortality rates between socioeconomic classes. Babies of poor families, regardless of ethnic or racial background, die at twice the rate of babies of nonpoor families (Boone, 1989; Kramer, 1988). Also, ethnic minorities have poorer mental health and more unsatisfied mental health needs than whites. Not surprisingly, they also receive less extensive and poorer quality mental health services (Jones & Korchin, 1982; Nickens, 1991).

THE INFLUENCE OF CULTURE ON FAMILY HEALTH

Culture, which is passed on from generation to generation, affects the health status of families. Moreover, a family's level of **acculturation** to the dominant culture in which they live makes a major difference in how important a family's cultural heritage is in shaping family behavior and health. "Acculturation comprises those gradual changes produced in a culture by the influence of another culture which results in an increased similarity of the two" (Kroeber, 1948, p. 425). In the case of ethnic minority families who immigrate to the United States, the influence is predominantly one way—the American culture exerts a greater influence on the ethnic group to conform to its cultural patterns than vice versa (Friedman, 1992). Kumabe, Nishida, and Hepworth (1985) suggest acculturation occurs on a continuum that ranges from adhering to the traditional values of an individual's homeland, along with traditional religious practices and cultural artifacts, at one end (the unacculturated), to adopting the mainstream values of the dominant group at the other end (the acculturated).

Ethnic minority families who have recently immigrated to the United States or those who have remained immersed in the culture of their country of origin are often unacculturated to the dominant culture of the United States. That is to say, they have not integrated the dominant American core values and practices into their lives. Families' ethnic background, derived from their country of origin, is therefore much more important in shaping their beliefs and behavior than is the ethnic background of acculturated American families.

The effects of culture on family health status may be explored by looking at selected family structural dimensions such as family values, family roles, power, and communication patterns, and family coping. Culture also affects health beliefs and practices.

Health Beliefs and Practices

Every cultural group possesses a system of beliefs and practices about health and illness (Helman, 1990). These include beliefs about what a symptom is and what it means, when and to whom to go when one is ill, what symbolizes relief or cure, and so forth. Cultures provide explanatory models of health and illness, which include the meaning, cause, process, prognosis, and treatment of illness, as well as maintenance of health (Kleinman, 1980). Western societies typically root their explanations of disease, illness, and health in natural phenomena and scientific findings; that is, the causes of disease are considered to be infection, mechanical injury, tumor growth, or stress. In non-Western societies, families may have explanatory belief systems in which illness and disease are viewed as resulting from social or supernatural causes or from unbalances (like hot and cold) in the body. The view of what is an effective therapy generally is congruent with the beliefs about the cause of the health problem (Kleinman, 1980). If the root cause of disease is perceived as spiritual, prayer and other spiritual interventions are used. For example, spiritual interventions are sought by Mexican Americans for certain "folk" and mental illnesses. If the root cause of disease is believed to be a problem with social interaction, social interventions are favored. For example, Native Americans who believe that illness is a social phenomenon may execute elaborate, ritualized ceremonies such as "sings" and sand paintings for therapy (Adair, Deuschle, & Barnett, 1988).

Health beliefs are translated into health care practices, which then affect the health status of the family. What constitutes appropriate care for specific health conditions is bound by cultural and social class expectations.

Most traditional health beliefs and practices promote the health of the family because they are generally family and socially oriented. They reinforce family cohesion. For example, in many cultures, when a family member is seriously ill, family members expect to be present, supportive, and protective. This practice serves to bind the family together in an important task in which all family members take part. Less common is the situation in which cultural beliefs and values adversely affect an individual family member's health. For example, a Hispanic family may delay seeking Western medical treatment because its members have identified a health problem as a folk illness, which they expect to be alleviated by folk remedies. In this case, needed health care may be delayed. However, most traditional health beliefs and practices, if not effective in terms of cure, are benign enough and have no negative consequences, unless they delay the decision to seek effective professional help (Helman, 1990).

Conflicts between family members about health care beliefs and practices may adversely affect family health. These conflicts are often created by generational differences. The older generation in the family may maintain their traditional views of illness and appropriate interventions whereas the younger generation may adopt Western health notions and health care practices. The two sets of beliefs and practices may clash, leaving the family divided and less adaptive and able to care for a family member with a major illness.

Family Values

A family's values guide the development of its norms and rules and serve as general guides to its behavior. Values involve the time dimension, relationships between people, the relationship of human beings to nature, individuals' prevailing orientation in life activities (Kluckholm & Strodtbeck, 1961), and views of independence and interdependence (Lin & Liu, 1993). **Family values** refer to shared systems of ideas, attitudes, and beliefs about the worth or priority of entities or ideas that bind the members of a family in a common culture (Parad & Caplan, 1965). They are a reflection of the society and the subculture(s) with which the family identifies. In families that are not acculturated to the society's dominant culture, values are largely based on the family's cultural background, and these are referred to as "traditional" values. But even traditional values are not static; they are shaped and modified to fit social and economic conditions (Mirande, 1991).

Some values are more central and influential than others; given a competing set of demands, it is these central values that will typically determine a family's priorities. "A family's configuration of values ascribes meaning to certain critical events and at the same time suggests ways to respond to these situations" (Friedman, 1992, p. 240).

Culturally derived values influence family health by setting priorities for making decisions and coping with life's stressors. For example, the value placed on relationships between people in part determines how the family and its members will function in crisis. In some cultures family needs and goals take precedence over individual needs and goals. (The primacy of family needs over individual needs is referred to as familism in the Latino family literature). Members generally pull together, with primary and secondary kin supporting the family member(s) in need. Generally, this practice has positive effects on family functioning and health, although in some families there may be a dark side to familism. De Vore and London (1993) note that "while ethnicity provides individuals with a sense of cohesion and identity drawn from the strength of the group, it also may be the source of strain, discordance and strife" (p. 323). For instance, extended family obligations may reduce a nuclear family's ability to meet its own needs and goals.

Orientation to time may also affect family health. When present time is the focus — rather than future time — family members may find it hard to change their lifestyles to avoid a potential health problem. For example, when family members appear well and the consequences of an unhealthy lifestyle are likely to become apparent only years later, needed lifestyle modifications may be difficult to implement. A common example of this situation is the family in which the husband or father has essential hypertension. If the husband or father is from a culture that is primarily present-oriented, feels "well," and is able to function, he may deny the need to modify his dietary patterns and lifestyle and fail to adhere to his medication regimen.

A family's relationship to its community also affects family health and functioning. The greater the congruence between a family's values and the wider community's values, the easier it is for individuals and the family to adjust and the greater the family's success in relating to its community (Friedman, 1992). When family values clash significantly with the values of the community and society in which the family resides, the family's relationship to their community may be strained. In such cases, families may believe they cannot obtain needed health and welfare services from their communities, and then "ask and receive little." They also may be discouraged from applying for assistance from community agencies that see them as less deserving or in some way "ineligible" for services. With diminished health or welfare services, family and individual health eventually suffer.

Family Roles, Power, and Communication Patterns

The impact of culture on family roles, power, and communication patterns is considerable — particularly in unacculturated families. Culture dictates the roles family members play within and outside of the family. This is not to say that culture is static; it is not. Culture changes, and family norms, rules and associated roles, power, and communications are modified to meet the demands and challenges families face. Our culture has changed in response to technological innovation (Murray & Zentner, 1993) and rapid social and demographic changes. These changes have in turn affected family roles, power, and communication patterns.

The traditional culturally derived roles of men, women, and children in families have been and continue to be modified to adapt to new realities and challenges. Two trends that have had a great impact on family roles, power, and communication patterns are the increasing numbers of women who work and the increasing numbers of single-parent families (Rossi, 1986). Table 4–3 shows how family roles have changed as a result of technological changes and women's participation in work outside the home. These changes in roles, power relationships, and communication have occurred in all types of families — Anglo-American, Mexican-American, and African-American (Baca-Zinn, 1980; Mirande, 1991; Pleck, 1985; Spitze, 1988; Wilkinson, 1987).

In those families where marital partners are from the same cultural background and

TABLE 4–3

RECENT CHANGES IN TWO-PARENT NUCLEAR FAMILY ROLES AND POWER

Traditional Role/ Power Structure	Changes Due to Technological Innovations	Changes When Women Participate in the Labor Force
Husband seen as primary breadwinner		Husband and wife share breadwinner role in most families
Husband "wears pants in the family"		Shift from male (husband/father) domination to greater shared power between husband and wife
Wife's roles:		
Support husband's efforts and decisions		More egalitarian decision making in marriage
In charge of child care and household	Women have ability to plan family; reduction in length of childbearing and childrearing period	Greater spousal sharing of child care roles and, to a lesser extent, household roles
	Women's time doing household work substantially reduced	
Communication in the family more complementary and and hierarchical		Communication more egalitarian and open

SOURCE: Data from Baca-Zinn, 1980; Chilman, 1993; Erickson and Gecas, 1991; McAdoo, 1993b; Pleck, 1985; Spitze, 1988; and Wilkinson, 1987.

agree about family roles, family power distribution, and communication patterns, the common cultural understanding provides meaning, structure, and continuity. In families without this commonly accepted culture mates may have differing expectations about family roles, communication, and power relationships, and family functioning may be affected negatively.

Culturally based conflicts frequently arise when family members from immigrant families have differing degrees of exposure to the wider American culture. Children may become more quickly acculturated to "the American way" in school. What and how they are taught in school may conflict with what and how they have been taught at home. As a result, culturally based conflicts often occur between the generations (Larrabee, 1973; Friedman, 1992).

Family Coping

Culture also influences the ways in which families adapt to and cope with internal and external demands and changes. The strategies that families use to cope influence family health and family functioning. **Family coping** is defined as positive, problem-appropriate affective, cognitive, and behavioral responses that families and their subsystems use to solve a problem or reduce the stress produced by the problem or event (Friedman, 1992). Family coping strategies develop and change over time in response to the stressors and demands experienced (Menaghan, 1983) and also differ across the family life cycle (Schnittger & Bird, 1993).

Various coping strategies are used to either eliminate the stressor or demand, control the meaning of the stressor or demand, or reduce the stress or tension created by the stressor or demand. These behavioral, cognitive, and affective strategies are summarized in Table 4–4.

Traditional or unacculturated ethnic families make extensive use of culturally derived family coping strategies. Chinese and Vietnamese immigrant families provide a good example of ethnic differences in family coping patterns. Both Chinese and Vietnamese families commonly use the coping strategy of family group reliance and family cohesiveness. In China, families' social network connections have been essential for survival. Consequently, in the face of family stressors the extended family pulls together. Chinese families encourage interdependence and family loyalty, and the receiving and giving of help between the generations (Lin & Liu, 1993).

Immigrant Vietnamese families use similar coping strategies. Gold (1993) quotes one Vietnamese family member's explanation of how his family deals with problems:

> To Vietnamese culture, family is everything. There are aspects [coping strategies] which help us readjust to this society. . . . We solve problems because the family institution is a bank. If I need money—and my brother and my two sisters are working I tell them I need to buy a house. . . . Now I help them. They live with me and have no rent. The family is a hospital. If mom is sick, I, my children, and my brother and sister care for her. (p. 304)

Research on ethnic differences in family coping is limited. One study in this area was done by Friedman (1985), who looked at 55 families who had a child with cancer. Half of the families were Anglo and the other half Latino. Anglo families (mostly middle-class) reported that information seeking and the support of neighbors, friends, and spouse were the most helpful coping strategies, while Latino families (mostly working- and lower-class Mexican-American families) reported that extended family support and spiritual support were most helpful. Latinos relied heavily on religion to cope with their child's cancer. Because culture and religion are so closely intertwined in Latin culture and most of the Latino families in this study were recent immigrants and unacculturated, the differences in coping between the two cultural groups was quite pronounced.

TABLE 4–4

TYPES OF FAMILY COPING STRATEGIES

INTERNAL FAMILY COPING STRATEGIES

1. Family group reliance, including delegation
2. The use of humor and stress management tactics
3. Increased sharing together: maintaining cohesiveness
4. Controlling the meaning of the stressor/demand: cognitive refraining and passive appraisal
5. Joint family problem solving
6. Role flexibility
7. Normalizing
8. Limiting leisure-time and recreational activities

EXTERNAL FAMILY COPING STRATEGIES

1. Seeking information
2. Maintaining active linkages with community groups and organizations
3. Seeking and using social supports (informal and formal social support systems and self-help groups)
4. Seeking and using spiritual supports

SOURCE: Adapted from Friedman (1992).

The Latino families in Friedman's study depended on primary and secondary kin to assist and support them with the array of demands created by childhood cancer. In those families who had recently immigrated from El Salvador and had no extended family support, family functioning was poorer. Friedman concluded that the absence of the families' natural social support system (the extended family) left a vacuum for these families and reduced their ability to cope. The inaccessibility of culturally appropriate social support and the reluctance of family members to use substitute social supports (e.g., health personnel, neighbors, friends) created personal and interpersonal difficulties in handling the stress of childhood cancer.

THE INFLUENCE OF SOCIAL CLASS ON FAMILY HEALTH

Like all other industrialized nations, the United States is stratified by class. A stratified society is marked by inequality, by differences among people that rank them as higher or lower (Gilbert & Kahl, 1987). Although social classes may be distinguished from each other, the lines of demarcation are not clear-cut. Income or wealth is one indicator of social class, and life conditions are another. Available resources (natural, material, social, political, economic) determine a person's or family's life conditions. The extent to which persons and families have access to and use resources (which are called "life chances") in the literature reflects their social class. Power, prestige, and privilege are often manifestations of wealth and, hence, a family's social class (Ropers, 1991).

America's Social Class Structure

As the United States has been transformed from an agricultural to an industrial and then postindustrial, technological society, the class structure has correspondingly changed. The components of the new class structure — which came about because of shifts in the types of jobs needed to sustain a postindustrial society — are described by sociologists Gilbert and Kahl (1987): a national capitalist class built on corporate wealth; an upper-middle class of college-educated professionals and managers; a lower-middle class of technicians, semiprofessionals, blue-collar workers, and clerical and sales workers; and a lower class of people engaged in menial, unskilled jobs or unemployed. At the bottom of the lower class are an increasingly isolated underclass of families and individuals who are employed in unstable menial jobs or are not working.

Poverty in Families

Families with incomes below the poverty line make up an increasing proportion of families in the United States today. Over 12% of families in the country had incomes below the poverty line in 1987; this proportion is probably higher today. We need only to look at large cities to see how poverty has increased. Homelessness, a rare sight in the past, is now glaringly apparent (Berne, Dato, Mason, & Rafferty, 1990).

Who Are the Poor?

The individuals and families who have suffered most from deterioration or stagnation in the economy and reductions in the level of governmental assistance are children, youth, and young families; the poorly educated and unskilled; African-Americans, particularly black men; Hispanics, especially illegal immigrants; Puerto Ricans; families headed by women; families with only one employed member; and residents of central cities and economically depressed small towns and rural areas (Chilman, 1991; Wilson, 1987).

One popular misconception about the poor in America is that they are concentrated in inner cities. This is not true. In 1987, only 42% of the poor in the United States lived in central cities, while 28.5% lived in suburban areas within metropolitan areas and 29.5% lived in small towns or villages and rural areas. The majority of poor African-American (59.2%) and Hispanic (62.9%) families do, however, live in central city areas. Because poverty is as much a problem in rural areas as in inner cities, the problem of poverty and its consequences for health must be addressed in both types of areas (Winnick, 1991).

There are two groups of poor families — those in temporary poverty and those in persistent poverty. The majority of those who are in temporary poverty escape it by obtaining jobs with living wages or by forming extended family units to gain a combined income that will ameliorate the worst effects of poverty. Those in persistent poverty, who are primarily women and children, have a much more difficult time escaping from poverty.

The **underclass** represent those in persistent poverty. They are described as having attitudes, values, and lifestyles that do not conform to the values of mainstream American society (McAdoo, 1993a). Because of the clash in values and behaviors between underclass families and the mainstream dominant culture, these families have a strained relationship with the wider community. This conflict makes it difficult for underclass families, who are stigmatized by the wider society, to obtain the resources needed to function at even a minimally acceptable level. The poor, and particularly the underclass or persistently poor, are a vulnerable population — living in poverty conditions with multiple persistent stressors that undermine the physical, psychological, and economic health of the family and its members (Chilman, 1991).

Homelessness is a growing, significant family stressor. Homelessness includes doubling up with relatives during hard times as well as simply having no home. In the latter instance, families or individuals may or may not have temporary housing in a shelter. While in the past, that is, in the 1950s through 1970s, most of the homeless had some shelter — "flophouses," single-room-occupancy hotels, or mission shelters — many of the contemporary homeless are literally sleeping on the streets. Being homeless subjects family members to myriad physical and psychosocial stressors. Homeless families are likely to be socially isolated, with no regular or strong ties to family, friends, or other social networks. Their lack of social support magnifies their vulnerability to disabilities and deprivations (Rossi, Wright, Fisher, & Willis, 1987). Single-parent families with children are tragically an increasingly visible, vulnerable component of the homeless population. Single women and minorities are also particularly vulnerable groups among the homeless. Compared with those who have homes, the prevalence of mental illness is greater among homeless women while the prevalence of alcoholism and other forms of substance abuse is greater among homeless men (Aday, 1993).

Social Class Effects

Social class status is strongly correlated with health. The more affluent an individual or family, the better their life conditions, the greater their access to preventive and curative health care services and the better their health status. Further, families from the upper and middle classes, regardless of ethnic background, tend to have better self-care behaviors. Because of numerous stressors, the poor find it difficult to be future-oriented and concerned about healthy lifestyles.

The correlation between social class and health holds true for both adults and children, for example, Starfield found (1992) that poor children are more likely to become ill and to have serious illnesses than children from higher-income families. The higher rates of serious health problems and the increased death rates from disease in poor children of all ages reflect exposure to environmental hazards, poor nutrition, inadequate preventive care, and poor access to medical care — all part of social class inequalities in "life conditions" and "life chances." Research findings since the 1930s have consistently demonstrated that lower-class, economically distressed families are more likely to have poorer family health, less family stability, poorer marital adjustment, greater problems in family coping, and troubled family relationships (Voydanoff & Donnelly, 1988).

THE EFFECTS OF THE INTERACTION OF CULTURE AND SOCIAL CLASS ON FAMILY HEALTH

While the separate influences of culture (particularly ethnicity) and social class on family health are considerable, the influence of these two variables together may be profound. Certain groups in the United States, largely because of ethnic or racial inequalities and social stratification, have become entrenched in poverty. Institutional racism often locks families into a state in which social class mobility is practically nonexistent. As a result, these families tend to pass on their "inherited" class disadvantages from one generation to the next.

Gordon (1964) described the pronounced association between ethnic group membership and social class as **ethclass**. This intersection of ethnicity and social class produces identifiable dispositions and behavioral patterns in families and individuals. Social class and ethnicity in interaction define the basic conditions of life and simultaneously account for differences between ethnic groups with different social class positions. For instance, important commonalties are created among families because of their common cultural heritage and experiences by virtue of being black in America. Despite these important commonalties, lifestyles and life chances vary drastically between affluent African-American families and poor African-American families. Ethnic families, especially those of color, are much likelier to be poor than white families of European descent. Among the major ethnic and racial groups in the United States, the percentage of those persons living in poverty in 1991 varied from a low of 11.3% among non-Hispanic whites to 28.7% among Hispanics and 32.7% among African-Americans (US Bureau of the Census, 1992c).

Being from an ethnic family of color and being poor pose greater hazards to family and family members' health than being either from a nonpoor ethnic family of color or from a poor white family. African-American and Hispanic children are nearly three times more likely than Anglo-American children to live in poverty, and indicators of poorer health status are clustered among poor minority children (US Bureau of the Census, 1989).

However, it must be understood that race and ethnicity have a significant impact on health status primarily because ethnically and racially diverse families more frequently are disadvantaged socioeconomically (Cockerham, 1987). Hence, even though cultural background is linked to differences in individual health status, social class is more important in producing such variation.

The interaction of culture and social class may also substantially influence health care practices. For example, de la Torre (1993) speculates that ethnic families in the United States who are poor use folk medicine and home remedies more often than they would prefer, simply because they lack access to professional health care. One piece of evidence to support this comes from a large survey of Mexican-Americans in southern California

(Keefe, 1981). Among Keefe's sample of Mexican-Americans it was only the unacculturated, poor Mexican-Americans who still used folk medicine to any great extent, and this was primarily in the treatment of folk illnesses. Among the middle-class and more affluent Mexican-American families, the use of folk medicine had practically disappeared. Moreover, according to a recent national survey of health care and health insurance coverage, almost 40% of working-age Latinos have no health insurance (de la Torre, 1993), which significantly limits their access to health care.

IMPLICATIONS FOR FAMILY NURSING PRACTICE

The family's sociocultural background is central in shaping family values, beliefs, and behaviors, and in shaping specific health beliefs and practices. Social class and ethnic background, both singly and in combination, also affect families' health status. Because of the centrality of **sociocultural dimensions** to family life and health, sensitivity to both ethnicity and social class and cultural competence are imperative. In the words of De Vore and London (1993), "practice skills and techniques must be adapted to respond to the needs or dispositions of various ethnic [and class] groups" (p. 324). Further, cultural and socioeconomic assessments must be an integral component of family assessments (Table 4–5).

TABLE 4–5

CULTURAL ASSESSMENT GUIDELINES

Assessment Criteria	Questions
Ethnic/racial identity	How does the family identify itself in terms of ethnicity and racial background? Are the parents both from the same ethnic background?
Languages spoken	What languages are spoken in the home? And by whom? What language is preferred when speaking to outsiders?
Place of birth	Where were the parents and children born? If born in the United States, where were the parents born? If born out of the United States, how many years have parents lived in the United States?
Geographic mobility	Where have the parents lived? When did they move to their present residence?
Family's religion	What is the family's religion? Are both parents from the same religious background? How actively involved is the family in religiously based activities and practices?
Ethnic group affiliation	What are the characteristics of the family's friends and associations? Are they all from the family's ethnic group? Are recreational, educational, and other social activities within the ethnic reference group, the wider community, or both? To what extent does the family use services and shop within the family's neighborhood or within the wider community?
Neighborhood affiliation	What are the characteristics of the family's neighborhood? Is it ethnically heterogeneous or homogeneous? What are the family's dietary habits and dress?
Household appearance	Are the family's home decorations, art, and religious objects culturally derived?
Use of folk systems	To what extent does the family use folk healing practices/practitioners?
Acceptance by community	To what extent is the family affected by discrimination?

SOURCE: Friedman (1992), with permission.

Family nurses working with diverse ethnic and social class families must have a clear understanding of their own ethnic and social class identification and recognize their own potential and real biases (McAdoo, 1993a). They also need to remember that behaviors and values of families from different subcultures or social classes may be quite adaptive for the family's circumstances (Erickson & Gecas, 1991).

Health professionals are repositories of their own ethnic, religious, racial, and social class subcultures. As health professionals we often believe that we can nullify our biases; however, it is only with continuing self-exploration and awareness of our preconceptions, attitudes, values, and beliefs that we can develop understanding and sensitivity to culture and social class. Our awareness and sensitivity are never complete; interpretations will continue to arise that have cultural or social class connotations that may interfere with the process of providing services to clients (McAdoo, 1993a).

SUMMARY

The health status of individuals in the United States differs dramatically across cultural groups and social classes. Major indicators show that the health status of minority Americans compared with whites is substantially poorer. The same is true in terms of social class differences: health status is worse among poor Americans.

Whereas the separate influence of ethnicity and of social class on family health is considerable, the influence of the interaction of these two variables may be profound. Gordon (1964) describes the pronounced association between ethnic group membership and social class as "ethclass." Social class and culture, particularly ethnicity, interact to define the basic conditions of life and simultaneously account for differences between ethnic groups with different social class positions.

The major implication for nursing practice is that in order to provide quality professional nursing care to families, nurses must be sensitive and competent in working with families from various cultural and social classes.

STUDY QUESTIONS

1. The growing significance of cultural diversity in the United States is emphasized by the fact that more than one in four residents is nonwhite or of Hispanic origin.
   a. True
   b. False

2. The country of origin of an individual is primarily related to his or her:
   a. Racial classification
   b. Social class classification
   c. Ethnic classification
   d. Cultural classification

3. Factors that contribute to differences in health status in various cultural groups and social classes include all of the following *except:*
   a. Inadequate access to preventive and basic healthcare resources
   b. Family and personal lifestyle differences
   c. Exposure to environmental hazards
   d. Personality differences
   e. Income inequality and rising unemployment

4. Research findings indicate that lower-class, economically distressed families are more likely than middle class families to have poor family health.
   a. True
   b. False

5. Ethnic families that have integrated dominant American core values and practices in their lives are considered to be:
   a. Ethnocentric
   b. Enculturated
   c. Culturally competent
   d. Acculturated

6. Culturally derived family values influence family health by setting priorities with respect to making family decisions. "Familism" in the Latino culture is an example of which cultural orientation?
   a. Time orientation
   b. Family versus self-interest
   c. Active versus passive orientation
   d. Past versus present

7. Women's participation in the labor force has contributed to all of the following changes in family roles, power relationships, and communication patterns *except:*
   a. More open communication
   b. Greater sharing of child care roles in family
   c. Less sharing of power in marital relationships
   d. Sharing of breadwinner role between husband and wife

8. Ethnic differences in family coping patterns are seen among traditional or unacculturated families. Which of the following coping strategies would commonly be used by Chinese families? (You may choose one or more answers).
   a. Family group reliance
   b. Role flexibility
   c. Spiritual support
   d. Maintaining family cohesiveness

9. What percent of families have incomes below the poverty line in the United States?
   a. 5%
   b. 12%
   c. 20%
   d. 30%

10. Families who live below the poverty line are at greater risk than those living above the poverty line of experiencing which of the following? (You may choose one or more answers.)
    a. Homelessness
    b. Poorer health status
    c. Lack of access to health services
    d. Higher mortality rates

REFERENCES

Ablon, J., & Ames, G. M. (1989). Culture and family. In C. L. Gilliss, B. L. Highley, B. M. Roberts & I. M. Martinson (Eds.), *Toward a science of family nursing.* Menlo Park, CA: Addison-Wesley.

Adair, J., Deuschle, K. W., & Barnett, C. R. (1988). *The people's health: Anthropology and medicine in a Navaho community.* Albuquerque: University of New Mexico Press.

Aday, L. A. (1993). *At risk in America.* San Francisco: Jossey-Bass.

Baca-Zinn, M. (1980). Employment and education of Mexican American women: The interplay of modernity and ethnicity in eight families. *Harvard Educational Review, 50,* 47–62.

Berne, A. S., Dato, C., Mason, D. J., & Rafferty, M. (1990). A nursing model for addressing the health needs of homeless families. *Image: Journal of Nursing Scholarship, 22,* 813.

Boone, M. S. (1989). *Capital crime: Black infant mortality in America.* Newbury Park, CA: Sage Publications.

Braun, D. (1991). *The rich get richer.* Chicago: Nelson-Hall.

Chilman, C. (1991). Working poor families: Trends, causes, effects, and suggested policies. *Family Relations, 40,* 191–198.

Chilman, C. (1993). Hispanic families in the United States. In H. P. McAdoo (Ed.), *Family ethnicity: Strength in diversity* (pp. 141–163). Newbury Park, CA: Sage Publications.

Cockerham, W. L. (1987). *Medical sociology* (2nd ed.). Englewood Cliffs, NJ: Prentice-Hall.

de la Torre, A. (1993, March 31). Access is vital in health care reform. *Los Angeles Times,* p. B7.

De Vore, W., & London, H. (1993). Ethnic sensitivity for practitioners. In H. P. McAdoo (Ed.). *Family ethnicity: Strength in diversity* (pp. 317–331). Newbury Park, CA: Sage Publications.

Erickson, R. J., & Gecas, V. (1991). Social class and fatherhood. In F. W. Bozett and S. M. H. Hanson (Eds.), *Fatherhood and families in cultural context.* New York: Springer.

Falicov, C. J. (1988). Learning to think culturally. In D. C. Breunlin & R. C. Schwartz (Eds.), *Handbook of family therapy, training, and supervision.* New York: Guilford Press.

Friedman, M. (1985). *Family stress and coping among Anglo and Latino families with childhood cancer.* Unpublished PhD dissertation, University of Southern California, Los Angeles.

Friedman, M. (1992). *Family nursing: Theory and practice* (3rd ed.). Norwalk, CT: Appleton & Lange.

Gilbert, D., & Kahl, J. A. (1987). *The American class structure: A new synthesis* (3rd ed.). Chicago: Dorsey Press.

Gold, S. J. (1993). Migration and family adjustment: Continuity and change among Vietnamese in the United States. In H. P. McAdoo (Ed.) *Family ethnicity: Strength in diversity.* Newbury Park, CA: Sage Publications.

Gordon, M. M. (1964). *Assimilation in American life.* New York: Oxford University Press.

Helman, C. G. (1990). *Culture, health and illness: An introduction for health professionals.* London: Wright.

Henry, W. (1990, April 9). Beyond the melting pot. *Time,* 28–31.

Jones, E. E., & Korchin, S. J. (1982). *Minority mental health.* New York: Praeger.

Kavanagh, K. H., & Kennedy, P. H. (1992). *Promoting cultural diversity.* Newbury Park, CA: Sage Publications.

Keefe, S. E. (1981). Folk medicine among Mexican-Americans: Cultural persistence, change and displacement. *Hispanic Journal of Behavioral Science, 3,* 41–48.

Kleinman, A. (1980). *Patients and healers in the context of culture: An exploration of the borderland between anthropology, medicine, and psychiatry.* Berkeley: University of California Press.

Kluckholm, F., & Strodtbeck, E. (1961). *Variations in value orientations.* New York: Row, Peterson.

Kramer, J. M. (1988). Infant mortality and risk factors among American Indians compared to black and white rates: Implications for policy change. In W. A. Van Horne & T. V. Tonnesen (Eds.), *Ethnicity and health* (pp. 89 - 115). Milwaukee: University of Wisconsin Institute on Race and Ethnicity.

Kroeber, A. L. (1948). *Anthropology.* New York: Harcourt Brace.

Kumabe, K. T., Nishida, C., & Hepworth, D. H. (1985). *Bridging ethnocultural diversity in social work and health.* Honolulu: University of Hawaii School of Social Work.

Larrabee, E. (1973). Comments to Loretta Ford's research. An ethnic perspective. *Community nursing research: Collaboration and completion.* Denver, CO: Western Institute of Higher Education Commission.

Lin, C., & Liu, W. T. (1993). Relationships among Chinese immigrant families. In H. P. McAdoo (Ed.). *Family ethnicity: Strength in diversity* (pp. 271 - 286). Newbury Park, CA: Sage Publications.

McAdoo, H. P. (1993a). Ethnic families and conclusions. In H. P. McAdoo (Ed.), *Family ethnicity: Strength in diversity* (pp. 3 - 14 and 332 - 334). Newbury Park, CA: Sage, Publications.

McAdoo, J. L. (1993b). Decision making and marital satisfaction in African American families. In H. P. McAdoo (Ed.), *Family ethnicity: Strength in diversity* (pp. 109 - 119). Newbury Park, CA: Sage Publications.

McCubbin, H. I., & Patterson, M. (1983). The family stress process. The double ABCX model of adjustment and adaptation. In H. I. McCubbin, M. S. Sussman, & J. M. Patterson (Eds.), *Social stress and the family* (special issue). *Marriage and Family Review, 6* (112), 7 - 27.

McGoldrick, M. (1993). Ethnicity, cultural diversity and normality. In F. Walsh (Ed.), *Normal family processes* (2nd ed.) (pp. 331 - 360). New York: Guilford Press.

Menaghan, E. G. (1983). Individual coping efforts and family studies. Conceptual and methodological issues. In H. I. McCubbin, M. B. Sussman, & J. M. Patterson (Eds.), *Social stress and the family (special issue). Marriage and Family Review, 6* (112), 113 - 135.

Mirande, A. (1991). Ethnicity and fatherhood. In F. W. Bozett and S. M. H. Hanson (Eds.), *Fatherhood and families in cultural context* (pp. 53 - 82). New York: Springer.

Murray, R. B., & Zentner, J. P. (1993). *Nursing assessment and health promotion: Strategies across the life span* (5th ed.). Norwalk, CT: Appleton & Lange.

National Center for Health Statistics. (1992). *Health: United States, 1991.* Hyattsville, MD: US Public Health Service.

Nickens, J. W. (1991). The health status of minority populations in the United States. *Western Journal of Medicine, 155* (July), 27 - 32.

Parad, H. J., & Caplan, G. (1965). A framework for studying families in crisis. In H. J. Parad (Ed.), *Crisis intervention: Selected readings* (pp. 55 - 60). New York: Family Service of America.

Peterson, J. (1993, April 11). Life in the United States, graded on the curve. *Los Angeles Times*, pp. A1, A16.

Pleck, J. H. (1985). *Working wives/working husbands.* Beverly Hills, CA: Sage Publications.

Rix, S. E. (1990). *The American woman, 1990 - 1991: A status report.* New York: W. W. Norton.

Ropers, R. H. (1991). *Persistent poverty.* New York: Plenum Press.

Rossi, A. S. (1986). Sex and gender in the aging society. In A. Pifer & L. Bronte (Eds.), *Our aging society* (pp. 111 - 139). New York: W. W. Norton.

Rossi, P. H., Wright, J. D., Fisher, G. A., & Willis, G. (1987). The urban homeless: Estimating composition and size. *Science, 235,* 1136 - 1341.

Schnittger, M. H., & Bird, G. W. (1993). Coping among dual-career men and women across the family life cycle. *Family Relations, 39,* 199 - 205.

Spector, R. E. (1991). *Cultural diversity in health and illness* (3rd ed.). Norwalk, CT: Appleton & Lange.

Spitze, G. (1988). Women's employment and family relations: A review. *Journal of Marriage and the Family, 50,* 595 - 618.

Starfield, B. (1992). Child and adolescent health status measures. In Center for the Future of Children, *The future of children.* The David and Lucille Packard Foundation. *2*(2), 24 - 39.

United Press International (1990, February 6). Tax report says rich gained, poor lost during the 80's. *Los Angeles Times*, p A4.

US Bureau of the Census. (1983). *1980 census of population. General population characteristics.* (Part I, United States Summary PC 80 -1-61). Washington, DC: US Government Printing Office.

US Bureau of the Census. (1989). *Statistical abstracts of the United States* (109th ed.). Washington DC: US Government Printing Office.

US Bureau of the Census. (1992a). *Statistical Abstracts of the United States.* Washington, DC: US Government Printing Office.

US Bureau of the Census. (1992b): *1990 census of population. General population characteristics.* Washington, DC: US Government Printing Office.

US Bureau of the Census. (1992c). *Poverty in the United States: 1991 current population reports*, Series P-60, No. 181. Washington, DC: US Government Printing Office.

US Department of Health and Human Services. (1985). *Report of the secretary's task force on black and minority health, Vol. I. Executive summary.* Washington DC: US Department of Health and Human Services.

Valdez, R. B., & Dallek, G. (1991). Does the health care system serve black and Latino communities in Los Angeles County? Claremont, CA: Tomas Rivera Center.

Voydanoff, P., & Donnelly, B. W. (1988). Economic distress, family coping and quality of family life. In P. Voydanoff & L. C. Le Majka (Eds.), *Families and economic distress* (pp. 97–115). Newbury Park, CA: Sage Publications.

Wilkinson, D. (1987). Ethnicity. In M. B. Sussman & S. K. Steinmetz (Eds.), *Handbook of marriage and the family* (pp. 183–210). New York: Plenum Press.

Wilson, W. J. (1987). *The truly disadvantaged.* Chicago: University of Chicago Press.

Winnick, A. J. (1991). *Toward two societies.* New York: Praeger Press.

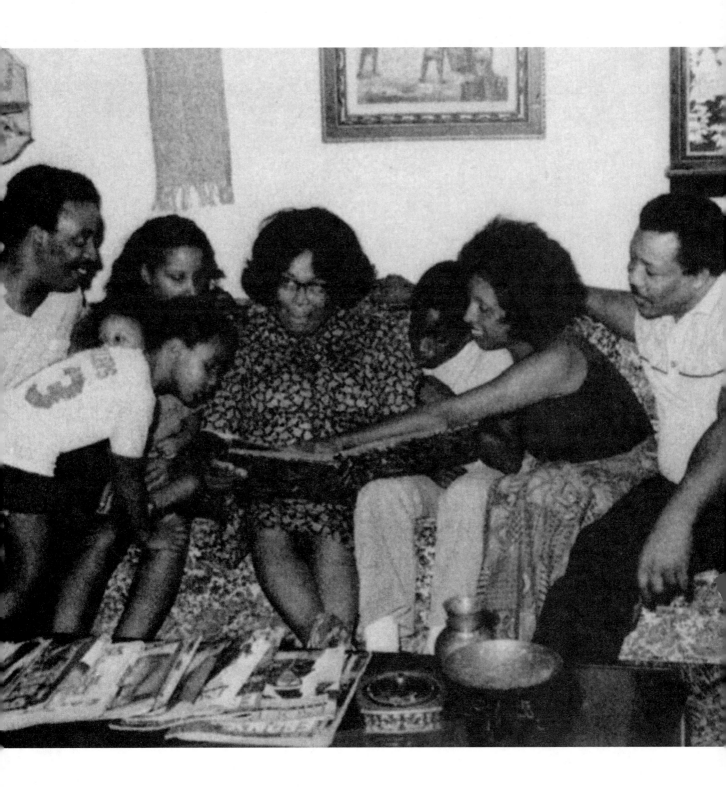

Factors Influencing Family Functioning and the Health of Family Members

This chapter approaches the family from a slightly different perspective than previous chapters. Here you will acquire an intimate view of family systems and health relationships and see how physical and psychological health factors within the family shape the health of individual members. In addition, you will see how the same factors within individual family members shape the health of the family as a whole.

This chapter also introduces nursing students to the Resiliency Model of Family Stress, Adjustment, and Adaptation (McCubbin & McCubbin, 1993). This useful model helps identify the factors that are important when evaluating how families adjust and adapt when faced with a member's illness; the accumulation of family stressors is explored and new family types are described. The importance of the family's appraisal of the illness situation, the coping strategies the family uses, as well as the family's typical communication patterns are some aspects of the model that are considered in depth. Understanding these factors provides nursing students with an additional tool for practice with families.

The importance of spirituality and religion to family health is also explored in this chapter. These sociocultural factors have been briefly discussed in Chapter 4, and their inclusion with the resiliency model is especially useful.

Legal affairs such as divorce decrees, child support arrangements, and visitation and custody issues have significant effects on the economic and social well-being of family members; and state and local courts make decisions every day that affect families. This chapter closes with a discussion of legal and ethical factors that will compel nursing students to examine their beliefs about government involvement in family health and family health policy.

CHAPTER 5

Factors Influencing Family Functioning and the Health of Family Members

Marilyn McCubbin, RN, PhD ■ *Marcia Van Riper, RN, PhD*

OUTLINE

FAMILY SYSTEM AND HEALTH RELATIONSHIPS
    Physical Health Factors
    Psychological Health Factors
    Application of a Family Stress Model in Illness of a Family Member
    Process of Family Adaptation to Illness
    Influence of Illness Characteristics on the Family
    Illness Time Phases and Family

SPIRITUALITY AND RELIGION

LEGAL AND ETHICAL FACTORS
    Legal Factors
    Ethical Factors

FAMILY POLICY
    What Is Family Policy?
    Pros and Cons of Family Policy
    The Family Medical Leave Act: A Policy Example
    The Role of Nursing in Family Policy and Health Care

OBJECTIVES   *Upon completion of this chapter, the reader will be able to:*
1. Examine the influence of family on the psychological and physical health of family members.
2. Describe the influence of spirituality and religion on family functioning.
3. Discuss legal and ethical factors that influence family functioning and the health of family members.
4. Explore the purpose of family health policy and how it may affect the family.
5. Examine the role of the nurse in advocating for social change that supports the family unit.

FAMILY SYSTEM AND HEALTH RELATIONSHIPS

The physical and emotional health of family members plays an important role in how the family functions on a day-to-day basis. If a family member is in bed with the flu, the chores and tasks which that individual usually performs for the family may need to be put on hold temporarily, or another family member may need to pitch in to keep things running smoothly until the flu has run its course. It also helps if another family member brings hot soup and a favorite magazine to read for the flu victim. Whereas acute illness usually requires only temporary alterations in family life, chronic illness may bring about more lasting changes. For example, when a family learns that Grandpa has been diagnosed with Alzheimer's disease, they have immediate questions: How long can Grandpa live alone? Will we need to have him move in with us? Where will we find the room? How will this affect the children's activities? Will we need to put him in a nursing home? How will we pay for his care? Many families face situations in which one member is dependent on alcohol or drugs, and they must ask themselves how they will manage this type of behavior. Do they ignore the problem and hope it will go away? Do they confront the member about it and insist that he or she seek help?

You can see from these examples that the family affects the individual's health and the individual's health affects the family (Doherty & Campbell, 1988). From family systems theory we know that family members are interconnected and dependent on one another. Thus, when there is a change in the health of one member, all family members will be affected and the family unit as a whole will be altered. The functioning of the family also influences the health and well-being of the family members.

Physical Health Factors

Research has consistently shown a positive relationship between marriage and physical health; poorer health outcomes are noted in never-married, divorced, or widowed persons than in those who are married. Although there may be a selection factor (many persons with major health problems do not get married or stay married), marriage appears to have a supportive and protective influence on physical health beyond any selection bias (Ross, Mirowsky, & Goldstein, 1990), and the additional support and higher incomes found in married households have both been associated with better physical health (Ross et al., 1990). If there are two incomes, these families have more economic resources and thus may have better access to health care. In addition, married persons are less likely to engage in risky lifestyle behaviors and more likely to live a healthier life (Venters, 1986). Husbands and wives are more likely to have nutritious diets, and are less likely to smoke, drink excessively, or take risks that increase the rate of accidents (Strong & DeVault, 1993). Although most relationships between marriage and physical health are positive, married persons are also more likely to be overweight and to exercise less (Venters, 1986).

A spouse or stable partner also may help to protect health. When one partner appears ill, the other partner may encourage seeking treatment and then support taking time off work to recover, using medication as prescribed, and resting. For example, a husband's encouragement to seek early treatment for a breast lump may make a big difference in the woman's prognosis if the mass turns out to be malignant.

Parenthood is generally viewed as desirable and healthy; however, children create economic burdens on the family and also decrease the amount of time parents have for each other (Ross et al., 1990). Thus, the addition of children to a family often creates tension and leads to a decline in the quality of the couple relationship (Belsky, Lang, & Rovine, 1985; Belsky, Spanier, & Rovine, 1983; White, Booth, & Edwards, 1986). Parents who have more economic resources, who support each other in work and parenting roles, and who have access to affordable child care and support from extended family tend to be healthier (Ross et al., 1990).

Psychological Health Factors

Most of the research to date on marriage, parenting, and the family has focused on psychological health. Marriage generally protects and improves psychological health, just as it does physical health (Ross et al., 1990). Unmarried individuals have more depression, anxiety, and other forms of psychological distress than those who are married (Gore & Mangione, 1983; Gove, Hughes, & Style, 1983; Mirowsky & Ross, 1989). One explanation for this is that married people are more likely to have consistent emotional support, and emotional support is associated with lower levels of depression and anxiety (Ross et al., 1990). Another explanation is that married people have higher household incomes, and economic well-being is related to psychological health (Kessler, 1979; Pearlin, Lieberman, Menaghan, & Mullan, 1981; Ross & Huber, 1985).

Marriage has a more positive impact on men's psychological health than on women's (Ross et al., 1990). Married women have more depression and anxiety than married men (Gove, 1984). Men seem to benefit most from the emotional support they gain in marriage, while women seem to benefit most from the economic support they gain. In a study by Gerstel, Riessman, and Rosenfield (1985), divorced men suffered from the loss of emotional support, whereas divorced women suffered from the loss of economic support.

There is increasing evidence that parents with children living at home experience more psychological distress than people without children or parents whose children have left home (Kandel, Davies, & Raveis, 1985; McLanahan & Adams, 1987; Ross et al., 1990; Umberson & Gove, 1989). According to McLanahan & Adams (1987), these differences may stem, in part, from pressures on married women who work and from the fact that many parents are single parents. Umberson and Gove (1989) noted that children have both positive and negative effects on parents. For example, parents report more psychological distress than nonparents, but they also indicate that life has more meaning. Psychological health appears to be strongly influenced by the age of children, whether the children are still living in the home, and whether the parents are married. Divorced parents find parenting more burdensome than married or widowed parents. Umberson (1989) noted that parents who feel burdened by their children experience less psychological well-being than parents who feel fewer demands.

Research on the family and psychological health is further advanced than research on the family and physical health (Campbell, 1986). In considering the relationship between the family and psychological health, From-Reichman's (1948) description of the schizophrenic mother stimulated a great deal of interest in the role of the family in schizophrenia and other forms of psychological distress. Since then, hundreds of studies on the family and schizophrenia have been carried out (see Goldstein & Strachan, 1987; Lukoff, Snyer, Ventura, & Nuechterlein, 1984). Researchers have found that poor parental communication (e.g., lack of commitment to ideas, unclear communication of ideas, disruptive speech, and closure problems) is common in families of schizophrenics and is present before the symptoms of schizophrenia appear (Doane, West, Goldstein, Rodnick, & Jones, 1981; Goldstein, 1985; Karon & Widener, 1994). Researchers have also found that the emotional climate of the family has a consistent and powerful effect on the course of schizophrenia (Brown, Birley, & Wing, 1972; Brown, Monck, Carstairs, & Wing, 1972; Vaughn & Leff, 1976; Vaughn, Snyder, Jone, Freeman, & Falloon, 1984). Individuals with schizophrenia appear to have difficulty tolerating critical comments by overinvolved family members.

When family interventions are successful in reducing overinvolvement and critical comments, individuals with schizophrenia have fewer relapses and they have less need for hospitalization (Anderson, Reiss, & Hogarty, 1986; Basolo-Kunzer, 1994; Bernheim & Lehman, 1985).

While much of the research on the family and psychological health has focused on the family's role in schizophrenia, there has been growing interest in the family's role in depression (Kaufman, 1984; Bromet, May, & May, 1984; Parker, 1983; Stuart, Laraia, Ballenger, & Lydiard, 1990), alcoholism (Ablon, 1984; Jacob, Dunn, & Leonard, 1983; Kaufman, 1980, 1984; Kosten, Novak, & Kleber, 1984), and anorexia nervosa (Garfinkel & Garner, 1982; Stanton & Todd, 1982; Yager, 1982). Yet our understanding of the family's role in the development and course of these conditions remains very limited (Campbell, 1986). Much of what we know is based on informal reports by family members and clinicians.

According to Tseng and Hsu (1991), researchers and clinicians have typically viewed the family as either the system of pathology, the cradle of pathology, or the catalyst of pathology. When the family is viewed as the system of pathology, the individual's psychopathology is considered to be a display of the total family psychopathology. Individual psychopathology therefore receives little attention. The primary focus is on identifying dysfunctions in family relationships, such as overprotectiveness, rigidity, or lack of conflict solution. When the family is viewed as the cradle of pathology, early family relationships are thought to be the source of vulnerabilities that appear as pathologies later in life. Researchers and clinicians direct much of their attention to early family relationships and their impact on the individual. When the family is viewed as the catalyst of pathology, the environment provided by the family is thought to provoke, maintain, or aggravate individual psychopathology. Modification or removal of the individual from the family situation is strongly encouraged as a way to improve the individual's condition.

Much of the research on the family and psychological health has focused on psychological distress or pathology. In addition, the research has looked at only one side of the problem. For example, some clinicians and researchers are still trying to identify the characteristics of the schizophrenic family or the alcoholic family. This simple one-to-one correspondence between a particular type of family and a particular type of psychological distress can no longer be assumed; rather researchers need to look at multidirectional interactions.

Application of a Family Stress Model in Illness of a Family Member

Family theories and models (see Chapter 2) can be helpful in providing a set of lenses through which to see how the physical and psychological health of family members affects family functioning and how the family, in turn, affects the health of its members. The Resiliency Model of Family Stress, Adjustment, and Adaptation (McCubbin & McCubbin, 1993) can provide insight into the factors that are important for evaluating how families adjust and adapt when faced with a member's illness (Fig. 5–1). In this model, families are considered more likely to adapt successfully to an illness if:

1. They are less vulnerable because fewer other **stressors** or family changes are occurring at the same time

2. They have patterns of functioning that are more adaptive (e.g., there is more emotional closeness among family members and they are more flexible and able to change roles, boundaries, and rules when necessary)

3. They define the situation positively and view it as something they can master and have some control over

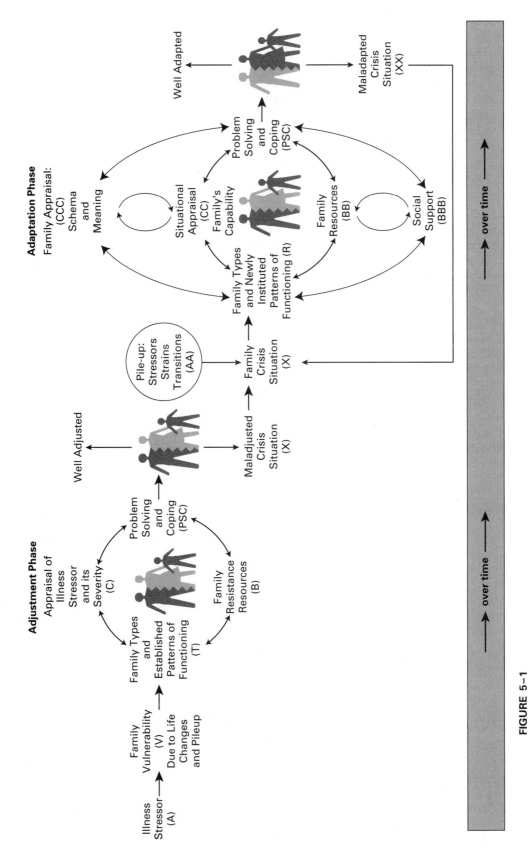

FIGURE 5–1

The Resiliency Model of Family Stress, Adjustment, and Adaptation. (From McCubbin, M. & McCubbin, H. [1993], with permission.)

4. They have good coping and communication skills (Danielson, Hamel-Bissell, & Winstead-Fry, 1993)

A short-term acute illness with a predictable course and cure is usually less difficult for the family to manage than longer illnesses, because the changes are not permanent and the family may be able to manage without drastically altering its usual patterns of functioning. When the illness is chronic or in a terminal stage, the family usually needs to alter its ways of functioning in order to accommodate the more severe and long-lasting sequelae of the illness. Let us look at the factors in the resiliency model that may influence how the family will respond to a member's illness.

Accumulation of Family Stressors

Families are more vulnerable if they experience other changes at the same time that a member becomes ill. Such changes may include financial problems; work stresses; conflicts among family members, with the extended family, or with former spouses; childbearing or child care strains; transitions of members in and out of the family; other illness or family care strains, such as care of an aging parent; recent losses of close relatives or friends; or legal violations (family member being arrested, sent to jail, or running away from home). Families rarely have to deal only with a member's illness; they also need to manage other normal expected transitions, as well as work and family demands. Existing strains in the family such as spousal conflicts or parent-child tensions may be exacerbated by illness. In addition, the illness itself brings new demands and changes. Negotiation with the health care system and decisions about treatment can go smoothly or become agonizingly difficult. There may be uncertainty about the diagnosis, the treatment options, and the prognosis. Complex conditions may require many types of helpers, who may offer conflicting opinions about what the patient and family should do.

Family Types

The resiliency model depicts several family types, which represent patterns of family behavior associated with better physical and psychological health for family members and more adaptive functioning of the family as a unit:

1. The **regenerative family type**, which is characterized by **family hardiness** (internal strength and a sense of control) and coherence (view of the situation as manageable and meaningful). These families are more likely to view the illness as a challenge, something to be managed and mastered, and they are committed to working together to solve problems that arise.

2. The **resilient family type**, which is characterized by greater emotional closeness among family members and by flexibility and ability to shift roles, rules, and boundaries. These families have strong connections among the members, with feelings of support and affirmation for one another, as well as an ability to take over roles and duties for the ill member, alter family rules of operation, and obtain outside help and information in order to manage the illness.

3. The **rhythmic family type**, which focuses on maintaining and valuing family time and routines that provide stability and predictability in times of illness. These families have established patterns of spending time together at meals, bedtime routines for children, ways of letting members know where they are, and so on. While these routines may be interrupted in times of illness, family time and routines provide a sense of security and consistency in stressful situations.

Family Appraisal

The **family appraisal** of the illness, that is, the way the family sees the illness, is also a critical factor in **family adaptation**. How do family members define the illness, and what does the illness mean to them? Do they see the illness as having an impact on them? Do they believe they have the resources and capabilities to handle what is happening? Are the family's goals, priorities, and expectations changed by the illness? Are these changes viewed as temporary or more permanent? Family members will appraise the situation differently depending on their age, gender, role in the family, and prior experience. Coming to a shared understanding of the situation is difficult and demanding and it is achieved only through perseverance, patience, negotiation, understanding, and shared commitment (McCubbin & McCubbin, 1993).

Coping and Communication

Coping and problem-solving communication skills are also important in the family adaptation process. Families need to balance coping efforts in three areas:

1. Maintaining the functioning of the family unit and optimism about the situation

2. Managing the tensions of individual members and maintaining their self-esteem, support, and psychological stability

3. Understanding the health care situation and any treatment regimens for the ill member (McCubbin, 1991)

Nurses and other health care professionals often focus on the third area of **family coping** by providing education about the disease and its treatment and emphasizing the need to comply with a prescribed regimen. Surprisingly, however, results in a study by Reiss, Gonzalez, and Kramer (1986) found that patients with end-stage renal disease undergoing center-based dialysis, who were more compliant with their regimen, died sooner. The authors concluded that family members had disengaged from the seriously ill member in an effort to prepare for the anticipated death; the excluded patient then turned to health care professionals for acceptance and was compliant in order to receive positive feedback from the health care team. Yet, because these patients lacked support from family members, their compliance was not enough to keep them alive. Those patients on dialysis who lived longer were not totally noncompliant. They generally followed the regimen but also allowed themselves a day off from diet restrictions and fluid limitations to enjoy a meal out or participate in a family celebration. Thus, these individuals remained more involved with their families and, therefore, they survived longer.

It is important for families who have an ill member to try to balance coping efforts in all three areas to maintain the family as a unit, to maintain the health and well-being of all the members, and to maintain care and support for the ill member. This may be difficult for families if the health care system emphasizes only the care of the ill member, to the detriment of the health of other members and the health of the family unit.

Family problem-solving communication also plays a role in family adaptation to illness. Two types of family communication have been found to predict family adaptation following the diagnosis of a child's congenital heart condition (McCubbin, 1993). **Incendiary communication** is characterized by bringing up old unresolved issues, failing to calmly talk things through to reach a solution, yelling and screaming at other family members, and walking away from conflicts without much resolution. This type of communication increases the stress. **Affirming communication**, as the name implies, is more supportive. It is characterized by being careful not to hurt other members emotionally or physically, taking time to hear what others have to say, conveying respect for others' feelings, and ending conflicts on a positive note. Families with more affirming communication and less incendiary communication are better able to adapt to the demands created by a member's illness.

Process of Family Adaptation to Illness

Families make trial-and-error efforts to sort out all the information they receive and decide on strategies to manage the illness situation. All families rely on previously established ways of functioning and coping to manage the initial crisis of a family member's illness. This period is the **family adjustment** phase in the Resiliency Model. Initially the family may totally reorganize around the member's illness, focusing only on the illness and neglecting other family needs. For short-term acute conditions, where recovery is predictable and complete, this adjustment on the part of the family system can work. In chronic illnesses and acute illnesses with prolonged recovery times, what seems to work at first may be detrimental over the long haul to meeting the needs of family members and the family unit as a whole. Thus, more fundamental changes in the family's way of operating may need to be made. This is called the **family adaptation phase** in the model (Fig. 5–1). For example, a mother may take time off from work to spend most of her time at the hospital bedside with an ill child while the father tries to manage his work and the other children at home. This approach may work at first; but if the child's illness is prolonged, the workplace may not continue to tolerate the mother's absence, problems of reduced income and potential job loss may surface, and the other children may begin to feel neglected. Further, both parents can become exhausted with this arrangement. The family system is then in a state of crisis. This does not mean the family is sick and needs fixing; however, it indicates that change is needed and new patterns of functioning need to be tried. Thus, the mother may return to work part-time; the father may spend more time at the hospital; both parents may try to spend time with the siblings left at home; additional help from relatives may be sought to ease the burden on the parents; and if financial resources permit, outside help with household tasks and chores may be obtained. The family thus tries to achieve adaptation. In the Resiliency Model this adaptation represents a fit at two levels of functioning: a fit of the individual and the family system (i.e., ensuring the care and well-being of family members and the family unit) and the fit of the family system with the community (including satisfactory relationships with the workplace, hospital, etc.).

Influence of Illness Characteristics on the Family

The characteristics of the illness itself also influence how the family responds. We have already noted that acute illness usually requires only temporary changes in how the family functions. Chronic illness requires more lasting alterations in how the family operates day to day. Rolland (1988) has proposed that four characteristics of an illness (onset, course, outcome, and degree of incapacitation) and three phases of illness (crisis, chronic, and terminal) should be examined in order to understand the relationship between the chronic illness, the affected family member, and the family unit.

The onset of chronic illness can be sudden (e.g., a burn injury) or gradual (e.g., AIDS). Although both illnesses may require considerable alterations in family functioning, a gradual onset of illness allows family members more time to mobilize their resources and develop ways to cope. Families who experience the sudden onset of a chronic illness in a family member must immediately try to manage their anxiety and tension, alter roles, and try to find ways to manage the situation.

The course of a chronic illness can be progressive, constant, or relapsing/episodic (Rolland, 1988). In progressive illnesses such as Alzheimer's disease or lung cancer, the affected family member deteriorates over time. The deterioration may occur quite rapidly or very slowly. Caretaking demands increase as the individual's condition worsens, and family caregivers may become exhausted, with deleterious effects on their health. In illnesses with a constant course such as spinal cord injury or stroke, the family must adapt to the reduced but relatively stable, predictable functioning of the affected family member. Here, too, however, stress on family caregivers is a concern, because the illness brings a permanent change in the individual's functioning. In relapsing/episodic illnesses such as many cancers or multiple sclerosis, the ill individual and the family as a whole experience relatively stable and normal periods interspersed with flare-ups or exacerbations. This requires a great deal of flexibility so that the family can move into a crisis mode when necessary and then revert back to previous patterns of functioning when all is going well. Because the family needs to be ready to respond to the next relapse, family members are often in a constant state of alertness and tension.

The outcome for the family is affected by whether the illness is inevitably fatal, as AIDS is, or may be fatal (as cancer may be), whether it shortens the expected life span (as in diabetes or emphysema) or has a minimal effect on the life span (arthritis, asthma). Rolland (1988) notes that it is the *initial expectation* of whether the disease is likely to be fatal that is critical. The family's perception of whether the illness represents an inevitable loss or a possible loss (Rolland, 1990) influences how the family includes the affected member in or excludes him or her from day-to-day family interactions and decision making.

The degree of incapacitation also influences the family response (Rolland, 1988). The family member can be incapacitated in various ways: cognition (Alzheimer's disease), sensation (blindness, deafness), motor functioning (stroke, spinal cord injury), energy level (cardiovascular disease, multiple sclerosis), or through social stigma (mental illness, AIDS) (Rolland, 1988). These different kinds of incapacitation require different adaptive strategies by the family. A cognitive deficit is usually considered difficult to manage because the family member cannot communicate or take part in decision making effectively. The individual's behavior also may be quite unpredictable and disturbing, which can isolate the family from the community. Some conditions such as stroke may involve both cognitive and motor impairment. Thus the chronic illness characteristics of onset, course, outcome, and degree of incapacitation all must be considered when examining how an illness influences the family.

Illness Time Phases and Family

Time phases of the illness include the initial crisis, the chronic or long-term care phase, and the terminal or final phase (Rolland, 1988). The initial crisis period includes the time preceding an actual diagnosis and confirmation of the illness, as well as time covered by the expected course of treatment. The family member and the family unit must mourn the loss of health, reorganize to accommodate the changes brought about by the illness, appraise how the illness affects each member and the family unit as a whole, and establish relationships with the health care system and any other outside systems (e.g., special education, insurance providers, vocational rehabilitation, etc.) needed to manage the illness. The chronic phase can be prolonged and last many years or be quite short, as in a fulminating fatal illness. This is the stage where permanent alterations are made in family functioning to accommodate the changes brought about by the chronic illness, though most families try to maintain some normality in family life if possible. The last phase or terminal stage of illness involves coming to grips with the death of a family member, grieving, and letting go. This can be an extremely stressful time, particularly if the family member's death is premature. While the family may feel some relief because the individual is no longer suffering and family caretaking demands have ceased, the irreversible nature of the loss and the permanent change it brings in the family system often require an enormous effort to accept.

SPIRITUALITY AND RELIGION

Another factor that influences the health of family members and the functioning of the family is spirituality and religion. Indeed, spirituality and religion can influence every aspect of family life. Transitions in the family life cycle (marriage, birth, death) are marked by religious ceremonies, observances, and traditions. Many families report new meaning in life and increased depth of spirituality after experiencing a significant illness in a family member. Spirituality and religion also can play a significant role in coping with a family member's death and helping the family to heal following such a loss. Spiritual hope and peace, and belief in the promise of eternal life after the temporary earthly journey, can help ease the trauma following the death of a family member (Thomas & Henry, 1984). Although spirituality and religion generally are viewed as having a positive impact on families, they also can be detrimental to the health of family members and family functioning. When families interact with nurses and the health care system, they bring to these interactions a set of beliefs and values that often reflect their religious background and spirituality. "Religion," "religiousness," "spirituality," and "spiritual well-being" are terms frequently used in discussions about spiritual issues. **Religion** has been defined as "any source of transcendent meaning from which people derive a sense of purpose and values that become the standards by which they direct actions and define, interpret, and judge the activities of human life" (Brigman, 1992, p. 39). Religion thus provides the beliefs and values that help families determine how they will act in various situations and how they will evaluate the actions of others. **Religiousness**, originally associated with church attendance and involvement in formal religious activities, has now been defined as adherence to the beliefs and practices of an organized church or religious institution (Shafranske & Maloney, 1990). Religiousness reflects how closely a family believes in and practices the beliefs of a particular religious group such as Roman Catholicism, Judaism, Islam, or various Protestant Christian denominations. Thus, both religion and religiousness provide a framework of values, beliefs, and actions that can influence the functioning of the family and the way the family responds to illness.

Spirituality is a broader term that has been defined as those more personal practices of a religious nature that may or may not emanate from a particular religious institution (Shafranske & Maloney, 1990). Spirituality encompasses a sense of relation or connectedness within oneself, with others, and with a higher, unseen power of God (Reed, 1992). **Spiritual well-being** is defined as a sense of inner peace, compassion for others, reverence for life, gratitude, and appreciation of both unity and diversity (Vaughn, 1986, pp. 20–21); it includes the conviction that there is a purpose and meaning in life, a relationship with God, and realistic views of adversity and loss (Moberg, 1974). Spirituality and spiritual well-being may not be linked to a specific religious institution or group.

Research on family strengths has confirmed the importance of religion and spirituality in strong families. DeFrain and Stinnett (1992) note that strong families are not perfect but they can effectively manage the challenges in their lives. After asking over 3500 family members, over a period of 16 years, about their family's strengths, DeFrain and Stinnett

(1992) concluded that spiritual well-being was one of six critical qualities of strong families. This spiritual well-being was reflected by family members' sense of optimism, hope, and meaning in their lives. These strong families had a spirituality that went deeper than church attendance and participation in religious activities. Awareness of a higher power gave them a sense of purpose, strength, and support that helped them to be more patient with each other, more forgiving, quicker to get over anger, more positive, and more supportive in their family relationships (Stinnett, 1979). This quality also allowed family members to find goodness and purpose in both the joys and sorrows of daily living and family life.

A shared religious core was found to be one of 15 traits of a healthy family by Curran (1983) in her survey of professionals in education, church, health, family counseling, and voluntary organizations. Two other healthy family traits, a sense of right and wrong and valuing service to others, also were linked to the role of religion and spirituality in the family. Curran stresses that the specific religion a family belongs to is not the important issue. Instead there are three hallmarks that identify a family with a shared religious core. These are (1) a faith in God, which plays a role in family life by giving it purpose, stability, and meaning; (2) a strengthened family support system that encourages nurturing and affirming relationships among family members; and (3) the feeling of parents that they have a strong responsibility for passing on the faith, which they do in positive and meaningful ways (Curran, 1985).

The aspects of religion and spirituality that contribute to more positive family functioning include religious beliefs related to love, faith, hope, forgiveness, reconciliation, and the worth of human beings; a lifestyle that emphasizes commitment, responsibility, giving, and caring for others; shared beliefs and values; shared religious and church activities; reverence for marriage and family; and affiliation with a support group or network that provides a sense of belonging (Brigman, 1992). Some aspects of religious and spiritual beliefs and values may also be detrimental to families. What constitutes a family may be narrowly defined by religions, with a clear preference for a nuclear family (husband, wife, and children all living together). Many religions have become more liberal about nontraditional families, sexuality, contraceptive use, divorce, and remarriage. Some religious groups, however, still strongly support only heterosexual unions, consider marriage a lifetime commitment, encourage childbearing, discourage regulation of fertility, and support traditional gender roles. For families whose situation is not congruent with the beliefs and values of their religion, this can be a source of stress rather than support and comfort. Also, a religious emphasis on sin and judgment may produce feelings of guilt and low self-esteem (Brigman, 1992).

The fit between the family's religious beliefs and values and the family's situation is critical. Although the inclusion of religious values and beliefs in the health care assessment may seem to be an invasion of the family's privacy, it is important for the nurse to be sensitive to how these beliefs and values influence a family's response in illness situations. Even if the family has no formal religious affiliation, it is important to know its world view and to work with it when delivering nursing care.

LEGAL AND ETHICAL FACTORS

Legal and ethical factors also influence family functioning and the health of family members. Legal factors include (1) legal definitions of what constitutes a family; (2) the federal government's involvement in family issues; and (3) decisions made by state and local courts about family issues (Liss, 1987). Ethical factors include three principles that provide a framework for determining how people should behave, or what behavior is morally right, in specific situations (Rhodes, 1993). These principles are (1) beneficence; (2) autonomy or self-determination; and (3) justice or equity (Rogers, 1988; Starck, 1991; Thompson, 1987).

Legal Factors

Legal Definitions of Family

The question of what constitutes a family has proved very perplexing to the courts (Liss, 1987). Prior to the 1960s, legal definitions of the family typically reflected the prevailing views of the nuclear family (Liss, 1987; Yorker, 1993). However, with the rapid proliferation of other family forms (e.g., single-parent families, unmarried adults with or without children, stepfamilies, and multigenerational communes), more and more people started to question these legal definitions of family. For example, in *Palo Alto Tenants Union v. Morgan* (1970), members of a communal living group challenged a zoning ordinance that defined the family as one person living alone or two or more persons related by blood, marriage, or legal adoption, or a group not exceeding four persons living in a single housekeeping unit. In *Moore v. City of East Cleveland, Ohio* (1977), a city ordinance was struck down because it made it a crime for a grandmother to live with her grandsons, who were first cousins rather than brothers.

Today, the nuclear family accounts for only 26% of all households in the United States (US Bureau of the Census, 1991). While there have been many attempts to change the way family is legally defined, definitions that reflect the traditional nuclear family still exist in state and local ordinances. Because of this, nontraditional families may have difficulty finding appropriate housing. In addition, they may be denied food stamps and other welfare benefits (Liss, 1987). This may have a negative effect on family functioning and the health of individual family members.

It has been suggested that the definition of family used to determine which families qualify for the Aid to Families with Dependent Children (AFDC) Program has been instrumental in breaking up many families (Liss, 1987). While the definition used is not the definition of a nuclear family, it is based on beliefs about the nuclear family; that is, the program's man-in-the-house rule assumes that when no breadwinner (i.e., father) is present, the government should take over the father's role of breadwinner and the mother should be able to stay home with the children (Johnson & Ooms, 1985; Liss, 1987). The man-in-the-house rule has become a built-in incentive for some poor fathers, even those who are very caring and hardworking, to desert their families. It has been estimated that over 80% of the children who receive welfare benefits do so because their father has left the family, not because their father is dead or disabled (Liss, 1987). Children who have been deserted by their fathers often find it necessary to take on additional roles in the family. This, in turn, may have negative effects on individual as well as family functioning.

Involvement of the Federal Government in Family Issues

The U.S. Constitution has very little to say about the rights of the family. According to Liss (1987), this omission by our founding fathers may have been intentional, because a basic assumption of the American system is that the rights of the individual outweigh those of the family. In addition, the family has traditionally been viewed as a bastion of privacy, not to be intruded on by the federal government.

Prior to the twentieth century, laws affecting family issues were relatively noninterventionist (Yorker, 1993). The few legal restrictions that existed were based on biblical sanctions (e.g., adultery) and social taboos (e.g., incest). During the late 1800s and early 1900s, state laws that had protectionist and regulatory effects on families were enacted. Many of these laws were paternalistic and based on prevailing notions of morality. Courts at the state and local levels used these laws to guide their decisions about family issues such as marriage, divorce, child support, child custody, and family violence. Ultimately, a confusing patchwork of government actions and services was created (Liss, 1987). The rights extended to the family vary from state to state. This makes it very difficult when state courts are asked to decide on family issues involving individuals living in different states. If there is a question about whether a state law or lower court decision is, in fact, constitutional, the matter goes to the United States Supreme Court (Myers, 1992).

In 1973, the Supreme Court made a landmark decision in *Roe v. Wade* (Liss, 1987). This decision protected the right of women to decide whether to bear a child and thus has had a major impact on family health. Over the last 20 years, there have been many unsuccessful attempts to overturn this decision. In 1977 the Supreme Court heard three cases challenging lower courts' decisions that states participating in the Medicaid program could refuse to pay the expenses incidental to nontherapeutic abortions while paying the expenses incidental to childbirth. The court ruled that these lower court decisions were not unconstitutional. Three of the Supreme Court justices disagreed with this decision on the grounds that it showed a distressing insensitivity to the plight of impoverished pregnant women. They also noted that it actually forced impoverished women to bear unwanted children. Forcing impoverished women to bear unwanted children is likely to have a negative impact on family functioning and the health of individual family members. An unwanted pregnancy is a very stressful experience for the pregnant woman and for her family. In addition, unwanted children typically receive less than adequate care and attention, which places them at increased risk for physical and psychological problems.

According to Liss (1987), there are three areas of family-related behavior that have been challenged in the courts, have been reviewed by the highest state courts or the Supreme Court, and have been denied constitutional protection. They are support obligations in marriage, the right to marital privacy in the bedroom, and homosexual relations, including same-sex marriage. Failure of the Supreme Court to intervene in these areas of family life may ultimately lead to poorer individual and family functioning. For example, if one spouse has total control of the family income and refuses to provide other family members with adequate food, shelter, and health care, failure of the court to intervene may further jeopardize the health and well-being of the family members who lack income and power. Ironically, it is only at divorce that the unemployed spouse can claim a proportion of the employed spouse's income.

State and Local Courts Decisions About Family Issues

State and local courts are routinely asked to make decisions on family issues such as marriage, divorce, child support, child custody, and family violence (Walker, 1992). The way in which these decisions are made can have a profound impact on family functioning and the health of family members. For example, until 1970, when California instituted the first no-fault divorce law, divorce could be obtained only if one party committed a marital offense (e.g., desertion, cruelty, adultery, insanity, or impotence) giving the other partner a legal basis or grounds for divorce (Weitzman & Dixon, 1989). The plaintiff's success in obtaining a divorce depended on the ability to prove the defendant's fault for having committed the marital offense. Fault-oriented divorce proceedings were stressful for everyone involved (Strong & DeVault, 1993). In most cases, the proceedings were very time-consuming, and they involved highly charged feelings about custody, property, and children (Liss, 1987; Raschke, 1987; Weitzman & Dixon, 1989). There is growing evidence that the adversarial nature of these proceedings had a negative impact on the psychological health of the children involved (Saayman & Saayman, 1988/1989; Schwartzberg, 1981). At present, 48 states have adopted no-fault divorce (Strong & DeVault, 1993). While no-fault divorce has been successful in eliminating much of the acrimony and shame that resulted from fault-oriented divorce (Dixon & Weitzman, 1980), there is little research to indicate whether no-fault divorce reduces the distress and conflict of divorcing couples (Kitson & Morgan, 1991). More research is needed to understand how, and under what conditions, legal factors affect the adjustment to divorce (Raschke, 1987).

Recently, concern about infants born to drug-addicted women has led a number of state and local prosecutors to attempt to impose criminal penalties for maternal substance abuse (Kocsis, 1991; Rhodes, 1992). The typical strategy is to charge the mother with the crime of delivering a controlled substance to the fetus, either before birth, or after birth before the umbilical cord is cut. To date, most courts have ruled that the state statutes related to child endangerment and delivery of controlled substances do not apply to the unborn child of a pregnant substance abuser, and the criminal charges against the pregnant women have been dismissed (Rhodes, 1992). However, there appears to be growing interest in the use of criminal sanctions to deter drug use among pregnant women. Many health care providers are concerned that this approach may actually have a negative impact on the health of unborn infants because women who use drugs will fail to seek prenatal care out of fear that they will be subject to criminal charges. Clearly, this is a medical-legal dilemma with ethical implications (Kocsis, 1991).

Ethical Factors

Ethical factors may also influence family functioning and the health of family members. Three major principles are typically encountered in the literature on ethics: beneficence, autonomy or self-determination, and justice or equity (Rogers, 1988; Starck, 1991; Thompson, 1987). Beneficence involves benefiting others or promoting their good (Aroskar, 1989; Jenkins, 1989). Autonomy, also known as self-determination, is a form of personal liberty in which the individual chooses his or her own course of action (Rogers, 1988). Justice or equity involves the fair distribution of benefits and burdens among all members of society (Rogers, 1988; Starck, 1991). These three principles may have important influences on family functioning and the health of family members. For example, the principle of beneficence requires that health care providers take positive steps to help patients and their families and to prevent harm to them, which is sometimes called nonmaleficence (Thompson, 1987). For example, when a community health nurse identifies and reports a possible case of child neglect, the nurse is taking steps to prevent harm to the child. When the nurse works with the family on issues such as proper nutrition, growth and development, age-appropriate discipline, and problem-solving skills, the nurse is taking steps to promote family functioning and the health of individual family members. If the nurse chooses to ignore the signs and symptoms of child neglect, the principle of beneficence has not been upheld and the nurse's action, or lack of action, may negatively affect the child's physical and psychological health.

The principle of autonomy or self-determination dictates that health care providers respect and support the right of families to choose their own course of action. Supporting a family's decision to refuse extraordinary life-saving measures for a critically ill family member is an example of action based on this principle. In contrast, pressuring a family to institutionalize their child with Down syndrome, despite the family's desire to raise the child in the family home, is an example of action contrary to the principle of autonomy.

According to the principle of justice or equity, everyone should be treated equally; in addition, goods and services should be provided first to those who have the greatest need (Churchill, 1987). Health care resources are very scarce at the present time, so this principle has become very important. Health care providers are constantly being confronted with issues such as: Who should receive services first? What type of services should patients and their families receive? Under what circumstances should families be denied services?

These are very difficult questions. The way in which they are answered will have a powerful impact on family functioning and the health of individual family members. For example, a decision to deny a patient a heart transplant may result in death for the patient and decreased psychological well-being for other family members. A decision to approve a heart transplant may result in improved health for the patient, but over time, it may still result in decreased psychological well-being for family members because of the additional stressors associated with the chronic condition.

The principles of beneficence, autonomy or self-determination, and justice or equity need to be considered as decisions are made about families at all levels: in a particular health care setting; at the local community level of providing health care; and at the larger state and national levels, where all types of health care services are organized and funded.

FAMILY POLICY

What Is Family Policy?

Policy involves a set of choices or decisions that are made to reach an overall goal through a specific type of action (Zimmerman, 1992). Values and the political process play an important role in setting policies. For example, in the United States, taxes are levied to reach the goal of providing to citizens certain services such as police and fire protection, road building and maintenance, libraries, schools, and public recreational facilities. Societal values and the negotiation and compromise involved in the political process play a critical role in determining how much tax individuals and businesses have to pay and how the tax dollars are spent.

The use of the term "family policy" is somewhat inappropriate since the United States has no overall official family policy. Zimmerman (1992, p. 3) broadly defines **family policy** as everything that governments do that affect families, directly or indirectly. Using this definition, any policy that has an impact on families, including those related to housing, health, income maintenance (e.g., Aid to Families with Dependent Children, Social Security), education, social services, or employment can be broadly termed a family policy. Aldous and Dumon (1990) refer to family policy as objectives concerning family well-being and the specific measures taken by governmental bodies to achieve them. This definition, however, limits family policy to those policies designed to positively benefit families (Aldous & Dumon, 1990). Regardless of the specific definition used, it is generally agreed that the overall goal of family policy is to enhance the well-being of individual family members and the family unit (Zimmerman, 1992). This has been defined as individual and family satisfaction with life, meeting the needs of families in the community, reducing the stress of families, providing additional resources to families, and matching resources to the needs of families (Zimmerman, 1988).

Pros and Cons of Family Policy

There has been ongoing debate about whether to establish specific family policies in the United States. Some argue that there is no need because all policies affect families in some way. Certainly policies related to family planning, abortion, termination of life support, child support, welfare reform, and benefits for the elderly — to name but a few — all affect families in some way. Others fear that a family policy will be intrusive and allow government to regulate what many consider to be a very private domain — one's family life. Furthermore, in establishing a family policy, the definition of what constitutes a family becomes quite controversial. If the definition of family is narrow, many individuals in nontraditional family situations will be excluded. For example, many health insurance policies do not recognize domestic partners as family, so these persons are not eligible for coverage under these policies. Cost is always a major concern in the design and execution of any policy, especially if it involves family issues because of the privacy issue and the many types of family structure that may need to be included. Thus some consider that an overall family policy would be entirely too expensive to implement and maintain, while others maintain that failure to support families in carrying out their societal roles will cost more in the long run.

Supporters of family policy for the United States note that without federal legislation, policies are piecemeal and not equitable across the country. Without comprehensive family policies, we leave to chance the care of some of the most vulnerable members of society — children, the elderly, the mentally ill, the disabled. On the other hand, American culture values individualism, or the notion that people need to work hard and be responsible for their own success; that they should rely on family help for assistance and use governmental resources only as a last resort; and that they should be able to live their lives with minimal governmental influence and interference (Zimmerman, 1988). These values have limited the development of an overall family policy.

The Family and Medical Leave Act: A Policy Example

Let us look at some recent legislation and its impact on the family. For many years now we have been aware that family members who need to take time off from work to give birth to a child, adopt a child, or care for an ill family member run the risk of losing their job. If they return to their place of employment, they may find that they have been demoted to a lower position with less pay. After considerable debate and controversy, the federal Family and Medical Leave Act was passed and went into effect in August 1993, during the first months of the Clinton administration. The bill had been vetoed during the previous administration, primarily based on cost. The new law provides 12 weeks of leave annually to employees for the birth or adoption of a child; to care for a newborn; to care for a child, parent, or spouse with a serious illness; or to recuperate from a serious illness that does not permit the employee to work. Employees are eligible for this benefit if they have worked at least 1250 hours during the past year (about 25 hours per week). The act applies to companies who have 50 employees or more. Companies do not have to pay workers during this leave but they can allow workers to use their paid vacation and sick leave during this time. For anticipated events (e.g., birth, adoption, scheduled surgery), 30 days notice to the employer is required. The leave need not be taken all at once but can be used in segments — for example, to accommodate renal dialysis treatments. While legal challenges to the benefits under this new law are expected (Saltzman, 1993), the legislation recognizes the need for family leave in parenting and serious illness situations. Thus, it is a policy that promotes both individual and **family well-being**.

Nurses can play a key role in informing clients and their families about this new legislation. Many individuals are not aware that they have a right to this leave. Workers who believe their old job will not be available to them on their return need to discuss this with their supervisor or the owner of the company before taking a leave. Complaints about violation of the policy must be filed within 2 years with a private attorney or with the local or regional office of the US Department of Labor's Wage and Hour Division, Employment Standards Administration (Saltzman, 1993).

This is just one example of how policy may influence family functioning and the health of individual family members. What is the future for family policy in the United States? The enactment of family policies is closely tied to the political atmosphere (Zimmerman, 1992). President Carter convened a White House conference on families during his administration in the late 1970s, but fighting between conservatives and liberals on family policy derailed all efforts at establishing family policy goals (Wilcox & O'Keefe, 1991). During the 1980s a more conservative political ideology prevailed and the administration supported reducing benefits such as AFDC, reducing funding for family planning and abortions, and decreasing Medicare expenditures through the use of Diagnosis Related Groups (DRGs). When the use of DRGs was instituted, many elderly patients were discharged earlier from the hospital, and the family was expected to care for these individuals and take over many complex care regimens that had previously been carried out only in the hospital. Thus, while these cost-cutting measures were not family policies per se, they did have a significant impact on the daily lives of families.

The political climate changes from administration to administration in the United States. Health care reform has been a major issue. How any health care reform debate and the response of the health care delivery system to any proposed changes could affect families remains to be seen. It is clear that any major initiative to change health care delivery and reimbursement will have important implications for families.

The Role of Nursing in Family Policy and Health Care

Nurses need to recognize how health care financing and delivery policies influence family functioning. Meister (1989) recommends that nurses analyze how health and social welfare policies are affecting the families they work with. First the economic and social status of each family member should be identified, including the educational level of the family members, the sources and amounts of income, and whether the family can meet their basic needs and unexpected emergencies (e.g., sudden illness, loss of job, etc.). The next step is to determine the family's dependence on Medicaid, Social Security, or AFDC; what health services they use; and their social vulnerabilities, such as unemployment, lack of insurance, or lack of a fixed income. Meister (1989) notes that this analysis helps the nurse to identify possible problem areas and risks for families, and to determine what policies and programs (or lack of these) are affecting families' well-being. Steps can then be taken to improve an individual family's access to services. This analysis also serves to identify families' common needs that may deserve further attention for policy development (Meister, 1989).

SUMMARY   This chapter has addressed some of the factors that influence the health of family members and family functioning. These include both factors within the family (illness in a family member, spiritual beliefs and values) and factors outside the family (legal and ethical decisions and public policies). Although illness in a family member may be viewed as something happening within the family, the family also is affected by how that illness is treated in the health care system, what resources are available for financing health care services, and how policies determine who is eligible for these services based on legal and ethical principles. Not only are family members interdependent, but so are the family and the community.

What is the role of the nurse in relation to all of the factors discussed in this chapter? The nurse has a role not only in managing health and illness situations in the individual families but also in advocating for social change that supports family integrity. As you work with individuals and families, you will recognize how the health of the individual family members influences the family unit and the influence of the family unit on the health of the individual members, and incorporate these into your plan of care. For example, how is a mother's depression affecting the care of the children? How does the father respond to the mother's depression? Does he help out or completely take over the mother's role? Does he stay aloof and criticize the way the children are being raised? How is the family functioning affected by the mother's depression? Is the family willing to use community resources that might be of help?

The legal, ethical, and public policy influences on individual families also need to be addressed at a larger societal level. Changing policies at this level is a challenging task; however, evidence from the nurse's experience with families can be a powerful tool for informing and influencing policy makers and the legal system. Nurses need to become more politically active, to provide testimony about needed changes in health care delivery, and to advocate for families who may be too vulnerable to speak for themselves, in order to promote positive policy changes that will benefit families and the society as a whole.

STUDY QUESTIONS

1. Match the following characteristics with family type:
   a. Flexibility is a strength
   b. Values family time
   c. Family hardiness
   d. Emotional closeness within family
   e. Views illness as a challenge
   f. Routines provide sense of security
      i. Regenerative family
      ii. Resilient family
      iii. Rhythmic family

2. Describe how the course of a family member's illness (progressive, constant, or episodic) may affect the functioning of the family.

3. List three characteristics of a family that indicate a shared religious core.

4. The United States Constitution provides a guideline for establishing the rights of the family within society.
   a. True
   b. False

5. Legal definitions of the family have been challenged as family structures have changed over the past two decades.
   a. True
   b. False

6. The principle of beneficence supports the decision to ignore signs of neglect until physical abuse has occurred.
   a. True
   b. False

7. Identify a family policy currently being debated within the state where you reside.

REFERENCES

Ablon, J. (1984). Family research and alcoholism. *Recent Developments in Alcoholism, 2*, 383–395.

Aldous, J., & Dumon, W. (1990). Family policy in the 1980s: Controversy and consensus. *Journal of Marriage and the Family, 52*, 1136–1151.

Anderson, C., Reiss, D., & Hogarty, B. (1986). *Schizophrenia and the family.* New York: Guilford Press.

Aroskar, M. (1989). Community health nurses: Their difficult ethical decision making problems. *Nursing Clinics of North America, 24*, 967–975.

Basolo-Kunzer, M. (1994). Caring for families of psychiatric patients. *Mental Health Nursing, 28*, 73–79.

Belsky, J., Lang, M., & Rovine, M. (1985). Stability and change in marriage across the transition to parenthood: A second study. *Journal of Marriage and the Family, 47*, 855–865.

Belsky, J., Spanier, G., & Rovine, M. (1983). Stability and change in marriage across the transition to parenthood. *Journal of Marriage and the Family*, *45*, 567 – 577.

Bernheim, K., & Lehman, F. (1985). *Working with families of the mentally ill.* New York: W. W. Norton.

Brigman, K. (1992). Religion and family strengths: Implications for mental health professionals. *Topics in Family Psychology and Counseling*, *1*, 39 – 52.

Bromet, E., & May, V., & May, S. (1984). Family environments of depressed outpatients. *Acta Pscyhiatrica Scandinavia*, *69*, 197 – 200.

Brown, G., Birley, J., & Wing, J. (1972). Influence of family life on the course of schizophrenic disorders: A replication. *British Journal of Psychiatry*, *121*, 241 – 258.

Brown, G., Monck, E., Carstairs, G., & Wing, J. (1972). The influence of family life on the course of schizophrenic illness. *British Journal of Preventive Social Medicine*, *16*, 55 – 68.

Campbell, T. (1986). Family's impact on health: A critical review. *Family Systems Medicine*, *4*, 135 – 327.

Churchill, L. (1987). *Rationing health care in America.* Notre Dame, IN: University of Notre Dame Press.

Curran, D. (1983). *Traits of a healthy family.* San Francisco: Harper & Row.

Curran, D. (1985). *Stress and the healthy family.* San Francisco: Harper & Row.

Danielson, C., Hamel-Bissell, B., & Winstead-Fry, P. (1993). *Families, health & illness: Perspectives on coping and intervention.* St. Louis, MO: Mosby.

DeFrain, J., & Stinnett, N. (1992). Building on the inherent strengths of families: A positive approach for family psychologists and counselors. *Topics in Family Psychology and Counseling*, *1*, 15 – 26.

Dixon, R., & Weitzman, L. (1980). Evaluating the impact of no-fault divorce in California. *Family Relations*, *29*, 297 – 307.

Doane, J., West, K., Goldstein, M., Rodnick, E., & Jones, J. (1981). Parental communication deviance and affective style: Predictors of subsequent schizophrenia spectrum disorders in vulnerable adolescents. *Archives of General Psychiatry*, *38*, 679 – 685.

Doherty, W., & Campbell, T. (1988). *Families and health.* Newbury Park, CA: Sage Publications.

From-Reichman, F. (1948). Notes on the development and treatment of schizophrenics by psychoanalytic psychotherapy. *Psychiatry*, *11*, 263 – 273.

Garfinkel, P., & Garner, D. (1982). *Anorexia nervosa: A multidimensional perspective.* New York: Brunner/Mazel.

Gerstel, N., Riessman, C., & Rosenfield, S. (1985). Explaining the symptomatology of separated and divorced women and men: The role of material conditions and social networks. *Social Forces*, *64*, 84 – 101.

Goldstein, M. (1985). Family factors that antedate the onset of schizophrenia and related disorders: The results of a fifteen-year prospective longitudinal study. *Acta Psychiatrica Scandinavia*, *319* (Suppl), 7 – 18.

Goldstein, M., & Strachan, A. (1987). The family and schizophrenia. In T. Jacob (Ed.), *Family interaction and psychopathology.* New York: Plenum Press.

Gore, S., & Mangione, T. (1983). Social roles, sex roles, and psychological distress. *Journal of Health and Social Behavior*, *24*, 300 – 312.

Gove, W. (1984). Gender differences in mental and physical illness: The effects of fixed roles and nurturant role. *Social Science and Medicine*, *19*, 77 – 84.

Gove, W., Hughes, M., & Style, C. (1983). Does marriage have positive effects on the psychological well-being of the individual? *Journal of Health and Social Behavior*, *24*, 122 – 131.

Jacob, T., Dunn, N., & Leonard, K. (1983). Patterns of alcohol abuse and family stability. *Alcoholism: Clinical and Experimental Research*, *7*, 382 – 385.

Jenkins, H. (1989). Ethical dimensions of leadership in community health nursing. *Journal of Community Health Nursing*, *6*, 108 – 112.

Johnson, A., & Ooms, T. (1985). The pressures of government on families. In K. Powers (Ed.), *Lives of families* (pp. 179 – 187). Atlanta: Humanics.

Kandel, D., Davies, M., & Raveis, V. (1985). The stressfulness of daily social roles for women: Marital, occupational, and household roles. *Journal of Health and Social Behavior*, *26*, 64 – 78.

Karon, B. (1994). Is there really a schizophrenogenic parent? *Psychoanalytic Psychology*, *11*, 47 – 61.

Kaufman, E. (1980). Myth and reality in the family patterns and treatment of substance abuse. *American Journal of Drug and Alcohol Abuse*, *7*, 257 – 279.

Kaufman, E. (1984). Family system variables in alcoholism. *Alcoholism: Clinical and Experimental Research*, *8*, 4 – 8.

Kessler, R. (1979). Stress, social status, and psychological distress. *Journal of Health and Social Behavior*, *20*, 259 – 272.

Kitson, G., & Morgan, L. (1991). Consequences in divorce. In A. Booth (Ed.), *Contemporary families: Looking forward, looking back.* Minneapolis, MN: National Council on Family Relations.

Kocsis, M. (1991). Pregnant women abusing drugs: A medical-legal dilemma. *Medical Trial Technique Quarterly*, *37*, 496 – 527.

Kosten, T., Novak, P., & Kleber, H. (1984). Perceived marital and family environment of opiate addicts. *American Journal of Drug and Alcohol Abuse, 10,* 491–501.

Liss, L. (1987). Families and the law. In M. Sussman & S. Steinmetz (Eds.), *Handbook of marriage and the family* (pp 767–794). New York: Plenum Press.

Lukoff, D., Snyer, K., Ventura, J., & Neuchterlein, K. (1984). Life events, familial stress, and coping in the developmental course of schizophrenia. *Schizophrenia Bulletin 10,* 258–292.

McCubbin, M. (1991). CHIP—Coping health inventory for parents. In H. McCubbin & A. Thompson (Eds.), *Family assessment inventories for research and practice* (pp. 175–194). Madison: University of Wisconsin Press.

McCubbin, M. (1993). *Predicting family adaptation following diagnosis of child's congenital heart disease.* Paper presented at the Annual Meeting of the American Educational Research Association, Atlanta, Georgia.

McCubbin, M., & McCubbin, H. (1993). Families coping with illness: The Resiliency Model of Family Stress, Adjustment, and Adaptation. In C. Danielson, B. Hamel-Bissell, & P. Winstead-Fry (Eds.), *Families, health & illness: Perspectives on coping and intervention* (pp 21–63). St. Louis, MO: Mosby.

McLanahan, S., & Adams, J. (1987). Parenthood and psychological well being. *Annual Review of Sociology, 13,* 237–257.

Meister, S. (1989). Health care financing, policy and family nursing practice. In C. Gilliss, B. Highley, B. Roberts, & I. Martinson (Eds.), *Towards a science of family nursing* (pp. 146–155). Menlo Park, CA: Addison-Wesley.

Mirowsky, J. & Ross, C. (1989). *Social causes of psychological distress.* New York: Aldine-de Gruyter.

Moberg, D. (1974). Spiritual well-being in late life. In J. Gubrium (Ed.), *Late life: Communities and environmental policy* (pp. 256–279). Springfield, IL: Charles C. Thomas.

Moore v. City of East Cleveland, Ohio (1977). 431 U.S. 494.

Myers, J. (1992). *Legal issues in child abuse and neglect.* Newbury Park, CA: Sage Publications.

Palo Alto Tenants Union v. Morgan (1970). 321 F. Supp. 908. 1970, N.D. Cal. aff d 487 F. 2d 883 (9th Cir, 1973).

Parker, G. (1983). Parental affectionless control as an antecedent to adult depression: A risk factor delineated. *Archives of General Psychiatry, 40,* 956–960.

Pearlin, L., Lieberman, M., Menaghan, E., & Mullan, J. (1981). The stress process. *Journal of Health and Social Behavior, 22,* 337–356.

Raschke, H. (1987). Divorce. In M. Sussman & K. Steinmetz (Eds.), *Handbook of marriage and the family* (pp. 597–624). New York: Plenum Press.

Reiss, D., Gonzalez, S., & Kramer, N. (1986). Family process, chronic illness, and death: On the weakness of strong bonds. *Archives of General Psychiatry, 43,* 795–804.

Reed, P. (1992). An emerging paradigm for the investigation of spirituality in nursing. *Research in Nursing and Health, 15,* 349–357.

Rhodes, A. (1992). Criminal penalties for maternal substance abuse. *Maternal Child Nursing, 18,* 311.

Rhodes, A. (1993). Law versus ethics. *Maternal Child Nursing, 18,* 311.

Rogers, B. (1988). Ethical decisions in occupational health nursing. *AAOHN Journal, 36,* 100–104.

Rolland, J. (1988). Family systems and chronic illness: A typological model. In F. Walsh & C. Anderson (Eds.), *Chronic disorders and the family* (pp. 143–168). New York: Haworth Press.

Rolland, J. (1990). Anticipatory loss: A family systems developmental framework. *Family Process, 29,* 229–244.

Ross, C., & Huber, J. (1985). Hardship and depression. *Journal of Health and Social Behavior, 26,* 312–327.

Ross, C., Mirowsky, J., & Goldstein, K. (1990). The impact of the family on health: The decade in review. *Journal of Marriage and the Family, 52,* 1059–1078.

Saayman, G., & Saayman, R. (1988/1989). The adversarial legal process and divorce: Negative effects upon the psychological adjustment of children. *Journal of Divorce, 12,* 329–348.

Saltzman, A. (1993, August 2). Time off without pain. *U.S. News and World Report, 115,* 52–55.

Schwartzberg, A. (1981). Divorce and children and adolescents: An overview. *Adolescent Psychiatry, 9,* 119–132.

Shafranske, E., & Maloney, H. (1990). Clinical psychologists' religious and spiritual orientations and their practice of psychotherapy. *Psychotherapy, 27,* 72–78.

Stanton, M., & Todd, T. (1982). *The family therapy of drug abuse and addiction.* New York: Guilford Press.

Starck, P. (1991). Health care under siege: Challenge for change. *Nursing and Health Care, 12,* 26–30.

Stinnett, N. (1979). Strengthening families. *Family Perspective, 13,* 3–9.

Stuart, G., Laraia, M., Ballenger, J., & Lydiard, R. (1990). Early family experiences of women with bulimia and depression. *Archives of Psychiatric Nursing, 9,* 43–52.

Strong, B., & DeVault, C. (1993). *Essentials of the marriage and family experience.* St. Paul, MN: West Publishing.

Thomas, D., & Henry, G. (1984). The religion and family connection: Increasing dialogue in the social sciences. *Journal of Marriage and the Family, 47,* 369–379.

Thompson, I. (1987). Fundamental ethical principles in health care. *British Medical Journal, 295,* 1461–1465.

Tseng, W., & Hsu, I. (1991). *Culture and family: Problems and therapy.* New York: Haworth Press.

Umberson, D. (1989). Relationships with children: Explaining parents psychological well-being. *Journal of Marriage and the Family, 51,* 999 – 1012.

Umberson, D., & Gove, W.R. (1989). Parenthood and psychological well-being: Theory, measurement, and stage in the family life course. *Journal of Family Issues, 10,* 440 – 462.

US Bureau of the Census (1991, February). *Census and You, 26.* Washington, DC: US Government Printing Office.

Vaughn, C., & Leff, J. (1976). The influence of family and social factors on the course of psychiatric illness: A comparison of schizophrenic and depressed neurotic patients. *British Journal of Psychiatry, 129,* 125 – 137.

Vaughn, C., Snyder, K., Jone, S., Freeman, W., & Falloon, I. (1984). Family factors in schizophrenia relapse: Replication in California of British research on expressed emotion. *Archives of General Psychiatry, 41,* 1169 – 1177.

Vaughn, F. (1986). *The inward arc: Healing and wholeness in psychotherapy and spirituality.* Boston: New Science Library.

Venters, M. (1986). Family life and cardiovascular risk: Implications for the prevention of chronic disease. *Social Science and Medicine, 22,* 1067 – 1074.

Walker, T. (1992). Family law in the fifty states: An overview: *Family Law Quarterly, 25,* 417 – 515.

Weitzman, L. & Dixon, R. (1989). The transformation of legal marriage through no-fault divorce. In A. Skolnick & J. Skolnick (Eds.), *Family in transition,* (pp. 315 – 327). 6th ed. Glenview, IL: Scott, Foresman & Company.

White, L., Booth, A. & Edwards, J. (1986). Children and marital happiness: Why the negative correlation? *Journal of Family Issues, 7,* 131 – 147.

Wilcox, B. & O'Keefe, J. (1991). Families, policy, and family support policies. In D. Unger & D. Powell (Eds.), *Families as nuturing systems: Support across the life span,* (pp. 109 – 126). New York: Haworth Press.

Yager, J. (1982). Family issues in the pathogenesis of anorexia nervosa. *Psychosomatic Medicine, 44,* 43 – 59.

Yorker, B. (1993). Family law. In C. Fawcett (Ed.). *Family psychiatric nursing.* St. Louis: Mosby.

Zimmerman, S. (1988). *Understanding family policy: Theoretical approaches.* Newbury Park, CA: Sage.

Zimmerman, S. (1992). *Family policies and family well-being: The role of political culture.* Newbury Park, CA: Sage.

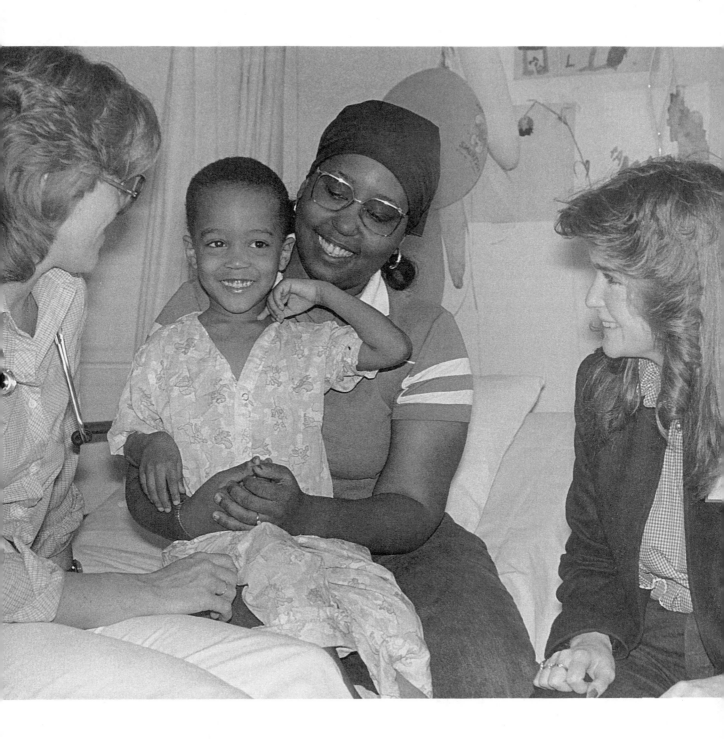

Nursing Process and Family Health Care

You have heard about nursing process since you began your nursing education and are probably asking, "Why more of it?" At this point in your education you are familiar with the use of this problem-solving process with individual clients. This chapter builds on your previous learning and challenges you to expand your understanding of nursing process and its application to the family client.

Nurses work with different family members, ancillary caregivers, and new technologies in a rapidly changing health care delivery system. They must be prepared to offer support, information, and direct care services to families. The professional nurse's use of a logical, systematic approach to the family client is essential if care is to be appropriate. Nursing process provides that approach.

This chapter describes the five-step nursing process — assessment, analysis, planning, implementation, and evaluation — and how to apply it in family situations.

Following this brief review, the complex role of the professional nurse with families is explored, and each step of the nursing process with the family is comprehensively addressed. The student is encouraged to use increasingly sophisticated assessment instruments in providing professional nursing care to family clients. In the analysis section both the NANDA diagnostic framework and the Omaha classification system are described. Students are referred to resources for additional details of these methods of labeling family problems that are amenable to nursing intervention.

The importance of working in partnership with the family is emphasized in the section dealing with implementing family health care. Here, too, the need for culturally sensitive interventions is discussed, as is the evaluation of family nursing care based on criteria jointly determined by the family and the nurse. Finally, a case study of the Jinks family provides nursing students with a clinical example of the cyclic and dynamic application of the nursing process.

CHAPTER 6

Nursing Process and Family Health Care

Beverly J. Ross, RN, MANEd, MSEd

OBJECTIVES   *Upon completion of this chapter, the reader will be able to:*

1. Define the nursing process.
2. Describe the five steps of the nursing process.
3. Discuss the application of the nursing process to the care of families.
4. Contrast the application of the nursing process to the care of families with its application in the care of individuals.
5. Describe the importance of family involvement in each step of the family nursing process.

Florence Nightingale (1969) wrote, in the conclusion to her *Notes on Nursing,* "nothing but observation and experience will teach us the ways to maintain or to bring back the state of health" (p. 133). The importance of that statement has not diminished over time. Nurses have continued to make every effort to improve their ability to observe, to analyze, and to understand how to best meet the needs of clients. The nursing process developed to enhance these essential skills is a problem-solving approach based on the scientific method. Nursing process can be used by any nurse in any setting, and can be applied to the care of individuals, families, groups, or communities. The reader is urged to "think family" as the following overview of the nursing process is presented. The remainder of the chapter will be devoted to the application of the nursing process to the family as client, the family nursing process. The five steps of the process are assessment, analysis, planning, implementation, and evaluation. A brief review of each step will follow.

OVERVIEW OF THE NURSING PROCESS

Yura and Walsh (1988) initially defined **nursing process** using four steps: assessment, planning, implementation, and evaluation. Ross and Cobb (1990) delineated a five-step process that included analysis as the second step. Gordon (1982, 1987) described a six-step process: assessment, analysis, outcome projection, planning, implementation, and evaluation. The five-step process seems to be the most commonly used at this time. The key concern is that, regardless of the number of steps, the process should embody a systematic approach to identify needs and concerns, to take appropriate action to assist the client in problem resolution, and to assess the degree to which those needs and concerns are met. Nursing process is an essential component in the delivery of comprehensive care to all clients, including families.

Assessment

Assessment is the first step in the nursing process and is possibly the most critical (Shaw, 1993). Yura and Walsh (1988) describe "assessing" as the act of reviewing a human situation to obtain data about the client for the purpose of affirming an illness state, diagnosing a client's problems, and determining the strengths and health promotion needs of the client. Data collection involves both subjective and objective data; both data verbally shared with the nurse by the client, and data obtained by direct observation and examination, or in consultation with other health care providers. Many sources may be used, and physical assessment is an essential element to validate history and identify areas in need of further exploration (Chitty, 1993).

There are many guidelines available to assist the nurse in data collection and to help organize that information. It is extremely important that assessment instruments be selected with care. Instruments must be appropriate for the purpose for which they are intended. For instance, an assessment instrument designed to facilitate the identification of medical problems will gather medical data. Such an instrument will not necessarily uncover concerns and problems amenable to nursing intervention. Thus, care must be taken to select an instrument with an underlying conceptual framework that guides assessment activities toward the identification of nursing phenomena.

Analysis

Chitty (1993) described **analysis**, the second step in the nursing process, as using knowledge from the biological and social sciences, as well as nursing, to analyze the data collected, that is, to note and cluster together those pieces of information that attest to a particular problem or concern. Yura and Walsh (1988) stress the importance of noting gaps in information, or contradictory information, and of seeking out additional data as needed in order to assure accuracy. The desired outcome of the analysis step is the identification of client concerns for which some intervention is needed. In any given situation, a client may have concerns that are medical in nature and require referral. There may be needs that will require collaboration and cooperative action by the nurse and another health care professional. In such instances the nurse works with the involved discipline to solve the identified problem. Those problems that are amenable to nursing intervention, independently of other health care disciplines, are nursing diagnoses. It is the nursing diagnoses that form the foundation for the nursing care plan.

Nursing Diagnosis

Gordon (1982, 1987) states that the act of making nursing diagnoses goes back to the founding of modern nursing. Although **nursing diagnosis** as a term is relatively new, Florence Nightingale and her colleagues diagnosed nutritional deficits as they cared for Crimean War casualties, and this "nursing diagnosis" led to interventions designed to correct the system of care in military hospitals to improve nutrition. Gordon described nursing diagnosis as creating the link between collecting information and care planning.

The current list of nursing diagnosis labels accepted for clinical testing by NANDA are included in Table 6–1. During the proceedings of the Ninth National Conference, NANDA adopted the following definition of nursing diagnosis:

> A nursing diagnosis is a clinical judgment about individual, family, or community responses to actual or potential health problems/life processes. Nursing diagnoses provide the basis for se-

TABLE 6–1

NANDA NURSING DIAGNOSES APPROVED FOR CLINICAL USE AND TESTING ORGANIZED ACCORDING TO THE NANDA TAXONOMY CLASSIFICATION SYSTEM

Pattern 1: Exchanging

Nutrition, altered, more than body requirements
Nutrition, altered, less than body requirements
Nutrition, altered, potential for more than body
  requirements
Infection, risk for
Body Temperature, altered, risk for
Hypothermia
Hyperthermia
Thermoregulation, ineffective
Dysreflexia
*Constipation
Constipation, perceived
Constipation, colonic
*Diarrhea
*Bowel Incontinence
Urinary Elimination, altered
Incontinence, functional
Incontinence, reflex
Incontinence, stress
Incontinence, total
Incontinence, urge
Urinary Retention
*Tissue Perfusion, altered (specify): cerebral,
  cardiopulmonary, renal, gastrointestinal,
  peripheral

Fluid Volume Excess
Fluid Volume deficit
Fluid Volume deficit, risk for
*Cardiac Output, decreased
Gas Exchange, impaired
Airway Clearance, ineffective
Breathing Pattern, ineffective
#Spontaneous Ventilation, inability to sustain
#Ventilatory Weaning Response, dysfunctional
  (DVWR)
Injury, risk for
Suffocation, risk for
Poisoning, risk for
Trauma, risk for
Aspiration, risk for
Disuse Syndrome, risk for
Protection, altered
Tissue Integrity, impaired
*Oral Mucous Membrane, altered
Skin Integrity, impaired
Skin Integrity, Impaired, risk for
*Decreased adaptive capacity: intracranial
†Energy disturbance

Pattern 2: Communicating

Communication, impaire verbal

Continued

TABLE 6–1

NANDA NURSING DIAGNOSES APPROVED FOR CLINICAL USE AND TESTING ORGANIZED ACCORDING TO THE NANDA TAXONOMY CLASSIFICATION SYSTEM *(Continued)*

Pattern 3: Relating

Social Interaction, impaired
Social Isolation
†Risk for loneliness
*Role Performance, altered
Parenting, altered
Parenting, altered, risk for
†Risk for altered parent/infant/child attachment
Sexual dysfunction
Family Processes, altered
#Caregiver Role Strain
Caregiver Role Strain, risk for
†Altered family process: Alcoholism
Parental Role conflict
Sexuality Patterns, altered

Pattern 4: Valuing

Spiritual Distress (distress of the human spirit)
†Potential for enhanced spiritual well-being

Pattern 5: Choosing

Coping, individual, ineffective
Adjustment, impaired
Coping, defensive
Denial, ineffective
Family Coping, ineffective: compromised
Family Coping, ineffective: disabling
Family Coping: potential for growth
†Potential for enhanced community coping
†Ineffective community coping
#Therapeutic regimen: Individual, ineffective
    management
†Ineffective management of therapeutic regimen:
    Community
†Effective management of therapeutic regimen:
    Individual
Noncompliance, (compliance, altered)
Decisional Conflict (specify)
Health-Seeking Behaviors (specify)

Pattern 6: Moving

Physical Mobility, impaired
#Peripheral Neurovascular Dysfunction, risk for
†Risk for perioperative positioning injury
Activity Intolerance (specify level)
Fatigue
Activity Intolerance, risk for
Sleep Pattern disturbance
Diversional Activity deficit

Home Maintenance Management, impaired
Health Maintenance, altered
†Health Maintenance, altered, disabling
Self Care deficit (specify): feeding, bathing/
    hygiene, dressing/grooming, toileting
Swallowing, impaired
Breastfeeding, ineffective
#Breastfeeding, interrupted
Breastfeeding, effective
#Infant Feeding Pattern, ineffective
Growth and Development, altered
#Relocation Stress Syndrome
†Risk for disorganized infant behavior
†Disorganized infant behavior
†Potential for enhanced organized infant behavior

Pattern 7: Perceiving

*Body Image disturbance
*Self Esteem disturbance
Self Esteem, chronic low
Self Esteem, situational low
*Personalt Identity disturbance
Sensory/Perceptual alterations (specify): visual,
    auditory, kinesthetic, gustatory, tactile, olfactory
Unilateral Neglect
Hopelessness

Pattern 8: Knowing

Knowledge deficit [Learning Need] (specify)
†Impaired environmental interpretation syndrome
†Acute confusion
†Chronic confusion
Thought Processes, altered
†Impaired memory

Pattern 9: Feeling

*Pain [acute]
Pain, chronic
Grieving, dysfunctional
Grieving, anticipatory
Violence, risk for, directed at self/others
#Self-Mutilation, risk for
Post-Trauma Response
Rape-Trauma Syndrome
Rape-Trauma Syndrome: compound reaction
Rape-Trauma Syndrome: silent reaction
Anxiety (specify level)
Fear

*Categories with modified label terminology.
†Diagnostic categories approved 1994.
#Diagnostic categories approved 1992.
SOURCE: *NANDA Nursing Diagnoses: Definitions and Classification, 1992–1993 (1993).*

lection of nursing interventions to achieve outcomes for which the nurse is accountable (*NANDA, Nursing Diagnosis: Definitions and Classification 1992 - 1993*, 1993).

Gordon used the NANDA nursing diagnoses in much of her work with nursing process, nursing diagnosis, and care planning. Gordon stated (1976, 1982, 1987) that there are three essential components in a nursing diagnosis. These three components are the problem (P), the etiology (E), and the defining cluster of signs and symptoms (S). They are often referred to as the P.E.S. format. The problem statement describes a problem or health state of the client, who might be an individual, a family, or a community. An example of a problem statement for a family might be noncompliance with immunization requirements for their school-age children. The problem statement represents a concise term for a cluster of signs or symptoms indicating a specific concern or health need. The NANDA labels accepted for clinical use and testing may be used as problem statements. *In many instances greater specificity is required.* A number of labels are followed by the term "specify" in parentheses. In instances where that particular label is used (see Table 6 - 1, e.g., decisional conflict or knowledge deficit), the specific area in which the problem has occurred must be included. In the example given above, the family was noncompliant with the school district immunization requirements. The term "noncompliant" alone is not sufficiently clear to communicate the problem.

The etiology or probable cause is the second component of any given nursing diagnosis statement. It identifies the factors that are believed to be causing or maintaining the health problem. The etiology may involve the environment, client behaviors, interactions between client and environment, or external factors. The family described above may be noncompliant with immunization requirements because of lack of understanding of the importance and availability of immunizations. Another family might have home maintenance deficits because they lack the money to obtain proper equipment for home upkeep. A category label can be used to communicate or describe the cause. The term used in the cause statement summarizes the cluster of cues or data that indicate the particular phenomenon sustaining or causing the identified problem. The problem itself, and the factors believed to be the primary cause or sustaining factors for that problem, taken together, become the diagnostic statement. (See Table 6 - 2 for a sample diagnostic statement.)

Finally, Gordon describes the third component of the nursing diagnosis as the cluster of signs and symptoms supporting the diagnosis. Each diagnostic label or title has a set of signs and symptoms that permit discrimination between health problems. When the client receiving care manifests the signs and symptoms that indicate the presence of a particular diagnostic label or title, the use of that label to define the presenting problem is appropri-

TABLE 6-2

NURSING DIAGNOSIS FORMAT AND SAMPLE DIAGNOSIS STATEMENT

Nursing Diagnosis Format	
_____ Related to	_____
Problem or Title	Cause or Etiology
Sample Nursing Diagnosis Statement	
Deficit, home maintenance/management	*Limited financial resources and knowledge deficit of available community resources*
_____ Related to	_____
Problem or Title	Cause or Etiology

ate. Evaluation of client outcomes as care progresses may well be based on ascertaining to what degree these presenting signs and symptoms have been relieved or improved.

Planning

Planning is the third step of the nursing process. Ross and Cobb (1990) discuss the planning step as "the process by which objectives are determined, interventions selected or designed, and the care plan written . . ." (p. 134). A clear plan of action is essential to the accomplishment of a complex task. The higher the degree of difficulty, the more important it is to plan carefully. Thus, the nurse must consider a number of elements in the task at hand. Priorities must be set; multiple concerns may need to be addressed. Those concerns considered most crucial at a given point in time must be dealt with first, and ascertaining what is important to the client is vital to successful planning. If the nurse and client do not agree on which concerns are primary, little headway will be made. Moreover, as conditions change, priorities may change.

Because the availability of resources, including time, support systems, and financial resources, will influence priority setting and the types of interventions selected, resources must be identified as a part of the planning process. "Although one might like to think finances need not be considered . . . in reality the lack of finances is one of the major reasons families neglect to follow through with mutually agreed upon plans of care" (Ross & Cobb, 1990, p. 135). Thus, it is essential to guard against recommending activities, equipment, and placements that clients cannot afford, and if the client is not personally able to pay for the interventions being suggested and financial assistance cannot be found, another option must be sought.

Outcome Determination

Planning involves the determination of possible outcomes for the defined nursing diagnosis. In order to establish realistic, attainable objectives, the nurse must determine both the probable outcome and the best possible recovery or state of health, given optimal care in light of the presenting circumstances. A time frame for achievement must also be determined. How much time is required to achieve the identified objective? As indicated previously, conditions do change. Clients may progress more quickly or slowly than expected, or achieve at levels of ability above or below that anticipated. Nevertheless, identifying potential outcomes increases the possibility of establishing achievable goals or objectives (Ross & Cobb, 1990).

Writing the Plan of Care

An essential and often neglected part of the planning process is writing the plan of care. It is this portion of the planning process that provides the means of communicating the care plan for this particular client to all those involved in care delivery. The written plan should include the specific concerns or nursing diagnoses being addressed. In order to assure ongoing evaluation of progress, the specific objectives to be achieved by the care provided should be written in clear, measurable terms, with time frames for the achievement of the projected outcomes. Finally, the plan should include the nursing interventions selected or designed to assist this client in moving toward achievement of the mutually defined goals and objectives. The written nursing interventions direct the care providers to initiate or carry out specific actions or activities, and specify how, when, and where these activities are to be completed. Yura and Walsh (1988) described the care plan as "the blue print for action, providing the direction for implementing the plan and providing the framework for an evaluation" (p. 39).

Implementation

The fourth step of the nursing process is implementation. **Implementation** is initiating or putting into effect the plan of care and completing the actions necessary to accomplish the defined objectives. The implementation phase of the process involves both critical and creative thinking, strong interpersonal skills, and technical expertise. As Yura and Walsh summarized, "Decision making, observation, and communication are significant skills. These skills are utilized with the client, the nurse, the nursing team members, and health team members . . ." (Yura & Walsh, 1988, p. 154). Throughout the implementation phase the nurse must work interdependently with others to encourage and support the client and significant others; to assist, guide, and support ancillary workers; and to keep other health team members informed of the type or degree of progress. The nurse must make the decisions as to which interventions can or should be delegated to others, and how to best incorporate other persons in care delivery.

Throughout the implementation process, data gathering continues. New information is obtained with each contact with the client, and this additional information must be incorporated into the current data base; then it must be analyzed for relevance and importance; and decisions must be made as to whether to proceed as originally planned or to modify the plan of care. As indicated previously, nursing process is not static. In practice, there is a constant flow among the components. The cycle continues as long as interaction with the client occurs.

Evaluation

The fifth step of the nursing process is evaluation. **Evaluation** requires that the nurse determine to what degree the client has achieved the expected outcomes. It is concerned with the ongoing assessment of progress as well as the degree to which the plan of care has been effective in solving the identified problem. As care is delivered, changes occur in the ability of clients to retain and use information, perform tasks, and to assume necessary roles or adopt required behaviors. As knowledge and behaviors change, status changes. The status of the client involves the current physical, emotional, social, and economic conditions, and how that client's circumstance has improved, remained the same, or deteriorated. The evaluation component has been the most neglected part of the nursing process and it may be perceived as the most difficult. It remains true that "Identification of the progress that has been made, or remains to be made to meet a specific standard is an important element in health care" (Martin & Scheet, 1992, p. 174).

FAMILY NURSING PROCESS

The nursing process that has been presented is a systematic approach to the design and delivery of nursing care to clients. Family nursing process assists the nurse in providing the care needed to enhance the well-being of families, an invaluable task, because healthy families have the ability to provide the "nurturing" needed to produce healthy individuals and are essential to a healthy society.

According to Baldwin (1990) the decade of the 1990s will be critical for the family, as dramatic social changes continue. Among these many changes are the increase in the number of women who work outside the home and the increase in the number of men who are assuming traditional "women's" jobs in the home. The population continues to age, and an increasing number of nonbiological and intergenerational families live together. These changes influence who gives care and the place in which that care is given.

Nurses must be prepared to work with caregivers and family members to offer support, information, and direct care services. Berkey and Hanson (1991) view the family as an essential focus of "nursing process." These authors described a comprehensive approach to the family nursing process in which family is seen as an open system interacting in a larger society. The family, which is also seen as the nurturing place for its members, with specific functions and roles, must be viewed in terms of these functions and needs. The comprehensive approach demands that the whole family and each of its members must be assessed simultaneously. In this context, the "family" may be broader than just those persons identified as residing together in a particular household. Significant others may include not only friends and relatives who are located in close proximity to the household unit, but also those who reside some distance away.

Family nursing process is a very complex undertaking. The nurse is dealing with many individuals rather than a single person, and with the multiple relationships that exist between and among family members. According to Friedman (1992), "Comprehensive family nursing is a complex process, making it necessary to have a logical systematic approach for working with families and individual family members. This approach is the nursing process" (p. 39). Family structure, family development, and family dynamics are only a few of the concepts essential to understanding families. The family nursing process entails the assessment of the family's strengths and limitations in meeting its needs and the needs of each of its members. A pattern of open communication between nurse and family, a willingness to share and validate information, is crucial to determining the types of concerns and healthcare needs that the family is experiencing and to evaluating which of these are amenable to nursing intervention. Figure 6–1 depicts the ongoing process of bidirectional communication in the family—nurse interaction, which is fundamental to effective family nursing care. The five steps in the family nursing process described in the following pages—assessment, analysis, planning, implementation, and evaluation—are the basic steps of the nursing process. Each step is discussed in terms of its application to the family as client.

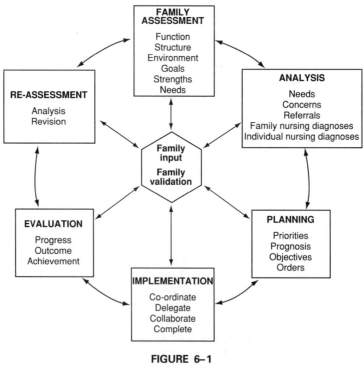

FIGURE 6–1
Family nursing process.

Family Assessment

The establishment of a solid foundation on which to build or design the plan of care is essential if comprehensive, effective care is to be provided for any client. This is especially true in caring for families. Successful data gathering is predicated on the establishment of a relationship with the client family that will facilitate an exchange of often sensitive information in as comfortable a manner as possible. As Martinson and Widmer (1989) stated, "A stage exists prior to assessment during which the nurse establishes rapport with and gains the trust of the patient. This is the necessary beginning of ongoing mutual respect and cooperation essential to the success of any intervention" (p. 50).

Providing holistic care carries with it the expectation that nurses will consider the patients' families, because the family is a system in which change in one member affects all the other members. The alteration in family function that can result from illness may result in feelings of anger and guilt. Nurses need to recognize the importance of assessing both "how the family is influencing the patient, and how they are influenced by the member who is ill" (Chitty, 1993, p. 338). In situations where family demands exceed coping resources, where family cooperation is unsteady or falters, where individuals express hurt feelings and pain in their interpersonal struggles, family nursing is always needed. Friedeman (1989) states that family health is a "state" that is dynamically balanced. It involves a process of weighing family togetherness and commitment to the family unit against individual achievement, the striving of individual family members to develop to their own personal potential. Assessing the family unit involves determining the ability of the family to function effectively in meeting the needs of its members.

Wasik, Bryant, and Lyons (1990) emphasized the importance of individualized approaches to family care needs. These authors recognized that today considerable diversity exists among families. This is true even among families of similar sociocultural backgrounds. The recognition of this diversity should lead to an acknowledgment of the importance of assessing each family's needs and priorities individually. Cantor (1991) described the American family as undergoing transformation. As the population ages, the ability to care for the elderly members of families will be challenged due to a number of factors. For example, individual family units are smaller; kin networks are multigenerational, but narrow, in the sense that there are fewer children, fewer uncles, aunts, and cousins. As more elderly persons need care, there are fewer siblings, aunts, and uncles to share the responsibilities of care (Cantor, 1991). Allen (1991) described a study which indicated that there was considerable aging not only of the general population but also of the most prominent caregivers of the elderly. The families showed considerable amounts of pain. There was evidence that there was "family feeling" existing beyond the actual caregiving situation, but that distance made it difficult for families to mobilize. As Allen saw it, the family was not organized to bear all burdens. It remains rather small and fragile in structure, yet it continues to be expected, at least in this country at this time, to care for all its members.

A variety of approaches are recommended in the assessment of the family, depending on the conceptual framework of the nurse. Lapp, Diemert, and Enestvedt (1990) describe the development of assessment guidelines based on a number of theoretical perspectives. Their guidelines emphasized the importance of "thinking" family and working with "the family as a partner" in making health care decisions. The guidelines do not prescribe questions, but allow an "exploratory and interactional experience in which the content and pace is mutually set" (p. 24). Many of these assessment techniques have been developed from family therapy and have been used in initial assessment by health care professionals. These include genograms and ecomaps. The genogram is a modified "family tree" diagram. It allows the health care professional to organize a large amount of information in a way that will allow intergenerational patterns in families to be more clearly visible. The ecomap is a diagram of a family's current connections with each other and with the environment, including the extended family. The diagram indicates strengths and weaknesses in a family's social support system (Paquin & Bushum, 1991). Genograms and ecomaps were described as allowing holistic and integrative analysis of behavior by the practitioner and the client. The activity was described as often positive for clients. The "drawing a picture" of the life situations was enlightening and helpful (Mattaini, 1990). Genograms and ecomaps will be discussed in greater detail in Chapter 7, Family Nursing Assessment and Intervention.

Analysis of Family Assessment Data

In the care of families as units, analysis involves clarifying and validating information in order to make accurate diagnoses that provide a focus for nursing intervention. Donnelly (1990) described this analytical process as diagnostic reasoning. Many health care professionals make judgments about the needs of clients, and many use the term "diagnosis." The physician, social worker, nutritionist, or professional nurse diagnose within their specific discipline or area of specialization.

The Diagnostic Process

Nursing is defined by the American Nurses Association as "the diagnosis and treatment of human responses to actual or potential health problems" (A Social Policy Statement, 1980). Donnelly sees the term diagnosis as significant to this definition. Nurses have always made judgments about client care needs, but the concept that diagnosis as an integral part of the definition of nursing is relatively new. Only recently has nursing begun the process of developing a classification system of nomenclature to facilitate its diagnosis and treatment of the phenomena unique to nursing. Diagnosis was seen by Donnelly as a critical aspect of the field.

Donnelly (1990) described the diagnostic reasoning process as a logical sequence that involves describing phenomena. The nurse is an observer of phenomena and describes those phenomena to identify signs and symptoms that might indicate problems or concerns. The family health care practitioner must then review the situation to identify the probable cause(s) for the identified problem(s). Practitioners working with families determine what information is significant, and assign meaning to the data, on the basis of their knowledge of baseline data and of established ranges of normal physical and emotional states. The conceptual perspective on the family as client, and on nursing goals and outcomes, strongly influences what kinds of information are gathered by the nurse. The nurse must develop a capacity to consider health as an effect and to reason out probable causes. The question is: How can family health be enhanced?

The NANDA System

At the current stage of development, the nurse may find the NANDA framework of nursing diagnosis shaping professional judgment. In view of the fact that a large part of the practice of community health nursing involves family health care, Donnelly (1990) expressed some concern that only seven of the approved diagnostic labels address family situations: (1) Family Coping, potential for growth; (2) Family Coping, ineffective: compromised; (3) Family Coping, ineffective: disabling; (4) Family Processes, altered; (5) Parenting, altered; (6) Parenting, altered, risk for; and (7) Parental Role conflict. Of particular concern is the fact that only one of the diagnoses identified—Family Coping, potential for growth—implies health promotion concepts. Donnelly strongly supported the importance of diagnosis as an essential step in the nursing process and as quite useful in the care of families. However, she saw the NANDA system as heavily weighted toward the indi-

TABLE 6–3

NANDA NURSING DIAGNOSES RELEVANT TO FAMILY NURSING

Altered Family Process

Alteration in Health Maintenance

Alteration in Nutrition: Less than Body Requirements

Alteration in Nutrition: More than Body Requirements

Alteration in Nutrition: Potential for More or Potential for
 Less than Body Requirements

Alteration in Parenting

Alteration in Patterns of Elimination: Inadequate Sanitary
 Disposal Conditions

Altered Role Performance

Altered Sexuality Patterns

Decisional Conflict (specify)

Family Coping: Potential for Growth

Health Seeking Behavior

Ineffective Family Coping: Compromised

Ineffective Family Coping: Disabling

Impaired Adjustment

Impaired Home Maintenance Management

Impaired Social Interaction

Knowledge Deficit (specify)

Noncompliance

Parental Role Conflict

Potential Altered Parenting

Potential for Trauma (injury)

Potential for Violence

Powerlessness

Social Isolation

SOURCE: From *Family Nursing—A Nursing Process Approach*,
 by B. Ross & K. L. Cobb, 1990, Redwood City, CA: Addison-
 Wesley. Copyright 1990 by Addison-Wesley. Reprinted with
 permission.

vidual. There are significant gaps in the current classification system, and an effort must be made to move forward more rapidly in the full development of a comprehensive set of family diagnostic categories. Donnelly (1990) saw the recent acceptance of a move toward diagnostic labels for health promotion nursing diagnoses as a positive sign.

Ross and Cobb (1990) discussed the use of the NANDA classification system in working with families. These authors identified 25 NANDA diagnostic labels that might be relevant to family nursing (Table 6–3). It might have been helpful if each NANDA category and title had been originally developed to address application to three kinds of clients — individuals, families, or communities. Progress in the development of nursing diagnosis specific to types of client is apparent, especially in the 1994 additions to the NANDA classifications. Common family nursing diagnosis were presented in table form by these authors and are included to illustrate one approach to the use of the NANDA system (Table 6–4). Possible nursing diagnosis titles that are relevant to families are listed on the left.

TABLE 6–4

COMMON NURSING DIAGNOSES AND ETIOLOGIES IN FAMILIES

Nursing Diagnosis	Possible Etiologies
Inability to manage home care activities secondary to	1. Lack of knowledge of time-management techniques 2. Lack of information related to community resources 3. Lack of support systems 4. Uncompensated physical limitations, family members
Ineffective parenting secondary to	1. Lack of knowledge of normal infant development and implications for care 2. Lack of available financial resources 3. Reactive depression (mother), perceived inadequacy postdivorce
Altered nutritional intake, less than requirements (family) secondary to	1. Lack of knowledge of appropriate food intake 2. Financial limitations and lack of knowledge of available resources 3. Limited availability of culturally preferred foods
Alteration in family processes: Inability to provide physical and emotional support to family member secondary to	1. Lack of knowledge of techniques of care delivery 2. Perception of self as incapable of learning complex tasks 3. Lack of available finances for needed equipment
Health management deficit: Lack of immunizations (children) secondary to	1. Lack of knowledge of importance of immunizations 2. Value belief conflicts/religious beliefs deny injections 3. Lack of access to financial resources and/or available well child care
Potential for injury secondary to	1. Uncontrolled refuse dumping and inadequate trash removal 2. Lack of awareness of lead paint present in housing units, local refuse used as fuel (e.g., lead batteries burned for heat) 3. Lack of knowledge of techniques to "toddler-proof" home environment 4. Inappropriate disposal of toxic waste materials

SOURCE: From *Family Nursing—A Nursing Process Approach*, by B. Ross & K. L. Cobb, 1990, Redwood City, CA: Addison-Wesley. Copyright 1990 by Addison-Wesley. Reprinted with permission.

The unique situation of each family requires that the nurse consider that the cause or sustaining factor will vary. Possible causes or etiologies are listed on the right.

The Omaha System

The Omaha system was designed to meet the challenge of describing the nursing needs of families. It was developed over a period of some 20 years and is based on the results of several major research projects. This effort, begun in 1970, was initiated by the Visiting Nurse Association (VNA) of Omaha, Nebraska. The need to effectively document community health nursing practice, particularly the care of families, was a major concern. Initiated in 1986, the system consists of three components: the Problem Classification Schema, the Intervention Schema, and the Problem Rating Scale. The Problem Classification Schema "is a taxonomy of nursing diagnosis, that provides a consistent language for collecting, sorting, classifying, documenting, and analyzing data about client concerns" (Martin & Scheet, 1992, pp. 19–20). It consists of 40 problems organized in four domains. Each problem may be made more specific by the use of modifiers. Of special note is the provision of a modifier that specifies a family focus. The definitions of the modifiers and the four domains, together with a sample problem, are presented in Table 6–5. The reader is referred to the comprehensive text by Martin and Scheet (1992) for a very thorough description of this unique system.

Family Care Planning

As was mentioned previously, the unique aspect of caring for families is the importance of including all members of the family in "the unit of care." Decisions made in regard to one family member will affect the entire family. Martinson and Widmer (1989) discussed the need to involve families in selecting or designing the interventions that will be most helpful to them. Planning should allow and encourage the family to make choices in order to assure that the types of intervention implemented will be accepted, supported, and carried out. When clients resist making choices, it is the nurse's role to help the family identify alternatives, understand consequences, and make the decision as to which options are most acceptable to them.

If the family is dealing with a significant loss or lifestyle change, values, priorities, capabilities, and potential problems will need to be explored. It is often difficult for a family to delineate clearly the impact of major change. Frequently the nurse assists the family to clarify needs and concerns and to establish priorities for problem solving. A thorough assessment that establishes the family's baseline functioning prior to the change allows the nurse to plan interventions that draw on family strengths.

Personal goals and values are important with all clients. It is essential that planning for care be a collaborative process between the family and the nurse. The family clearly knows best what their needs are as a family system and as an interactive unit. The professional nurse, in contrast, has an objective viewpoint that can be useful to clients. Although there are certainly situations when families need to step back and allow others to provide the care, or even to make certain decisions, the essence of the "healthy" family implies movement toward self-care. Family health care planning should encourage movement in the direction of independence (Martinson & Widmer, 1989).

Implementation of Family Health Care

Working with the Family

In implementation, the family and nurse work together to carry out the interventions designed to achieve the identified goals (Ross & Cobb, 1990). Interventions are outlined in the plan of care; actions are taken by designated team members to assist in moving the client from a current state of health to a desired state of health; and the nurse supports, guides, and advocates for the family during the implementation of the plan of care. In the course of intervention it may be necessary to seek assistance from other caregivers, family members, or community agencies; and throughout the process the nurse must evaluate progress in problem resolution and be alert for the emergence of new concerns with which the family must cope.

TABLE 6–5

THE OMAHA SYSTEM: DEFINITIONS OF MODIFIERS AND DOMAINS, AND A SAMPLE PROBLEM

Modifiers	Domains
Health Promotion. Client interest in increasing knowledge, behavior, and health expectations as well as developing resources that maintain or enhance well-being in the absence of risk factors, signs, or symptoms.	*The Environmental Domain* of the Problem Classification Scheme is defined as the material resources, physical surroundings, and substances both internal and external to the client, home, neighborhood, and broader community.
Potential Deficit/Impairment. Client status characterized by the absence of signs/symptoms and the presence of certain health patterns, practices, behaviors, or risk factors that may preclude optimal health.	*The Psychosocial Domain* is defined as patterns of behavior, communication, relationships, and development. The effects of situational and developmental crisis or stress are evident in the Psychosocial Domain.
Deficit/Impairment/Actual. Client status characterized by one or more existing signs and/or symptoms that may preclude optimal health.	*The Psychosocial Domain* is defined as activities that maintain or promote wellness, promote recovery, or maximize rehabilitation.
Family. A social unit or related group of individuals who live together and who experience a health-related problem.	*The Health-Related Behaviors Domain* is defined as functional status of processes that maintain life.
Individual. A person who lives alone or single family member who experiences a health-related problem.	

SAMPLE PROBLEM FROM THE ENVIRONMENTAL DOMAIN

Problem 03.

Residence. Place where individual/family lives

Modifier

Health Promotion	Family
Potential Deficit	Individual
Deficit	

Signs/Symptoms

01. structurally unsound	08. inadequate safety devices
02. inadequate heating/cooling	09. presence of lead-based paint
03. steep stairs	10. unsafe gas/electrical appliances
04. inadequate/obstructed exits/entries	11. inadequate/crowded living space
05. cluttered living space	12. homeless
06. unsafe storage of dangerous objects/substances	13. other
07. unsafe mats/throw rugs	

SOURCE: From *The Omaha System Applications for Community Health Nursing*, by K. S. Martin, & N. J. Schect, Philadelphia: W. B. Saunders. Copyright 1990 by W. B. Saunders. Reprinted with permission.

Smith, Smith, and Toseland (1991) worked extensively with family caregivers and found a number of concerns that needed to be dealt with in caring for elderly clients. As the process of providing care for their elderly relative continued, family members requested assistance with such concerns as improving coping skills, learning to meet the needs of their elderly dependent relative, dealing with issues surrounding spouses and siblings, dealing with concerns over the need for formal and informal support, feelings of inadequacy and guilt, and dealing with the necessary planning for their elderly relative's future. Two major themes seem to run through the comments of these family members: the need to maintain control, and the onus of increasing responsibility (Smith, Smith, & Toseland, 1991).

Whitlatch, Zarit, and Von Ege (1991) found that brief psychoeducational interventions may be more beneficial in working with family caregivers than previously thought and suggested that a program of individual and family counseling can have particular benefits in relieving stress. Wilson's experience with the families of hospice patients and their needs for assistance and support from hospice staff was especially helpful in describing the nature of support families found helpful (Wilson, 1992). The hospice staff enabled families to fulfill their roles as caregivers in several ways. They were extremely important in explaining to the caregivers the role they were undertaking and were available around the clock to families. Moreover, they made a conscious effort to give families recognition for the work they did as caregivers, and if family members were unable to continue the caregiving role, the hospice staff assisted families to make alternate arrangements.

Adaptation to the Family

The great value of family involvement in health behavior interventions was documented by Nader et al. (1992), who conducted a year-long study of a family-based cardiovascular disease risk reduction intervention that was to be used with Mexican-American and Anglo fifth and sixth graders and their parents. Cultural adaptations were made in the education sessions, which involved both parents and children and targeted dietary habits and physical activity. Follow-up, 3 years after the study, showed significant persistent changes in exercise and eating habits even though there had been no additional education and no environmental changes. These authors reported that families participated and that the outcomes were positive.

The significance of adaptation to meet the special needs of the family was well illustrated by the experience of Stephany, a hospice nurse, who found herself caring for a 6'3" "biker" who was dying of colon cancer. He was frequently a problem patient, not cooperative with care, and finally refused to return to the hospital. Stephany found herself trying to assist this terminally ill patient at home in a tiny, less than well equipped house, with only his alcoholic mother and a physically handicapped brother to provide care. After deterioration at home, and continued refusal to return to the hospital, Stephany contacted her patient's biker family, called a meeting and taught his friends and their girls how to provide the needed care, including administering medication. The concern and care of these caregivers and the gratefulness of her patient led her to believe she had mobilized this patient's unique community and family. He died a short time later, holding Stephany's hand (Stephany, 1990).

Implementation must involve the family, however defined, and the nurse, working together to carry out the plan of care to achieve the mutually established goals. One must always be alert to new information that may dictate adjustment or change of plans.

Evaluating Family Nursing Care

Achievement of Objectives

Evaluation of family nursing care is carried out in accordance with established objectives, outcomes, and identified criteria. The care provided is monitored from the initial implementation of the care plan, through achievement of the final outcome, and discharge of the client family from the facility or release from agency care. The written care plan with its specific nursing diagnoses and family care objectives, outcomes, and criteria provides the measures of success. Outcome evaluation refers to long-term individual client-centered goals in the situation involving an ill family member, and also the maintenance of the family's health. Quality care is delivered to the extent predefined goals and outcomes of care are met and family maintenance and growth needs are sustained (Keating & Kelman, 1988).

Evaluation is an ongoing process that continues throughout care delivery, and ends only when a final assessment by client and nurse determines that goals have been successfully met.

Termination with the Family

Termination of the therapeutic relationship is the final step. In the course of evaluating care delivery, the question of how and when to terminate with the family client does arise. Determining when the client family no longer is in need of the services of the nurse is part of evaluating outcomes. Fortune, Pearling, and Rocelle (1991) interviewed a number of practitioners about their reasoning in the decision to terminate family care. The practitioners identified the most important criteria as improvement in the family dynamics and family functioning, as well as the meeting of the specified treatment goals. They also reported that the family's wish to terminate was important. There was, in many instances, a change in the therapeutic content that signaled a readiness to end. Generally, "Practitioners waited for success before terminating and used both improved behavior and intrapsychic functioning to determine success" (Fortune et al., 1991, p. 369).

The following case study illustrates the family nursing process with a childbearing family.

Case Study: The Jinks Family

Family Assessment   The Jinks family is composed of Sarah and John Jinks, 36 and 42 years of age, and their children: John Jr., 11 years of age; Tony, 8 years of age; and a new infant girl, Susan. Susan was born at 35 weeks gestation, weighing 4 lb. 11 oz. All infants under the birth weight of 5 lb are automatically followed by the public health nurse, whose initial visit reveals a caring, supportive family with limited financial resources. The family live in a four-bedroom white frame house, which they are buying. Sarah is a teacher's assistant, and plans to return to work. John Sr. works in construction. They are of Italian and French ancestry, and attend the Lutheran church regularly. Sarah's parents live in the area and visit often. She reports her father to be in good health at 61 years of age. Her mother is 59 years of age, with well-controlled adult-onset diabetes. Sarah is an only child. John Sr. lost his father recently at age 69 years, to a heart attack. His mother, aged 67 years, has arthritis, hypertension, and adult-onset diabetes. She will be coming to live with her son and his family within the month. John Sr. has three siblings, but all live out of state. Sarah has primary responsibility for the household; John helps and participates in child care. Sarah describes herself as a "great cook." Family menus include both Italian favorites and "the best" French pastries. The family's activity together is largely sedentary, watching television, going to movies, and attending their son's sports events.

Both parents describe the family's health as "good." They go to a local clinic for "checkups" and "immunizations." Sara received prenatal care at the clinic of the community hospital. The family expressed several health concerns. Sarah worries about her "weight gain" during pregnancy. She reports a prenatal weight of 170 lb, weight gain of 40 lb, and a loss of 20 lb since Susan's birth. John sees himself as "healthy" although "a little overweight." Both parents describe the children as well, but are concerned about giving proper care to the new baby, "she's pretty small," and see busy times ahead with the active older children and having to care for John Sr.'s mother.

Analysis Issues that might be of concern include the following: The Jinks family is a strong, supportive family with limited financial resources. There is expressed concern regarding weight gain, a history of diabetes and cardiovascular disease, and potential stress due to the dual responsibilities of caring for an older parent with health problems and a new baby with a history of prematurity. The family will also be coping with active school-age children, one a preteen. Possible diagnostic statements might include:

> Potential ineffective family process related to ineffective coping with multiple care responsibilities of elderly parent, new infant (premature), school-age children, and limited financial resources.
>
> Alteration in nutrition: Excess caloric intake related to lack of knowledge of appropriate dietary adjustments and cooking techniques to reduce caloric intake.
>
> High risk for diabetes mellitus and cardiovascular disease related to lack of knowledge of risk factors and methods to reduce risk.
>
> Family coping: Potential for growth related to strong family support, readiness to seek assistance.

Planning The goals for the Jinks might include:

1. The family will report the ability to carry out multiple roles with minimal difficulty by second clinic visit and will demonstrate healthy interaction as evidenced by consistent weight gain and developmental progress of their newborn, positive school reports of children, and ability to involve grandparent in family life and in outside activity. Assess each visit.

2. Both parents will report commitment to a healthy eating and lifestyle program by third clinic visit and demonstrate positive results by minimum weight loss of 2 lb.

Interventions for the Jinks family might include:

1. Initial visit. Review infant development and follow-up needs, and respond to questions and concerns related to prematurity. Reinforce positive expectations.

2. Initial visit. Review diet history with Sarah, possible alternatives to reduce calorie count, including food selection and cooking techniques. Pay particular attention to retain cultural favorites. (Review and provide written material on "healthy" ethnic/cultural tools, consider referral to nutritionist.)

3. Second visit. Discuss possible activities of interest to family that will increase physical activity. Identify availability in neighborhood, participation of children, availability of child care for infant.

4. Second visit. Review available activities for older adults and transportation options. Discuss needed adjustments to family routines; offer assistance and guidance as requested.

5. Arrange periodic contact with family as acceptable and possible to continue support and assistance. Identify preference for telephone contact or home visit and best time for approach of choice.

Implementation The plan of care for this family must involve facilitating their contact with available resources and following through as needed. It is essential to identify and deal with problems and concerns as they arise, including access issues, financial need, and the stress of dealing with change. Continuing contact with the family is needed to assess their ability to use the information given or the resources available, and their effectiveness in solving identified problems.

Evaluation Both formative and summative approaches are required. As plans are implemented, to what degree are positive results beginning to appear? As contacts with the family are made, the nurse must monitor infant development, family dynamics, and parental weight gain and loss. Time frames established when the goals are agreed on with the family become the point at which summative evaluation occurs. To what degree have the goals been achieved? Is the family satisfied with the level of achievement? Do new goals or plans need to be devised? Is the family comfortable with the current level of function, ready to assume totally independent role, and terminate contact?

SUMMARY	Family nursing process is a systematic approach to identifying problems and initiating appropriate activities designed to meet the specified needs or concerns of the client family. It is an open approach that is dynamic and cyclic in nature, and is ongoing throughout the time the family receives care. The family is a partner in care design and delivery, and family input and family validation are essential. Nurses have the unique role of diagnosing and guiding human responses to life's changes. In this role, the nurse is assisted by the nursing process, which provides the decision-making framework for the delivery of comprehensive care to families.

STUDY QUESTIONS

1. In what way is the use of the nursing process unique in providing care for the family as client?

2. Describe two diagnostic classification systems that might be used in interpreting data and identifying the specific health care needs of families.

3. What are the limitations of the NANDA system in the defining of family health care needs?

4. What is an ecomap?

5. Discuss how family health care might be evaluated.

REFERENCES

Allen, C. V. (1991). *Comprehending the nursing process in workbook approach.* Nowalk, CT: Appleton & Lange.

Berkey, K. M., & Hanson, S. M. H. (1991). *Pocket guide to family assessment in intervention.* St. Louis, MO: C. V. Mosby.

Cantor, M. H. (1991). Family and community: Changing roles in an aging society. *Gerontologist, 31,* 337–346.

Chitty, K. K. (1993). *Professional nursing concepts and challenges.* Philadelphia: W. B. Saunders.

Donnelly, E. (1990). Health promotion, families, and the diagnostic process. *Family and Community Health, 12,* 12–20.

Fortune, A. E., Pearling, B., & Rochelle, C. D. (1991). Criteria for terminating treatment. *Families in Society: The Journal of Contemporary Human Services, 72,* 366–370.

Friedeman, M. L. (1989). Closing the gap between grand theory and mental health practice with families, part I. The framework of systematic organization for nursing of families and family members. *Archives of Psychiatric Nursing, 3,* 10 – 19.

Friedman, M. M. (1992). *Family nursing: Theory and practice* (3rd ed.). Norwalk, CT: Appleton & Lange.

Gordon, M. (1976). Nursing diagnosis and the diagnostic process. *American Journal of Nursing, 76,* 1276 – 1300.

Gordon, M. (1982). *Nursing diagnosis: Process and application.* New York: McGraw-Hill.

Gordon, M. (1987). *Nursing diagnosis: Process and application* (2nd ed.). New York: McGraw-Hill.

Keating, S. B., & Kelman, G. B. (1988). *Home health.* Philadelphia: J. B. Lippincott.

Lapp, C. A., Diemert, C. A., & Enestvedt, R. (1990). Family-based practice: Discussion of a tool merging assessment with intervention. *Family and Community Health, 12,* 21 – 28.

Martin, K. S., & Scheet, N. J. (1992). *The Omaha system: Applications for community health nursing.* Philadelphia: W. B. Saunders.

Martinson, L. M., & Widmer, A. (1989). *Home health care nursing.* Philadelphia: W. B. Saunders.

Mattaini, M. A. (1990). Contextual behavior analysis in the assessment process. *Family in Society: The Journal of Contemporary Human Services, 71,* 236 – 245.

Nader, P. R., Sallis, J. F., Abramson, L. S., Broyles, S. L., Patterson, T. L., Senn, K., Kupp, J. W., & Nelson, J. A. (1992). Family-based cardiovascular risk reduction education among Mexican and Anglo-Americans. *Family and Community Health, 15,* 57 – 74.

NANDA Nursing Diagnosis: Definitions and classification 1992 – 1993. (1993). Philadelphia: North American Nursing Diagnosis Association.

Nightingale, F. (1969). *Notes on nursing* (unabridged republication of original text published by Appleton-Century Crofts, 1860). New York: Dover Publications.

Paquin, G. W., & Bushum, R. J. (1991). Family treatment assessment for novices. *Families in Society: The Journal of Contemporary Human Services, 72,* 353 – 359.

Rosen, A. (1992). Facilitating clinical decision making and evaluation. *Families in Society: The Journal of Contemporary Human Services, 73,* 522 – 532.

Ross, B., & Cobb, K. L. (1990). *Family nursing: A nursing process approach.* Redwood City, CA: Addison-Wesley.

Shaw, M. (1993). (Senior Ed.). *Nursing progress in clinical practice.* Springhouse, PA: Springhouse.

Smith, G. C., Smith, M. F., & Toseland, R. W. (1991). Problems identified by family caregivers in counseling. *Gerontologist, 31,* 15 – 22.

Stephany, T. M. (1990). A death in the family. *American Journal of Nursing, 90,* 54 – 56.

Wasik, B. H., Bryant, D. M., & Lyons, C. M. (1990). *Home visiting: Procedures for helping families.* Newbury Park, CA: Sage Publications.

Whitlatch, C. J., Zarit, S. H., & Von Eye, A. (1991). Efficacy of interventions with caregivers: A reanalysis. *Gerontologist, 31,* 9 – 14.

Wilson, S. A. (1992). The family as caregivers: Hospice home care. *Family and Community Health, 15,* 71 – 80.

Yura, H., & Walsh, M. B. (1988). *The nursing process* (5th ed.). Norwalk, CT: Appleton & Lange.

BIBLIOGRAPHY

Baum, M., and Page, M. (1991). Caregiving and multigenerational families. *Gerontologist, 31,* 762 – 769.

Clements, S. D. (1992). When family caregivers grieve for the Alzheimer's patient. *Geriatric Nursing, 13,* 305 – 309.

Davidhizar, R. (1992). Understanding powerlessness in family member caregivers of the chronically ill. *Geriatric Nursing, 13,* 66 – 69.

Elston-Hurdle, B. J., & Poyzer, D. (1989). Fight over a critically ill patient. *American Journal of Nursing, 89,* 327 – 333.

Ernst, L. (1990). Value differences in families of differing socioeconomic status: Implications for family education. *Family Perspective, 24,* 401 – 410.

Ferris, M. (1992). Nursing interventions for families of nursing home residents. *Geriatric Nursing, 13,* 37 – 40.

Fisher, L. F., Terry, H. E., & Ransom, D. C. (1990). Advancing a family perspective in health research: Models and methods. *Family Process, 29,* 177 – 189.

Futcher, J. A. (1988). Chronic illness and family dynamics. *Pediatric Nursing, 14,* 381 – 385.

Glasser, M., Prohaska, T., & Roska, J. (1992). The role of the family in medical care seeking decisions of older adults. *Family and Community, 15,* 59 – 70.

Gillis, C. L. (1991). Family nursing research, theory and practice. *Image: Journal of Nursing Scholarship, 23,* 19 – 22.

Hanson, S., Helms, M., & Julian, D. (1992). Education for family health care professionals: Nursing as a paradigm. *Family Relations, 41,* 49 – 53.

Heiney, S. P. (1988). Assessing and intervening with dysfunctional families. *Oncology Nursing Forum, 15,*

585 – 590. Reprinted in G. D. Wegner & R. J. Alexander (Eds.). (1993). *Readings in family nursing* (357 – 367). Philadelphia: J. B. Lippincott.

Johnson, M. A., Morton, M. K., & Knox, S. M. (1992). The transition to a nursing home: Meeting the family's needs. *Geriatric Nursing, 13,* 299 – 302.

Klee, M. A. E. (1989). Family influences on home care. In L. M. Martinson & A. Widmer, *Home health care nursing* (pp. 151 – 162). Philadelphia: W. B. Saunders.

Kneeshaw, M. F., & Lunney, M. (1989). Nursing diagnosis: Not for individuals only. *Geriatric Nursing, 10,* 246 – 247.

Lemer, H., & Byme, M. W. (1991). Helping nursing students communicate with high-risk families. *Nursing and Health Care, 12,* 98 – 101.

Levin, L., & Trost, I. (1992). Understanding the concept of family. *Family Relations, 41,* 348 – 351.

Lynn-McHale, D. J., & Smith, A. (1991). Comprehensive assessment of families of the critically ill. *Critical Care Nurse, 2,* 195 – 209. Reprinted in R. J. Alexander & G. D. Wegner, *Readings in family nursing* (pp. 309 – 321). Philadelphia: J. B. Lippincott.

Martin, K. S., & Scheet, N. J. (1989). Nursing diagnosis in home health: The Omaha system. In L. M. Martinson & H. Widmer, *Home health care nursing* (pp. 67 – 72). Philadelphia: W. B. Saunders.

Moos, R. H. (1990). Conceptual and empirical approach to developing family-based assessment procedures: Resolving the case of the family environment scale. *Family Process, 29,* 199 – 208.

Novak, M., & Guest, C. (1989). Application of a multidimensional caregiver burden inventory. *Gerontologist, 29,* 798 – 803.

Roberts, F. B. (1983). An interaction model for family assessment. In L. W. Clements & F. B. Roberts (Eds.), *Family health: A theoretical approach to nursing care* (pp. 189 – 204). New York: John Wiley & Sons.

Silvia, L. Y., & Liepman, M. R. (1991). Family behavior loop mapping enhances treatment of alcoholism. *Family and Community Health, 13,* 72 – 83.

Swenson, V. M. (1989). Do you want everything done? *American Journal of Nursing, 89,* 1252.

Taylor, S. G. (1989). An interpretation of family within Orem's General Theory of Nursing. *Nursing Science Quarterly, 2,* 131 – 137. Reprinted in G. D. Wagner & R. J. Alexander (Eds.), *Readings in Family Nursing* (pp. 75 – 86). Philadelphia: J. B. Lippincott.

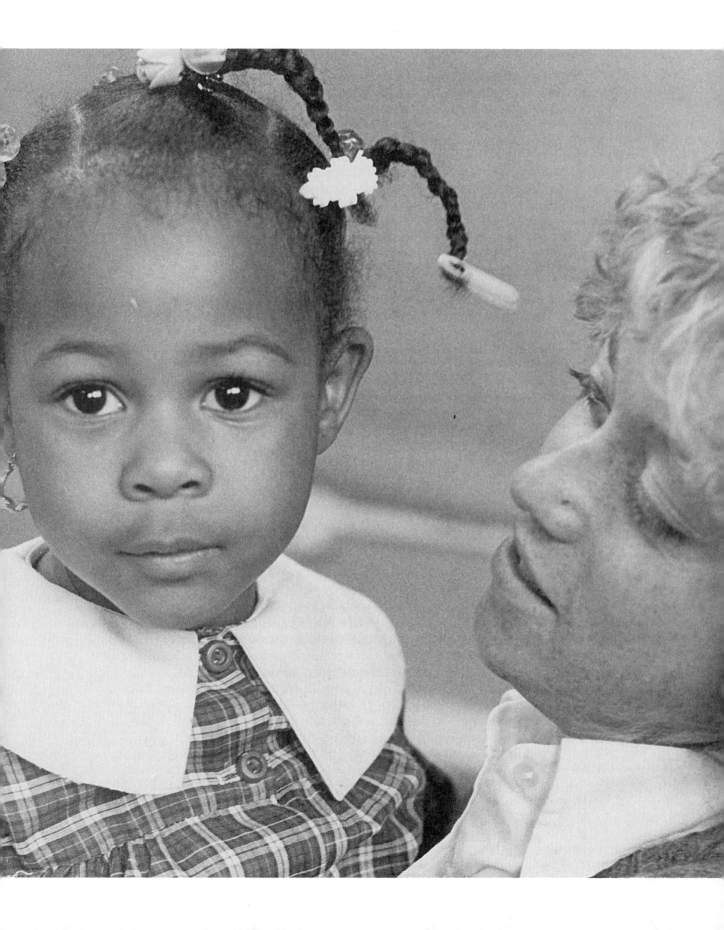

Family Nursing Assessment and Intervention

In previous nursing courses, the assessment of the individual client was emphasized; this chapter focuses on the accurate assessment of families. It is essential for students preparing for professional practice with families to be thoroughly conversant with the sophisticated assessment models in use today. Here students are provided with a comprehensive overview of family assessment models and their importance to professional practice in family nursing, and are exposed to the intricacies of systematic family assessment. While you may find this material particularly challenging, a careful reading of previous chapters provides a comprehensive foundation for understanding family assessment.

The family may be viewed as a context for individual development, as client, as system, and as a unit of society. Each view has a different philosophical base and a different set of operational assumptions that direct the assessment approach. An understanding of these views and their philosophical foundations will assist nursing students in selecting assessment models for use in practice.

This chapter emphasizes the scientific basis of family nursing and explains the differences between measurement and assessment, and describes how each is essential to professional nursing practice with families. A focus on the Family Assessment and Intervention Model and the Family System Stressor-Strength Inventory that accompanies it is followed by a discussion of the Friedman Family Assessment Model and Form and the Calgary Family Assessment Model. All of these models have a different focus and are useful in whole or in part for professional family nursing practice.

CHAPTER 7

Family Assessment and Intervention

Shirley May Harmon Hanson RN, PMHNP, PhD, FAAN

OUTLINE

FAMILY ASSESSMENT AND MEASUREMENT APPROACHES

FAMILY NURSING ASSESSMENT MODELS
The Family Assessment and Intervention Model and the Family System Stressor-Strength Inventory
The Friedman Family Assessment Model and Form
The Calgary Family Assessment Model

GENOGRAMS AND ECOMAPS
Genogram
Ecomap
Clinical Uses of Genograms and Ecomaps

CASE STUDY: FAMILY ASSESSMENT OF THE ANDERSONS

CURRENT STATUS OF FAMILY MEASUREMENT

OBJECTIVES

Upon completion of this chapter, the reader will be able to:
1. Explain how family assessment and intervention fit into the nursing process.
2. Distinguish between family assessment and family measurement.
3. Differentiate between qualitative and quantitative approaches in family measurement.
4. Summarize the current status of instrumentation for family nursing.
5. Compare three different models and approaches that can be used for family assessment and intervention.
6. Explain one assessment model and approach in detail.
7. Describe other resources for assessment techniques and instruments.

FAMILY ASSESSMENT AND MEASUREMENT APPROACHES

It is important to distinguish between assessment and measurement, and between qualitative and quantitative assessment strategies. **Assessment** is a continuously evolving process of data collection whereby the assessor, by drawing on the past and the present, is able to plan and predict for the future (Berkey & Hanson, 1991, p. 226). In contrast to assessment, **measurement** is defined as "the process of using a rule to assign numbers to objects or events which represent the amount and/or kind of specified attribute possessed" (Waltz, Strickland, & Lenz, 1991, p. 62). Measurement requires a formal instrument that gives numerical values to or *quantifies* the traits being measured and gives a quantitative result when a particular attribute is examined. It is often considered a narrower aspect of assessment, focusing on more specific concepts or traits.

Assessment is the first step in the family nursing process and the data it yields are often **qualitative** or descriptive in nature. Clinical assessment often involves the use of a qualitative interview guide, whereas measurement often involves the administration of scales and other instruments that yield **quantitative data**. During family assessment, data about the family are systematically collected using predetermined guidelines or questions, and then classified and analyzed according to their meaning (Friedman, 1992, p. 41).

In clinical practice, assessment involves collecting the information necessary to diagnose and treat presenting problems and evaluate the success of the intervention (Grotevant, 1989, p. 108; Carlson, 1989, p. 161). The initial assessment is often cursory. It is then conducted in more detail when potential problem areas are identified and continues throughout the provision of health care services to the family. The amount of detail is determined by the client, the clinician, the time available, and the instrument or guidelines used. Data can come from many sources — family members themselves, referrals, and community agencies working with the family. Structured and unstructured interview guides are generally used during the assessment process, but more structured quantitative instruments can also be employed. In this book, the term "assessment" includes the use of measurement instruments as well as both qualitative and quantitative data-gathering strategies and techniques.

FAMILY NURSING ASSESSMENT MODELS

Three family assessment models and approaches have been developed by family nurses: the Family Assessment and Intervention Model and the Family Systems Stressor-Strength Inventory (FS³I), the Friedman Family Assessment Model and Form, and the Calgary Family Assessment Model (CFAM). Nurses are encouraged to learn each of the three approaches and select the model that best fits their philosophy and practice. The following discussion of each model will assist in that process.

The Family Assessment and Intervention Model and the Family Systems Stressor-Strength Inventory

The Family Assessment and Intervention Model diagrammed in Figure 7–1 is based on Betty Neuman's Health Care Systems Model (Berkey & Hanson, 1991; Mischke-Berkey, Warner, & Hanson, 1989; Mischke & Hanson, in press; Neuman, 1989; Reed, 1993). Neuman's theoretical constructs were extended by Berkey and Hanson to focus on the family rather than the individual.

According to the Family Assessment and Intervention Model, families are subject to

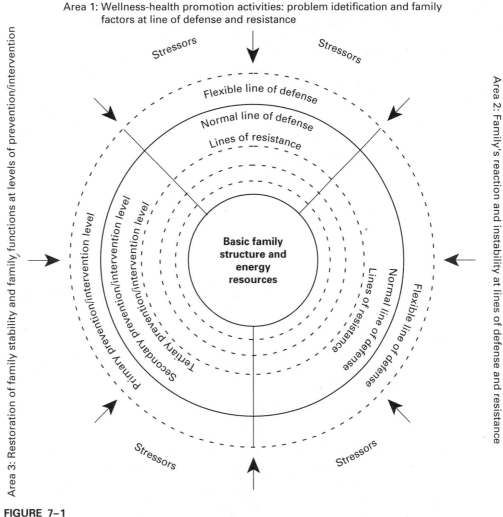

FIGURE 7–1

Family assesment intervention model. (From Mischke, KM and Hanson, SMH: Family health assessment and intervention. In Bomar, PJ (ed). Nurses and Family Health Promotion: Concepts, Assessment, and Interventions (2nd Ed). WB Saunders, Philadelphia, 1995, with permission.)

tensions when stressors, in the form of problems, penetrate their defense system. The family's reaction depends on how deeply the stressor penetrates the family unit and how capable the family is of adapting to maintain its stability. The lines of resistance protect the family's basic structure, which includes the family's functions and energy resources. The core contains the patterns of family interactions and unit strengths. The basic structure must be protected at all costs, or the family will cease to exist. Reconstitution or adaptation is the work the family undertakes to preserve or restore family stability after stressors penetrate the family lines of defense, altering usual family functions. The model addresses three areas: (1) health promotion, wellness activities, problem identification, and family factors at lines of defense and resistance; (2) family reaction and instability at lines of defense and resistance; and (3) restoration of family stability and family functioning at levels of prevention/intervention. The basic assumptions of this family-focused model are listed in Table 7–1.

TABLE 7-1

BASIC ASSUMPTIONS FOR FAMILY ASSESSMENT AND INTERVENTION MODEL

1. Though each family as a family system is unique, each system is a composite of common, known factors or innate characteristics within a normal, given range of response contained within a basic structure.

2. Many known, unknown, and universal environmental stressors exist. Each differs in its potential for disturbing a family's usual stability level, or normal line of defense. The particular interrelationships of family variables—physiological, psychological, sociocultural, developmental, and spiritual—at any time can affect the degree to which a family is protected by the flexible line of defense against possible reaction to one or more stressors.

3. Over time, each family/family system has evolved a normal range of response to the environment, referred to as a normal line of defense, or usual wellness/stability state.

4. When the cushioning, accordionlike effect of the flexible line of defense is no longer capable of protecting the family/family system against an environmental stressor, the stressor breaks through the normal line of defense. The interrelationships of variables—physiological, psychological, sociocultural, developmental, and spiritual—determine the nature and degree of the system reaction or possible reaction to the stressor.

5. The family, whether in a state of wellness or illness, is a dynamic composite of the interrelationships of variables—physiological, psychological, sociocultural, developmental, and spiritual. Wellness is on a continuum of available energy to support the system in its optimal state.

6. Implicit within each family system is a set of internal resistance factors, known as lines of resistance, which function to stabilize and return the family to the usual wellness state (normal line of defense), or possibly to a higher level of stability, following an environmental stressor reaction.

7. Primary prevention relates to general knowledge that is applied in family assessment and intervention in identification and mitigation of risk factors associated with environmental stressors to prevent possible reaction.

8. Secondary prevention relates to symptomatology following reaction to stressors, appropriate ranking of intervention priorities, and treatment to reduce their noxious effects.

9. Tertiary prevention relates to the adjustive processes taking place as reconstitution begins and maintenance factors move the client back in a circular manner toward primary prevention.

10. The family is in dynamic, constant energy exchange with the environment.

SOURCE: From *Pocket Guide to Family Assessment and Intervention* (pp. 23–24), by K.M. Berkey, & S.M.H. Hanson, 1991, St. Louis: C. V. Mosby. Reprinted with permission.

An assessment instrument based on this model is titled the *Family Systems Stressor-Strength Inventory (FS³I)* (Berkey & Hanson, 1991; Hanson & Mischke, in press; Hanson & Kaakinen, in press). (Appendix C contains an updated copy of the instrument with instructions for administration and a scoring guide). The FS³I elicits both qualitative and quantitative information about family health, and particularly about family stressors and strengths. The instrument provides direction for nurses (and other clinicians) in planning interventions to enhance or restore family functioning and growth. The FS³I is simple to administer and interpret, obtains both qualitative and quantitative data, focuses on individuals and the family simultaneously, and incorporates family strengths as well as stressors. It is intended for use with multiple family members who may be assessed collectively or individually. It helps to identify stressful situations occurring in families and the strengths families use to maintain healthy functioning despite their problems. The FS³I is divided into three sections: (1) Family Systems Stressors: General, (2) Family Stressors: Specific, and (3) Family System Strengths. Family members are asked to complete the instrument prior to an interview with the clinician. Questions can be read to members unable to read. Individual members can complete the FS³I or the whole family can sit together and complete the instrument. Both types of data are useful.

The interview with the clinician clarifies perceived general stressors, specific stressors, and family strengths as identified by family members. The clinician evaluates family members on their stressors and strengths, as well as overall family functioning and stability.

Family stability is assessed by gathering information on family stressors (Curran, 1985) and strengths (Curran, 1983). The assessment of general, overall stressors is followed by an assessment of specific problems. Family strengths are identified to give an indication of the potential and actual problem-solving abilities of the family system, and the use of their strengths to deal with their problems. Nurses have a history of asking people about their problems (stressor), but often they have not identified the strengths and resources of the family for dealing with their problems.

The clinician records family members' scores on the Quantitative Summary. A different color code may be used for each individual member. The graph on the quantitative summary sheet (Appendix D) gives a visual representation of family health, and variations in how individuals or the clinician view the situation. The clinician also completes the Qualitative Summary (Appendix D), synthesizing the information gleaned from all participants.

The quantitative and qualitative data help determine the level of prevention/intervention needed: primary, secondary, or tertiary (Pender, Barkauskas, Hayman, Rice, & Anderson, 1992). Primary prevention focuses on moving the individual and family toward a state of improved health or toward health promotion activities. Primary interventions include providing families with information about their strengths, supporting their coping and functioning capabilities, and encouraging movement toward health through family education. Secondary prevention is designed to attain system stability after the family system has been invaded by stressors or problems. Secondary interventions include helping the family to handle their problems, helping them find and use appropriate treatment, and intervening in crises. Tertiary prevention is designed to maintain system stability. Tertiary intervention strategies are initiated after treatment has been completed and may include, for example, coordination of care following discharge from the hospital or rehabilitation services.

Data on family stressors and family strengths are used to complete the Family Care Plan. This plan requires the clinician to prioritize diagnoses; set goals; develop primary, secondary, or tertiary intervention activities; and evaluate outcomes (see Figs. 7-7 to 7-10 for examples).

In summary, the Family Assessment and Intervention Model extends the Neuman Health Care Systems Model to focus on the family as client. The FS³I was developed as one way of assessing families using this model. This approach focuses on family stressors and strengths, and provides the nurse with data useful for nursing interventions.

The Friedman Family Assessment Model and Form

The Friedman Family Assessment Model and Form (Friedman, 1992) draw heavily on the structural-functional framework, as well as on developmental and systems theory. This model takes a macroscopic approach to family assessment (as compared with the microscopic approach of the FS³I), viewing families as subsystems of the wider society. That is, the family is viewed as just one of the basic units of society, along with the institutions devoted to religion, education, health, and so on. This model views the family as an open social system and focuses on the family's structure (organization) and functions (activities and purposes), and the family's relationships with other social systems. This framework is commonly used when the family in community is the setting for care — for example, in community/public health nursing. This approach enables family nurses to assess the family system as a whole, as a subunit of the society, and as an interactional system. The general assumptions of this model are contained in Table 7–2 (Friedman, 1992, p. 74).

Structure refers to how a family is organized and how the parts relate to each other. The four basic structural dimensions are role structure, value systems, communication processes, and power structure (Friedman, 1992). These dimensions are interrelated and interactive and they may differ in single-parent and two-parent families. For example, a single mother may be the head of the family but she may not necessarily take on the authoritarian role that a traditional man might in a two-parent family. In turn, the value systems, communication processes, and power structures may be quite different in the single-parent and two-parent families as a result of these structural differences.

Function refers to how families go about meeting the needs of individuals and meeting the purposes of the broader society. The functions of the family have historically been to:

■ Pass on culture (e.g., religion, ethnicity)
■ Socialize young people for the next generation (e.g., to be good citizens, to be able to cope in society through going to school)
■ Exist for sexual satisfaction and reproduction
■ Provide economic security
■ Serve as a protective mechanism for family members against outside forces
■ Provide closer human contact and relations

The Friedman Family Assessment Model consists of six broad categories of interview questions: (1) identifying data, (2) developmental stage and history of the family, (3) environmental data, (4) family structure (role structure, family values, communication patterns, and power structure), (5) family functions (affective functions, socialization, health care), and (6) family coping. Each category has several subcategories. Friedman's family assessment guide exists in both a long form and a short form. The short form in Appendix E simply outlines of the types of questions the nurse can ask. The long form is quite extensive, providing nine pages of questions and can be found in Friedman's book (Friedman, 1992, p. 399).

Friedman's assessment model was developed to provide guidelines for family nurses in interviewing a family. The guidelines list categories of information about which the interviewer asks questions in order to gain an overall view, in descriptive terms, of what is going on in the family. The list is quite extensive and it may not be possible to collect all of

TABLE 7–2

ASSUMPTIONS UNDERLYING FRIEDMAN'S FAMILY ASSESSMENT MODEL

1. The family is a social system with functional requirements.
2. A family is a small group possessing certain generic features common to all small groups.
3. The family as a social system accomplishes functions that serve the individual in addition to the society.
4. Individuals act in accordance with a set of internalized norms and values that are learned primarily through socialization in the family.

SOURCE: Adapted from *Family Nursing: Theory and Practice* (3rd ed., p. 74), by M. M. Friedman, 1992, Norwalk, CT: Appleton & Lange. Copyright 1992 by Appleton & Lange.

the data in one visit. Also, all the categories of information listed in the guidelines may not be pertinent for every family. One problem with this approach is that it can generate large quantities of data with no clear direction as to how to use all this information in diagnosis, planning, and intervention. Like other approaches, this model has its strengths and weaknesses; it is one of many tools in the armamentarium of the family nurse.

The Calgary Family Assessment Model

The Calgary Family Assessment Model developed by Wright and Leahey (1984, 1994) blends nursing and family therapy concepts and is grounded in systems theory, cybernetics, communication theory, and change theory. Wright and Leahey (1994, pp. 15–21) set forth a number of concepts from general systems theory and family systems theory as a theoretical framework for the model:

1. A family system is part of a larger suprasystem and is also composed of many subsystems.
2. The family as a whole is greater than the sum of its parts.
3. A change in one family member affects all family members.
4. The family is able to create a balance between change and stability.
5. Family members' behaviors are best understood from a perspective of circular rather than linear causality.

A second theoretical foundation used in the model is cybernetics, or the science of communication and control theory. Cybernetics differs from systems theory: where systems theory helps change the focus of our conceptual lens from parts to wholes, cybernetics changes the focus from substance to form. "Both parts and whole are examined in terms of their patterns of organization" (Keeney, 1982, p. 155). Wright and Leahey (1994, p. 22) present two useful concepts from cybernetics theory:

1. Families possess self-regulating ability through the process of feedback.
2. Feedback processes can occur simultaneously at several different system levels with families.

A third theoretical foundation for the model is communication theory, based on the work of Watzlawick, Beavin, and Jackson (1967). Communication is how individuals interact with one another, so concepts derived from communication theory are used in the Calgary Family Assessment Model (Wright & Leahey, 1994, pp. 23–24). For example:

1. All nonverbal communication is meaningful.
2. All communication has two major channels for transmission: digital (verbal) and analogic (nonverbal).
3. A dyadic relationship has varying degrees of symmetry and complementarity.
4. All communication consists of two levels: content and relationship.

Because helping families to change is at the very core of family nursing interventions, change is also an important concept in this assessment model. Families need a balance between change and stability: change is required to make things better, and stability is required to maintain some semblance of order. Watzlawick, Weakland, and Fisch (1974) support the notion that persistence (stability) and change have to be considered concurrently despite their opposing natures. A number of concepts from change theory are important to family nursing (Wright & Leahey, 1994, pp. 25–33):

1. Change is dependent on the perception of the problem.

2. Change is dependent on context.

3. Change is dependent on coevolving goals for treatment.

4. Understanding alone does not lead to change.

5. Change does not necessarily occur equally in all family members.

6. Facilitating change is the nurse's responsibility.

7. Change can be due to a myriad of causes.

Figure 7–2 shows the branching diagram of the Calgary Family Assessment Model (Wright & Leahey, 1994, p. 38). The assessment questions with the model are organized in three major categories: (1) structural, (2) developmental, and (3) functional. Nurses examine a family's structural components to answer these questions: Who is in the family? What is the connection among family members? What is the family's context? Structure has internal, external, and contextual aspects. The internal aspects include family composition, gender, rank order, subsystems, and the boundaries of the family system. The external structure refers to the family of origin and family context. Strategies recommended to assess external structure include the genogram and the ecomap, which will be discussed later in this chapter.

The second major assessment category is family development, which includes assessment of family stages, tasks, and attachments. For example, nurses may ask, "Where is the family in the family life cycle?" Understanding the stage of the family enables nurses to as-

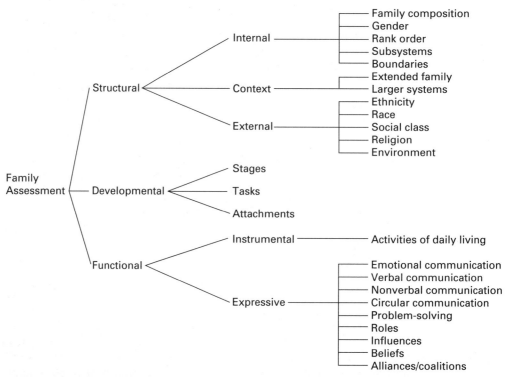

FIGURE 7–2

Branching diagram of the Calgary Family Assessment Model (CFAM). (From Wright, LM and Leahey, M: Nurses and Families: A Guide to Family Assessment and Intervention (2nd Ed). F.A. Davis, Philadelphia, 1994, p 38, with permission.)

sess and intervene in a more purposeful, specific, and meaningful way. There are no specific tools for assessing development, but developmental tasks can be used as guidelines. It is important to note here that there have been many alterations to the traditional family life cycle as a result of modern trends such as divorce, remarriage, single-parent or unmarried parent families, and childless families. Many families no longer fit the traditional family life cycle. Carter and McGoldrick (1980) discuss various "dislocations" of the family life cycle, which require additional steps to restabilize and proceed developmentally.

The third area for assessment in the CFAM model is family functioning, which includes both instrumental and expressive aspects. Family functioning reflects how individuals actually behave in relation to one another, or the "here-and-now aspect of a family's life" (Wright & Leahey, 1994, p. 80). Instrumental aspects of family functioning are activities of daily life such as eating, sleeping, meal preparation, and health care. Expressive aspects of family functioning are emotional functioning, verbal/nonverbal communication, problem solving, influence, beliefs, and alliances/coalitions. Wright and Leahey indicate that nurses may assess in all three areas (structural, developmental, functional) for a macro view of the family, or they can use any part of the approach for a micro assessment.

Wright and Leahey also have developed a companion model to the CFAM, the Calgary Family Intervention Model (CFIM) (1994). This intervention model provides concrete strategies by which nurses can promote, improve, and sustain effective family functioning in the cognitive, affective, and behavioral domains. More detail about this assessment model and intervention is available in Wright and Leahey's book *Nurses and Families: A Guide to Family Assessment and Intervention* (1994).

Each of these three family approaches is unique, and each creates a different data base on which to plan interventions. Berkey and Hanson's, Family Assessment and Intervention Model and the FS³I are used to measure specific family dimensions. The FS³I yields both qualitative and quantitative data. Friedman's Family Assessment Model and Short Form is broader and more general and is particularly useful for viewing families in the context of their community. This approach is enhanced by an interview guide (detailed in the long form), which lists specific categories for assessment. Wright and Leahey's CFAM and CFIM provides an approach for both assessment and intervention, though it is less specific than the other two approaches. The CFAM is broad in perspective though it focuses on internal relations within the family rather than the interface between the family and community. Finally, all three approaches can be used alone or in some combination. For example, the FS³I can be used for specific assessment, while either the Friedman Family Assessment Short or Long Form or the CFAM model is used for more global assessment.

GENOGRAMS AND ECOMAPS

The genogram and ecomap are essential components of any family assessment. They should be used concurrently with all three models and approaches previously described.

Genogram

The genogram is a format for drawing a family tree that records information about family members and their relationships over at least three generations (McGoldrick & Gerson, 1985). The genogram is a diagram, a skeleton, a constellation showing the structure of intergenerational relationships. The genogram has been commonly used in both genealogy and genetic charts, and it is now being used in family therapy and in health care settings. The genogram is a rich source of information for planning intervention strategies because

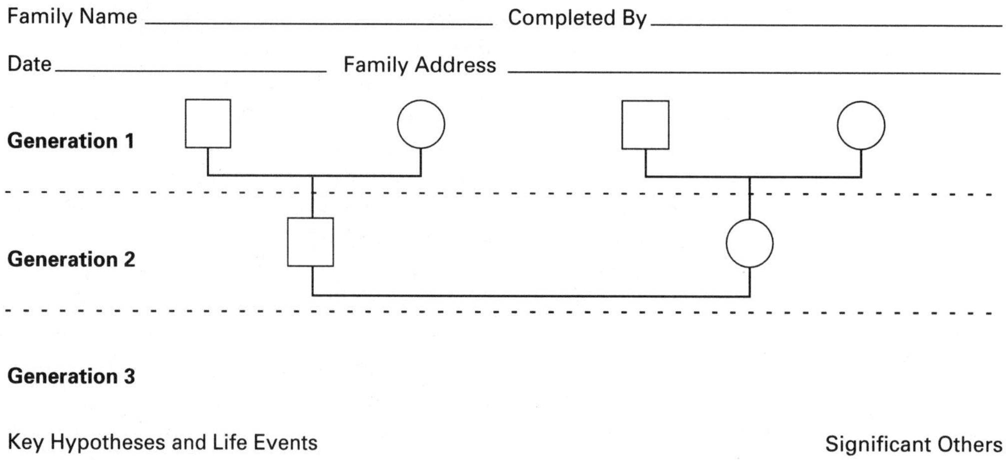

Family Name _____ Completed By _____

Date _____ Family Address _____

Generation 1

Generation 2

Generation 3

Key Hypotheses and Life Events   **Significant Others**

FIGURE 7–3
Genogram form. (From McGoldrick, M and Gerson, R: Genograms in Family Assessment. W.W. Norton, New York, 1985, p 156, with permission.)

it displays the family visually and graphically in a way that provides a quick overview of family complexities. The genogram was developed primarily out of the family systems theory of Murray Bowen (1978). According to Bowen, people are organized in family systems by generation, age, sex, and so on. Where a person fits into the family structure influences the person's functioning, relational patterns, and type of family he or she forms in the next generation. Bowen incorporated Toman's (1975) ideas about the importance of sex and birth order in shaping sibling relationships and characteristics. According to Bowen (1978), families repeat themselves over generations in a phenomenon called the transmission of family patterns. What happens in one generation repeats itself in the next, so the same issues are played out from generation to generation. These include psychosocial as well as health issues.

Figure 7–3 provides a basic genogram form from which the nurse can start plotting family members over the first, second, and third generations (McGoldrick & Gerson, 1985, p. 156).

Figure 7–4 shows symbols provided by McGoldrick and Gerson (1985, pp. 154–155) to describe basic family membership and structure, family interaction patterns, and other family information of particular importance, such as ethnic background, religion, education, health, drug and alcohol use, occupation, military service; and nodal events, such as retirement, trouble with the law, and family relocations.

The health history of all family members (morbidity, mortality, onset of illness) is very important information for family nurses and can be the focus of analysis of the family genogram. An example of a family genogram developed from one interview is contained in the case example shown in Figure 7–5.

During the assessment interview, the nurse asks the family for background information and then completes the genogram together with the family; it is a joint nurse-family endeavor. An outline for a brief genogram interview is given in Table 7–3, and genogram interpretive categories are contained in Table 7–4 (McGoldrick & Gerson, 1985, pp. 157–160). Most families are cooperative and interested in completing their genogram, which becomes a part of the ongoing health care record. The genogram does not have to be completed at one sitting. As the same or a different nurse continues to work with the family, data can be added to the genogram over time in a continuing process.

A

Symbols to describe basic family membership and structure. Include on genogram significant others who lived with or cared for family members and place them on the right side of the genogram with a notation about who they are.

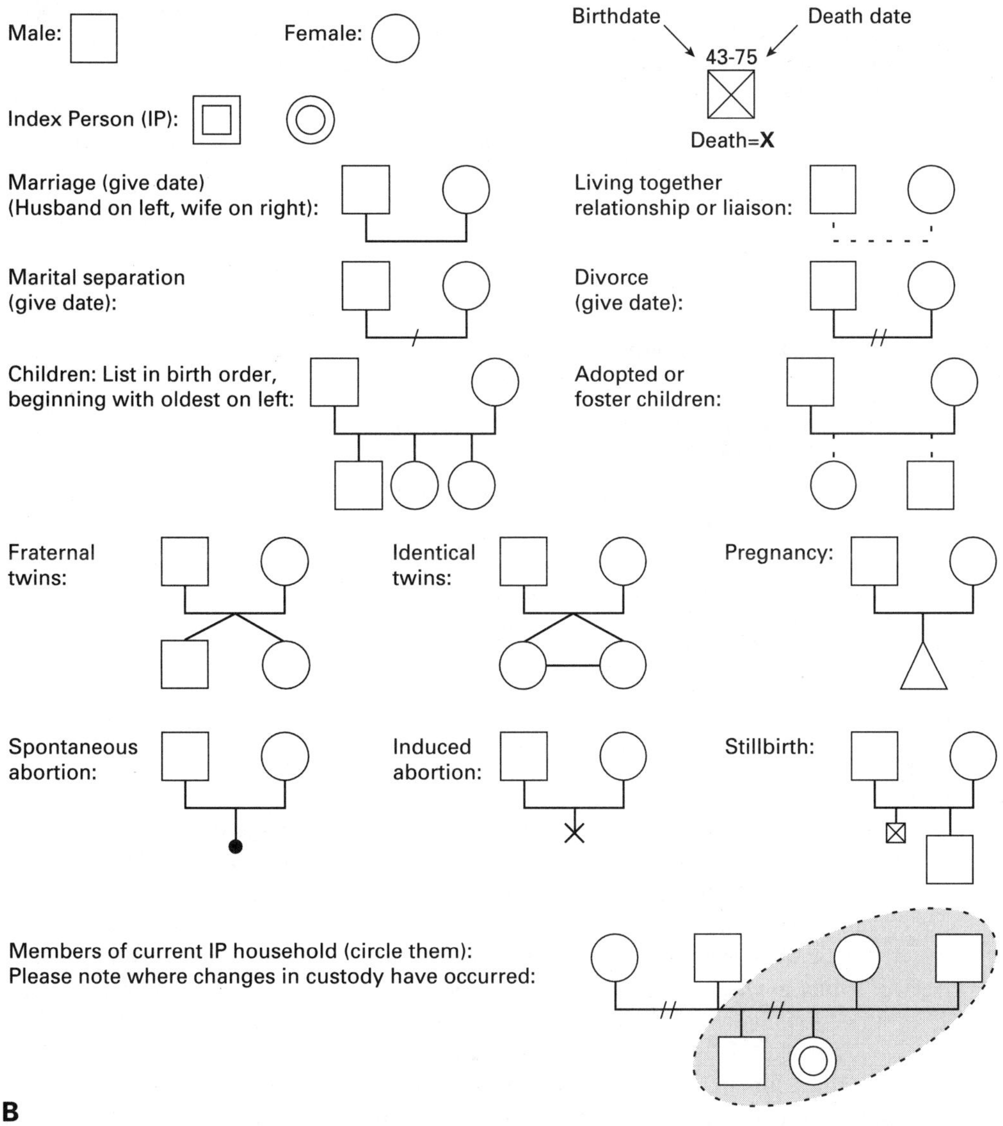

Male: ☐ Female: ○

Birthdate → 43-75 ← Death date
Death=X

Index Person (IP): ☐ ◎

Marriage (give date) (Husband on left, wife on right):

Living together relationship or liaison:

Marital separation (give date):

Divorce (give date):

Children: List in birth order, beginning with oldest on left:

Adopted or foster children:

Fraternal twins:

Identical twins:

Pregnancy:

Spontaneous abortion:

Induced abortion:

Stillbirth:

Members of current IP household (circle them):
Please note where changes in custody have occurred:

B

Family interaction patterns. The following symbols are optional. The clinician may prefer to note them on a separate sheet. They are among the least precise information on the genogram, but may be key indicators of relationship patterns the clinician wants to remember:

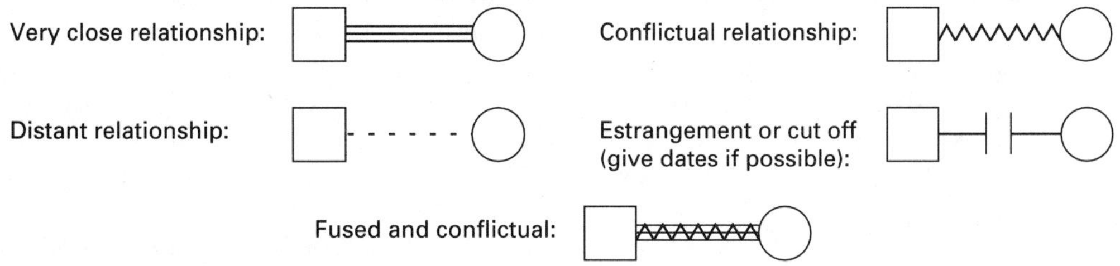

Very close relationship:

Conflictual relationship:

Distant relationship:

Estrangement or cut off (give dates if possible):

Fused and conflictual:

FIGURE 7-4

Genogram format. (From McGoldrick, M and Gerson, R: Genograms in Family Assessment. W.W. Norton, New York, 1985, pp 154-155, with permission.) *Figure 7-4 continues on next page.*

C

Medical history. Because the genogram is meant to be an orienting map of the family, there is room to indicate only the most important factors. Thus, list only major or chronic illnesses and problems. Include dates in parentheses where feasible or applicable. Use DSM-IIIR categories or recognized abbreviations where available (e.g., cancer: CA; stroke: CVA).

D

Other family information of special importance may also be noted on the genogram:
1. Ethnic background and migration date
2. Religion or religious change
3. Education
4. Occupation or unemployment
5. Military service
6. Retirement
7. Trouble with law
8. Physical abuse or incest
9. Obesity
10. Smoking
11. Dates when family members left home: LH '74
12. Current location of family members

It is useful to have a space at the bottom of the genogram for notes on *other key information*. This would include critical events, changes in the family structure since the genogram was made, hypotheses, and other notations of major family issues or changes. These notations should always be dated and kept to a minimum, since every extra piece of information on a genogram complicates it and therefore diminishes its readability.

FIGURE 7–4 *Continued*

Ecomap

Another useful approach in assessing families is the ecologic map, or ecomap. Ecology is a branch of science concerned with the interrelationships of organisms to each other in the environment. The ecomap is a visual representation of the family unit in relation to the community; it shows the nature of the relationships between family members and between family members and the world around them. The ecomap is thus "an overview of the family in their situation, picturing both the important nurturant and stress-producing connections between the family and the world" (Ross & Cobb, 1990, p. 176).

The blank ecomap consists of a large circle with smaller circles around it. To complete the ecomap, the genogram of the family is placed in the center of the large circle. This circle marks the boundary between the household and its external environment. The smaller outer circles represent "significant people, agencies, or institutions in the family's context" (Wright & Leahey, 1994, p. 56). Lines are drawn between the circles and the family members to depict the nature and quality of the relationships and to show what kinds of resources are going in and out of the family. Straight lines show strong or close relationships; the more pronounced the line, the stronger the relationship. Straight lines with slashes denote stressful relationships and broken lines show tenuous or distant relationships. Arrows show the direction of the flow of energy and resources between people, and between people and the environment. Figure 7–6 gives an example of a completed family ecomap.

The ecomap is a tool for organizing a great deal of factual information to give the nurse a more integrated perception of the family situation. Ecomaps not only can portray the present but also can be used to set goals, for example, to increase connections and exchanges with individuals and agencies in the community. More detailed discussions of

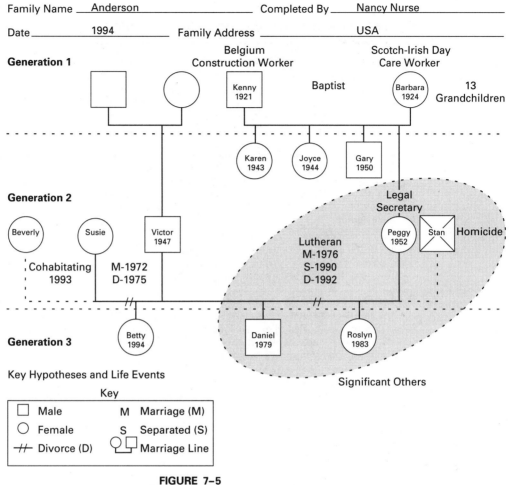

FIGURE 7–5
Example genogram of the Anderson family.

ecomapping can be found in Hartman and Laird (1983), McGoldrick and Gerson (1985), and Ross and Cobb (1990).

Clinical Uses of Genograms and Ecomaps

It is important to draw a key on both the genogram and the ecomap, because the data become a part of the official family health record and other professionals need to be able to interpret the meaning at another time. Families find it stimulating to help develop the genogram and ecomap depicting their family and their situation, and the process helps build a full family-nurse partnership, because everyone's voice is heard. Development of the genogram and ecomap are interventions in and of themselves and can also serve as useful teaching tools. Kissman and Allen (1993) describe a process that professionals can follow in ecomapping a single-parent family and using the information in therapeutic interventions. The case example below illustrates use of the genogram and ecomap.

TABLE 7–3

OUTLINE FOR A BRIEF GENOGRAM INTERVIEW

Index Person, Children, and Spouses

Name? Date of birth? Occupation? Are they married? If so, give names of spouses, and the name and sex of children with each spouse. Include all miscarriages, stillbirths, adopted and foster children. Include dates of marriages, separations, and divorces. Also include birth and death dates, cause of death, occupations, and education of the above family members. Who lives in the household now?

Family of Origin

Mother's name? Father's name? They were which of how many children? Give name and sex of each sibling. Include all miscarriages, stillbirths, adopted and foster siblings. Include dates of the parents' marriages, separations, and divorces. Also, include birth and death dates, cause of death, occupations, and education of the above family members. Who lived in the household when they were growing up?

Mother's Family

The names of the mother's parents? The mother was which of how many children? Give name and sex of each of her siblings. Include all miscarriages, stillbirths, adopted and foster siblings. Include dates of grandparents' marriages, separations, and divorces. Also include birth and death dates, cause of death, occupations, and education of the above family members.

Father's Family

The names of the father's parents? The father was which of how many children? Give name and sex of each of his siblings. Include all miscarriages, stillbirths, adopted and foster siblings. Include dates of grandparents' marriages, separations, and divorces. Also include birth and death dates, cause of death, occupations, and education of the above family members.

Ethnicity

Give the ethnic and religious background of family members and the languages they speak, if not English.

Major Moves

Tell about major family moves and migrations.

Significant Others

Add others who lived with or were important to the family.

For All Those Listed, Note Any of the Following:

Serious medical, behavioral, or emotional problems
Job problems
Drug or alcohol problems
Serious problems with the law

For All Those Listed, Indicate Any Who Were:

Especially close
Distant or conflictual
Cut off from each other
Overly dependent on each other

SOURCE: From *Genograms in Family Assessment* (pp. 157–158), by M. McGoldrick & R. Gerson, 1985, New York: W. W. Norton. Copyright by W. W. Norton. Reprinted with permission.

Case Study: Family Assessment of the Andersons

The Anderson family came to the attention of the nursing staff when Mrs. Anderson (Peggy) was hospitalized with a gunshot wound. The nurses cared for her first in the intensive care unit and then on the stepdown trauma unit. This mid-

TABLE 7–4

GENOGRAM INTERPRETATIVE CATEGORIES

Category 1: Family Structure
A. Household composition
  1. Intact nuclear household
  2. Single-parent household
  3. Remarried family household
  4. Three-generational household
  5. Household including non-nuclear family members
B. Sibling constellation
  1. Birth order
  2. Siblings' gender
  3. Distance in age between siblings
  4. Other factors influencing sibling constellation
    a. Timing of each child's birth in family history
    b. Child's characteristics
    c. Family's "program" for the child
    d. Parental attitudes and biases regarding sex differences
    e. Child's sibling position in relation to that of parent
C. Unusual family configiations

Category 2: Life Cycle Fit

Category 3: Pattern Repetition Across Generations
A. Patterns of functioning
B. Patterns of relationship
C. Structural patterns

Category 4: Life Events and Family Functioning
A. Coincidences of life events
B. The impact of life changes, transitions, and traumas
C. Anniversary reactions
D. Social, economic, and political events

Category 5: Relational Patterns and Triangles
A. Triangles
B. Parent-child triangles
C. Common couple triangles
D. Divorce and remarried family triangles
E. Triangles in families with foster children or adopted children
F. Multigenerational triangles
G. Relationships outside the family

Category 6: Family Balance and Imbalance
A. Family structure
B. Roles
C. Level and style of functioning
D. Resources

SOURCE: From *Genograms in Family Assessment* (pp. 159–160), by M. McGoldrick & R. Gerson, 1985, New York: W. W. Norton. Copyright by W. W. Norton. Reprinted with permission.

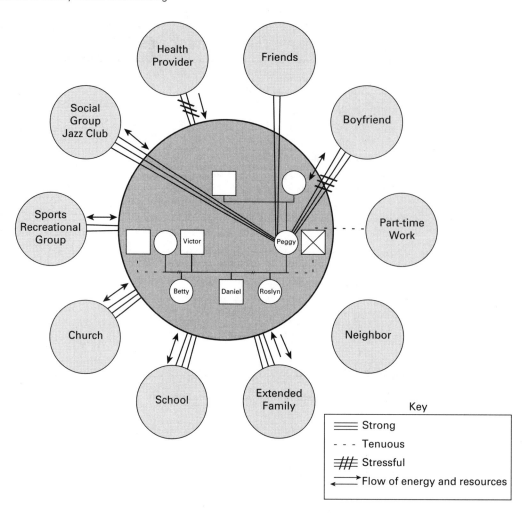

FIGURE 7–6
Example ecomap of the Anderson family.

dle-class white family consisted of Peggy (mother, age 42 years), Victor (father, age 47 years), Betty (daughter, age 20 years), Daniel (son, age 15 years), and Roslyn (daughter, age 11 years). (See Fig. 7-5 for the Anderson family genogram and Fig. 7-6 for the Anderson family ecomap.) Victor was originally married to Susie (in 1972), but they were divorced in 1975 after the birth of Betty, and Victor became the custodial parent for Betty. In 1976, Peggy and Victor were married and had two biological children, Daniel and Roslyn. Although Peggy was stepmother to Betty, she raised her as her own child, and they maintained a good relationship over the years. Victor graduated from law school and took his first job as an attorney after he and Peggy got married. The family relocated frequently (17 times), with Peggy serving as homemaker and legal secretary in various places while Victor pursued his dream of a perfect job, as an attorney, and a perfect location.

As the children grew up, Peggy and Victor "grew apart" and the relationship ceased to be mutually supportive. Peggy neglected her personal needs for growth and adult development and Victor sought sexual alliances outside of the marriage. Over time their relationship became stormy and they made a decision to separate in 1990. The court-mandated reconciliation counseling was merely a cursory review of the relationship difficulties and they were divorced in 1992, after 18 years of marriage.

Peggy received legal custody of the two younger children and Victor got the customary visiting privileges (every other weekend and every Wednesday), an arrangement to everyone's satisfaction. Victor was ordered to pay child support until the two younger children were 18 years of age and spousal support to Peggy for 2 years following the divorce. By the time of the divorce, Betty (Victor's daughter by his first marriage) had left home to go to college. Immediately following his divorce from Peggy, Victor moved in with his new girlfriend, Beverly. This event was a source of considerable pain for Peggy and added to her low self-esteem. Victor continued to have almost weekly contact with his children.

After the divorce, Peggy went to work and tried to get her life back together. For financial reasons, she and the children moved to a smaller house. She soon met Stan, a charming, socially adept, and seemingly supportive man with whom she became quickly infatuated. He moved into the family house with Peggy and the children soon after they met and initially brought an element of excitement and security to the home. As the realities of sharing a household emerged, Peggy noted some disturbing features about Stan: he became obsessive and possessive of her and the children. Peggy became extremely upset and decided she had moved too fast. She asked Stan to move out. Stan was furious; he became even more obsessed with Peggy and became hostile to her and the children after she asked him to leave.

Stan refused to leave and Peggy had to obtain a court order to remove him from the house. She was soon frightened to discover that Stan had been following her and asked for police support to reinforce the restraining order. One afternoon Stan took Peggy hostage at gunpoint at the door of her house. The neighbors called the police and within a couple of hours, a violent confrontation took place. During the shootout Peggy was shot in the shoulder by Stan, and Stan was killed by the police.

Peggy was hospitalized for multiple lacerations and a gunshot wound through the shoulder that resulted in nerve damage to her right arm. Peggy's parents came from out of town and moved into the house to take care of the children and support their daughter. The first hospitalization lasted 10 days and consisted primarily of surgery and wound care. Peggy was sent home with minimal discharge planning, and when she got home, she experienced intractable pain in her arm, hand, and shoulder. Peggy's parents took her back to the hospital, where she was admitted to the psychiatric unit for pain management, physical therapy, and treatment of posttraumatic stress disorder. The hospital course was uneventful and Peggy was discharged again after a month. By now her pain was under control and she had regained some use of her injured arm.

Getting back to "normal," or system stability, was the goal of the family members. Within the period of 1 year, the Anderson family had gone through divorce, relocation, and an episode of violence. The initial family assessment involved the use of all three approaches described previously in this chapter, and use of the genogram and ecomap. The findings from this assessment follow.

Family Systems Stressor-Strength Inventory   The FS³I was deemed most suitable to look at problems and resources the family had to cope with these problems. Peggy and her children were interviewed together by the nurse, but each person completed the FS^3I separately. Each person's score was computed using the scoring guide for the FS^3I. Figures 7-7 and 7-8 summarize the stressors and strengths perceived by the family members and the nurse. As shown on this summary, the general stressors were viewed differently by different family members and they were also assessed as more serious by the nurse than by the family. Everyone considered the general stress level as high, however, which was consistent with what the family was going through. In addition, the family members viewed their strengths as fairly good, as did the nurse.

The qualitative summary in Figure 7-9 served as the guide for the family care plan (Fig. 7-10). It summarizes general stressors, specific stressors, and family strengths, as well as the overall physical and mental health of the family. The

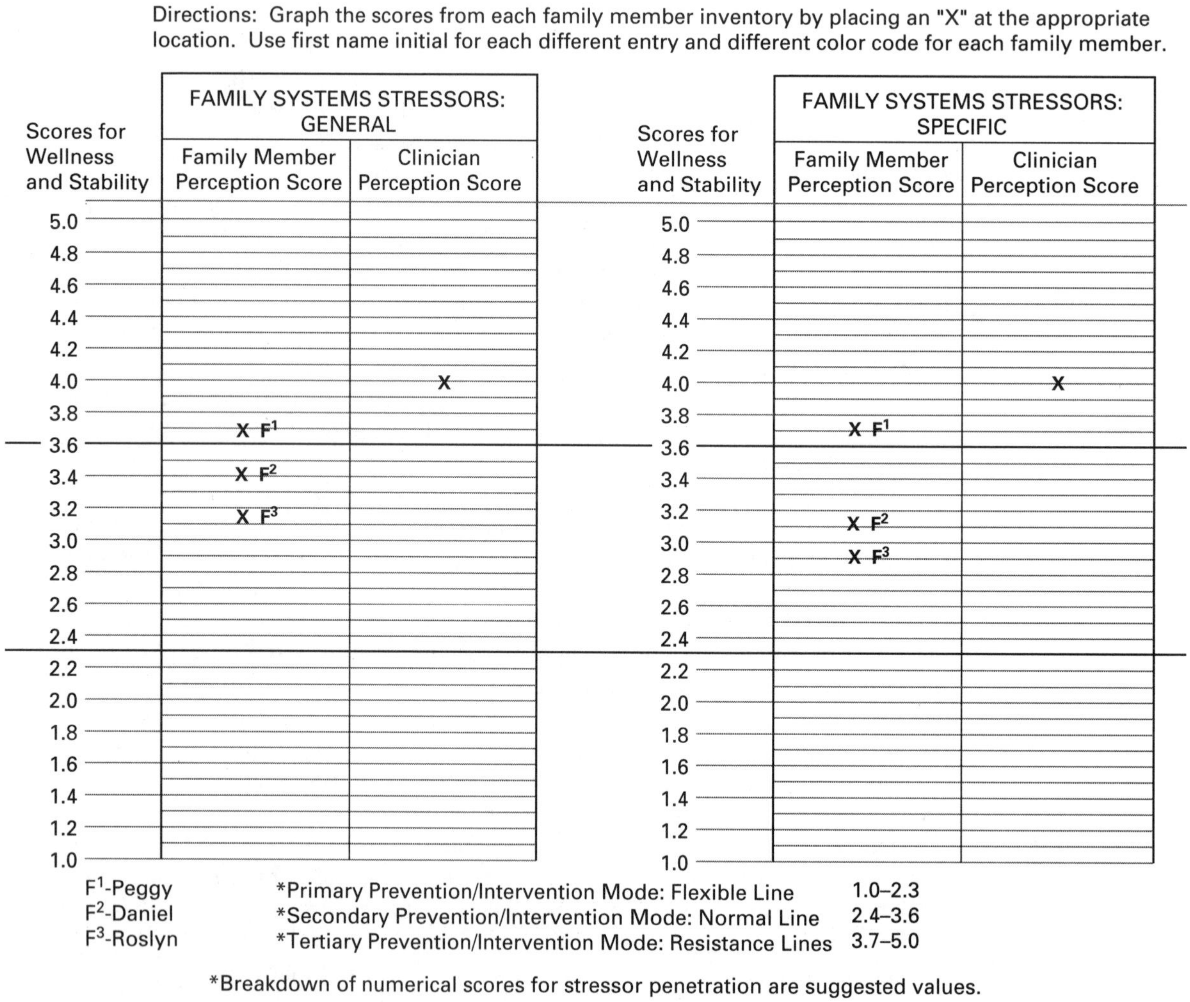
Directions: Graph the scores from each family member inventory by placing an "X" at the appropriate location. Use first name initial for each different entry and different color code for each family member.
FAMILY SYSTEMS STRESSORS: GENERAL
Scores for Wellness and Stability
Family Member Perception Score
Clinician Perception Score
FAMILY SYSTEMS STRESSORS: SPECIFIC
Scores for Wellness and Stability
Family Member Perception Score
Clinician Perception Score
5.0
4.8
4.6
4.4
4.2
4.0
3.8
3.6
3.4
3.2
3.0
2.8
2.6
2.4
2.2
2.0
1.8
1.6
1.4
1.2
1.0
X F1
X F2
X F3
X
F1-Peggy
F2-Daniel
F3-Roslyn
*Primary Prevention/Intervention Mode: Flexible Line 1.0–2.3
*Secondary Prevention/Intervention Mode: Normal Line 2.4–3.6
*Tertiary Prevention/Intervention Mode: Resistance Lines 3.7–5.0
*Breakdown of numerical scores for stressor penetration are suggested values.

FIGURE 7-7

Example of the Anderson family Family Systems Stressor Strength Inventory (FS^3I) quantitative summary of general and specific family systems stressors, including family and clinician perception scores.

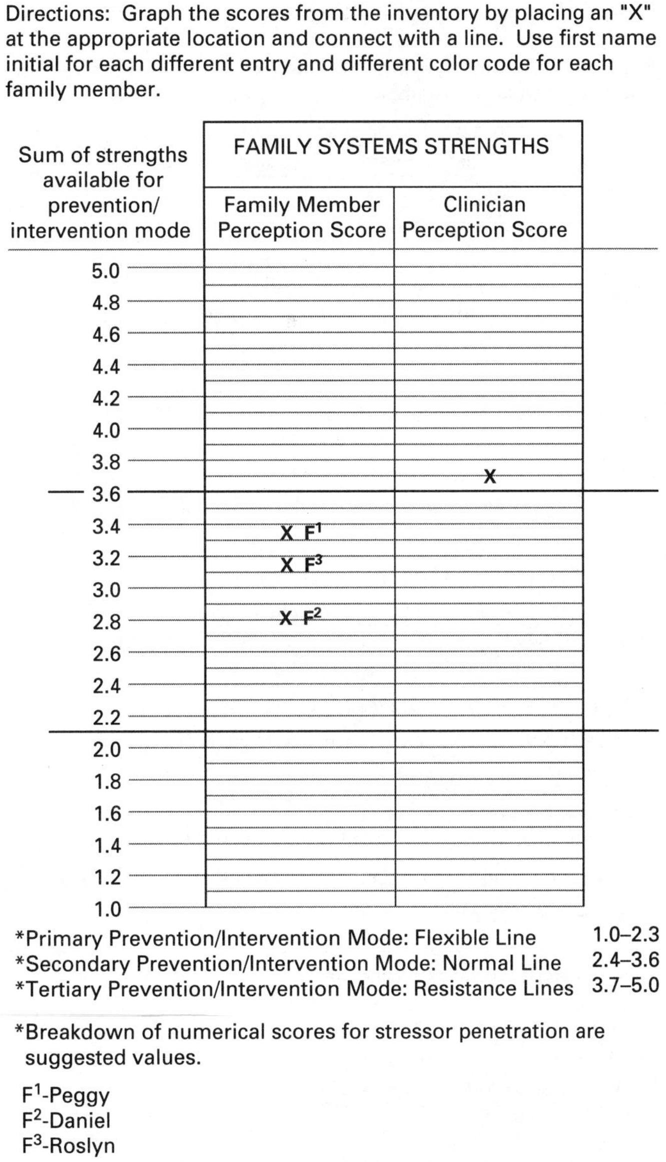

Directions: Graph the scores from the inventory by placing an "X" at the appropriate location and connect with a line. Use first name initial for each different entry and different color code for each family member.

Sum of strengths available for prevention/ intervention mode	FAMILY SYSTEMS STRENGTHS	
	Family Member Perception Score	Clinician Perception Score
5.0		
4.8		
4.6		
4.4		
4.2		
4.0		
3.8		X
3.6		
3.4	X F^1	
3.2	X F^3	
3.0		
2.8	X F^2	
2.6		
2.4		
2.2		
2.0		
1.8		
1.6		
1.4		
1.2		
1.0		

*Primary Prevention/Intervention Mode: Flexible Line   1.0–2.3
*Secondary Prevention/Intervention Mode: Normal Line   2.4–3.6
*Tertiary Prevention/Intervention Mode: Resistance Lines   3.7–5.0

*Breakdown of numerical scores for stressor penetration are suggested values.

F^1-Peggy
F^2-Daniel
F^3-Roslyn

FIGURE 7–8
Example of the Anderson family Family Systems Stressor Strength Inventory (FS^{3}I) quantitative summary of family systems strengths, including family and clinician perception scores.

nurse completed this summary using both verbal input and written data from the FS^{3}I. The family members and the nurse viewed the divorce, shooting, post-traumatic stress syndrome, and trauma surgery as general stressors. The family reported specific stressors as communication between the mother and children and the noncustodial father, finances, and lack of fun time. The nurse listed specific stressors as the aftermath of the divorce, single parenthood, and resource depletion. The strengths of the family were seen as communication between the mother and children, religious faith, the social support network, and good physical and mental health before the events. Overall the family members had similar

Part I: Family Systems Stressors: General

Summarize general stressors and remarks of family and clinician. Prioritize stressors according to importance to family members.

Divorce (visitation, custody, and child support issues)

Homicide of family friend. Post-traumatic Stress Syndrome

Post-trauma/surgery rehabilitation

Part II: Family Systems Stressors: Specific

A. Summarize specific stressor and remarks of family and clinician.

Family: Communication between divorced parents, economics, time for fun

Clinician: Divorce issues, single parenthood, resource depletion.

B. Summarize differences (if discrepancies exist) between how family members and clinician view effects of stressful situation on family.

Family and clinician see stressors about the same. Clinician views general and specific stressors higher than family. Clinician sees more family strengths than family members see in themselves.

C. Summarize overall family functioning.

Functioning quite well given recent traumatizing events and single parent structure. Physical health average and mental health good. Good social networks. Family adaptable.

D. Summarize overall significant physical health status for family members.

Physical health status of family members is good. Peggy is still recovering from nerve damage to arm and shoulder. Receiving physical therapy.

E. Summarize overall significant mental health status for family members.

Mental health appears fairly good at this time. Family well adjusted. Open and sharing feelings. Mother receiving counseling once a month.

Part III: Family Systems Strengths

Summarize family systems strengths and family and clinician remarks that facilitate family health and stability.

Family has been cohesive in time of trauma. Good communication patterns established earlier in family history helped family during this time. Religion and social support play important role in getting family through crisis.

FIGURE 7–9

Example of the Anderson family Family Systems Stressor Strength Inventory (FS³I) qualitative summary, including family and clinician remarks.

perceptions of their stressors and strengths and the nurse concurred with their perceptions; however, the nurse rated both stressors and strengths higher than the family members. The nurse concluded that they had the strengths they needed to deal with the stressors. The ecomap makes it apparent that the family was supported well by community resources, an important factor in coping with stress, and they used their resources to achieve a more positive health status than they had in the beginning.

Diagnosis General and Specific Family System Stressors	Family System Strengths Supporting Family Care Plan	Goals Family and Clinician	Prevention/Intervention Mode		Outcomes Evaluation and Replanning
			Primary, Secondary, or Tertiary	Prevention/Intervention Activities	
Divorce (custody, visitation, and child support) DX: Altered family processes	Religious faith Extended family support	Restoration of stability	Support family changes Children of divorce support group	Mother receive counseling	
Homicide of boyfriend Post-traumatic stress syndrome DX: Grieving, fear, powerlessness	Basic trust in one another Admit to and seek help with problems	Management of PTSD Healthy grieving process	Grief counseling Victim support group	Counseling Mother return to productive job that empowers her and strengthens her self-esteem	
Post-trauma surgery to arms and shoulders DX: Sensory-perceptual alterations	Seek help with problems Support one another Trust in family Trust health care professionals	Full arm and shoulder function without pain	Rehabilitation Physical therapy	Pain management	

FIGURE 7–10

Family Systems and Stressor Strength Inventory (FS³I) Family Care Plan. It is important to prioritize the three most significant diagnoses.

Friedman Family Assessment Form   Friedman's Family Assessment Short Form was also used with this family and was particularly helpful in planning for Peggy Anderson's discharge. This assessment provided data on the developmental stage and history of the family, the environment, the family structure, family functions, including health care, and family coping.

Developmental Stage and History of the Family   The family is in the developmental stage of childrearing family of adolescents. Betty was a college student and Daniel and Roslyn were teenagers. The children were age-appropriate in terms of their developmental tasks at the time of the divorce, but the divorce and shooting created some regressive behavior in Roslyn and some parentlike behavior in Daniel.

Environmental Data   The family lived in an upper-middle-class urban neighborhood at the time of the divorce. Afterwards, they were forced for economic reasons to move to a smaller three-bedroom house in a middle-class neighborhood. They were close to schools, church, and shopping areas, and the neighborhood was clean and safe. The family had a good network in the community, as the ecomap shows. The children were active in school, sports, and church activities. Victor lived in another part of the city with his new partner Beverly. The children were transported back and forth between their parents because their dad had visitation every other weekend. There were also frequent telephone calls between father and children.

Family Structure   The communication patterns in the family worked well, and the relationships between children and mother, and children and father were good, although the relationship between the two parents was tense at times. Peggy was quite verbal and expressive about her life and needs, which made for open and honest communication.

Peggy had always made the decisions around the home, even before she was divorced from Victor. Some of this power focus changed, however, as the children got older and participated more in decision making. The role structure in this single-parent family could also be considered binuclear, because the mother was in charge in one setting most of the time, but the father was the head of his own household when the children were with him.

Family Values   The mother, Peggy, was very clear about passing along her values to her children. The values she articulated included a Christian philosophy and action, a work ethic, open communication, learning, family cohesion, and trust in one another.

Family Functions: Affective Function   This single-parent family household was cohesive and close. Peggy was a responsive mother to her children and a child-centered parent in a healthy sense. She also stayed in contact with her extended family, and her parents were a great support to her and their grandchildren.

Family Functions: Socialization Function   The parents assumed the major role in socializing their children. Peggy in particular was involved in childrearing and was very involved with her children's friends as well. The children were doing well in school, at home, and at church in terms of performance, friendships, and adjustment.

Family Functions: Health Care   The family was connected with a primary physician and a major health center. They had good medical and dental care before the divorce and the shooting, and the care continued. Their physical and mental health appeared to be good in part because of their dietary practices, sleeping and resting habits, exercise and recreation, and other self-care practices. Peggy received tertiary care at a major medical center when she was hospitalized for the gunshot wound and posttraumatic stress syndrome. She continued to receive health care that included periodic counseling through the outpatient department of the medical center.

Family Functions: Family Coping   This family was seen shortly after the shooting, hospitalization, and discharge. At that time, they were coping remarkably well with familial stressors. They had some experience in dealing with crises in the past, which enabled them to hold together during this crisis in their lives. This effective coping was due in part to their financial stability, access to good health care resources, extended network and family support systems, and a past history of good physical and mental health.

Calgary Family Assessment Model   The CFAM was also used to assess the Anderson family, along with the FS³I and Friedman's family assessment form. The data obtained from the CFAM model on the structural, developmental, and functional components of the family were in many ways similar to the data obtained using Friedman's guidelines. However, the CFAM has a more expressive focus, and when the expressive segment of the CFAM tool was used with the Anderson family, more detailed information about emotional communication, verbal/nonverbal and circular communication, and family alliances/coalitions was obtained. For example, the verbal and nonverbal communications between Peggy and her children were congruent. The expressive nature of the family becomes more visible when more time is spent interviewing the family.

In summary, there is some overlap in the kind of information the nurse can glean using the three assessment models and approaches, especially because all three use the genogram and ecomap concurrently. Whatever approach the nurse uses, it needs to be consistent and systematic. Each approach may lead to different intervention strategies although they may be commonalities. Redundant information is less of a problem than missing information.

CURRENT STATUS OF FAMILY MEASUREMENT

Although general guidelines for family assessment have been published in a number of nursing textbooks in the past decade, instruments to measure family structure, function, and so on have only recently begun to be developed (Touliatos, Perlmutter, & Straus, 1990). Most instruments in the family literature were developed in other disciplines such as psychology, social work, and family social science. "There is a paucity of materials that speak specifically to family nursing measurement" (Berkey & Hanson, 1991, p. 228). Thus, most family instruments are "non-nursing" and may or may not be relevant to the phenomena of interest to family nurses. Of the three family-focused assessment models and approaches presented in this chapter (Berkey & Hanson, 1991; Friedman, 1992; Wright & Leahey, 1994), only the FS[3]I can be used both for general assessment and measurement of family dimensions.

Several major problems confront the nurse who tries to use family nursing assessment and measurement instruments. First, the instruments developed by nurses tend to be time-consuming to administer and they provide overwhelming information, which must then be summarized to set priorities for interventions. Second, the instruments make no clear link between assessment and intervention strategies. Third, the instruments have focused primarily on problems that families experience, rather than on family strengths on which nursing interventions can be built. Finally, the psychometric properties (reliability and validity) of family instruments are largely untested. Clearly, much work still needs to be done in to order to develop appropriate strategies and instruments to assess families.

SUMMARY

Many approaches, techniques, and models can be used to collect data on families. This chapter has presented three of the major models in the literature on family nursing assessment. None of the existing models or approaches suit all the needs of families and clinicians, in every situation. The advantage of learning and adopting one particular approach is that it then provides a framework for gaining expertise in systematically collecting data on the complex client nurses call "the family." Much work needs to be done in refining the assessment techniques and strategies available, and even more work needs to be done to make them efficient and effective in clinical settings. In particular, bridging the gap between assessment data and intervention strategies is critical. Assessment of the family as client is a challenging but rewarding part of nursing practice today and represents the practice of tomorrow.

STUDY QUESTIONS

1. Family assessment and family measurement mean the same thing.
   a. True
   b. False

2. Once the nurse assesses the family, they have all the information needed to develop a comprehensive care plan.
   a. True
   b. False

3. Match the following terms
   _____ a. Measurement   i. Systematic collection of data
   _____ b. Assessment   ii. Assigning numbers to an attribute
   _____ c. Qualitative   iii. Data that describe family characteristics
   _____ d. Quantitative   iv. Data that compare, measure, or count family properties

4. The Family Systems Stressor-Strength Inventory is a measurement instrument that evolved out of the model of the nursing theorist:
   a. Sister Callista Roy
   b. Dorthea Orem
   c. Madelaine Leininger
   d. Betty Neuman

5. Family stability is the goal of which model:
   a. Friedman's Family Assessment Model
   b. Calgary Family Assessment Model
   c. Family Assessment and Intervention Model

6. Friedman's model and the CFAM model yield substantially different kinds of information.
   a. True
   b. False

7. Friedman's model is based on which of the following theoretical frameworks? (You may choose more than one answer.)
   a. Structural-functional theory
   b. Systems theory
   c. Developmental theory
   d. Cybernetic theory

8. Wright and Leahey's model is based on which of the following theoretical frameworks? (You may choose more than one answer.)
   a. Structural/functional
   b. Systems theory
   c. Developmental theory
   d. Communications theory
   e. Change theory

9. Genograms and ecomaps should only be used with families if you are working with the whole group.
   a. True
   b. False

10. Nursing instrumentation is at an early stage of development.
    a. True
    b. False

11. How does family assessment fit into what we call nursing process?

12. How is family assessment different from individual assessment?

13. Give some examples of how qualitative measurement is used in your daily life. Quantitative measurement?

14. Compare measurement and assessment.

15. Discuss the current status of the development of family measurement.

16. Summarize the key parts of each family assessment model and discuss how they are different or overlap.

REFERENCES

American Nurses Association. (1980). *Social policy statement.* Kansas City, MO: Author.

Berkey, K. M., & Hanson, S. M. H. (1991). *Pocket guide to family assessment and intervention.* St. Louis, MO: Mosby Year Book.

Carlson, C. L. (1989). Criteria for family assessment in research and intervention contexts. *Journal of Family Psychology, 3,* 158–176.

Carter, E., & McGoldrick, M. (1980). The family life cycle and family therapy: An overview. In E. Carter & M. Mc-Goldrick (Eds.), *The family life cycle: A framework for family therapy* (pp. 3 - 28). New York: Gardner Press.

Curran, D. (1983). *Traits and the healthy family*. Minneapolis, MN: Winston Press.

Curran, D. (1985). *Stress and the healthy family*. Minneapolis, MN: Winston Press.

Feetham, S. (1983). *Feetham family functioning survey*. Available from Suzanne Feetham, National Center for Nursing Research, Office of Planning Analysis Evaluation, Building 31, Room 5BO9, Rockville Pike, Bethesda, MD, 20882.

Friedman, M. M. (1992). *Family nursing: Theory and practice* (3rd ed.). Norwalk, CT: Appleton & Lange.

Grotevant, H. D. (1989). The role of theory in guiding family assessment. *Journal of Family Psychology, 3*, 104 - 117.

Hanson, S.M.H, & Kaakinen, J. (1996). Family assessment. In M. Stanhope & J. Lancaster (Eds.) Community health nursing: process and practice for promoting health. St. Louis: CV Mosby.

Hanson, S. M. H., & Mischke, K. (1996). Family health assessment and intervention. In P. J. Bomar (Ed.), *Nurses and family health promotion: Concepts, assessment and interventions*. Philadelphia: W. B. Saunders.

Hartman, A., & Laird, J. (1983). *Family-centered social work practice*. New York: Free Press.

Keeney, B. (1982). What is an epistemology of family therapy. *Family Process, 21*, 153 - 168.

Kissman, K., & Allen, J.A. (1993). *Single-parent families*. Newbury Park, CA: Sage Publications.

McCubbin, M. A., & McCubbin, H. L. (1993). Families coping with illness: The resiliency model of family stress, adjustment, and adaptation. In C. B. Danielson, B. Hamel-Bissell, & P. Winstead-Fry (Eds.), *Families, health and illness: Perspectives on coping and intervention* (pp. 21 - 64). St. Louis, MO: C. V. Mosby.

McGoldrick, M., & Gerson, R. (1985). *Genograms in family assessment*. New York: W. W. Norton.

Mischke-Berkey, K., Warner, P., & Hanson, S. M. H. (1989). Family health assessment and intervention. In P. J. Bomar (Ed.), *Nurses and family health promotion: Concepts, assessment and interventions* (pp. 115 - 154). Baltimore: Williams & Wilkins.

Neuman, B. (1989). The Neuman systems model. In B. Neuman (Ed.), *The Neuman Systems Model* (2nd ed., pp. 3 - 50). Norwalk, CT: Appleton & Lange.

Pender, N., Barkauskas, V., Hayman, L., Rice, V., & Anderson, E. (1992). Health promotion and disease prevention: Toward excellence in nursing practice and education. *Nursing Outlook, 40*, 106 - 109.

Reed, K. S. (1993). *Betty Neuman: The Neuman systems model*. Newbury Park, CA: Sage Publications.

Ross, B., & Cobb, K. L. (1990). *Family nursing: A nursing process approach*. Redwood City, CA: Addison-Wesley.

Touliatos, J., Perlmutter, B. F., & Straus, M. A. (Eds.). (1990). *Handbook of family measurement techniques*. Newbury Park, CA: Sage Publications.

Waltz, C. F., Strickland, O. L., & Lenz, E. R. (1991). *Measurement in nursing research* (2nd ed.) Philadelphia: F. A. Davis.

Watzlawick, P., Beavin, J. H., & Jackson, D. D. (1967). *Pragmatics of human communication*. New York: W. W. Norton.

Watzlawick, P., Weakland, J., & Fisch, R. (1974). *Change: Principles of problem formulation and problem resolution*. New York: W. W. Norton.

Wright, L. M., & Leahey, M (1994). *Nurses and families: A guide to family assessment and intervention* (2nd ed.) Philadelphia: F.A. Davis.

Wright, L. M., & Leahey, M. (1993). Trends in nursing of families. In G. D. Wegner & R. J. Alexander (Eds.), *Readings in family nursing* (pp. 23 - 33). Philadelphia: J. B. Lippincott.

BIBLIOGRAPHY

Bomar, P. J. (Ed.). (in press). *Nurses and family health promotion: Concepts, assessment, and interventions* (2nd ed.). Philadelphia: WB Saunders.

Bowen, M. (1987). *Family therapy in clinical practice*. New York: John Wiley & Sons.

Clemen-Stone, S., Eigsti, D., & McGuire, S. (1991). *Comprehensive family community health nursing* (3rd ed.). St. Louis, MO: C.V. Mosby.

Danielson, C. B., Hamel-Bissell, B., & Winstead-Fry, P. (Eds.). (1993). *Families, health and illness: Perspectives on coping and intervention*. St. Louis, MO: C.V. Mosby.

Feetham, S. L., Meister, S. B., Bell, J. M., & Gilliss, C. L. (Eds.). (1993). *The nursing of families: Theory/research/education/practice*. Newbury Park, CA: Sage Publications.

Freeman, R. B., & Heinrich, J. (1981). *Community health nursing practice* (2nd ed.). Philadelphia: W. B. Saunders.

Gilliss, C. L., Highley, B. L., Roberts, B. M., & Martinson, L. M. (Eds.). (1989). *Toward a science of family nursing*. Menlo Park, CA: Addison-Wesley.

Hanson, S. M. H. (1985). *Family health inventory: A measurement*. Paper presented at the National Council of Family Relations, Dallas, TX.

Hanson, S. M. H. (1986). Healthy single parent families. *Family Relations, 35*, 125 - 132.

Hanson, S. M. H. (1987). Family nursing and chronic illness. In M. Leahey & L. Wright (Eds.), *Families and chronic illness* (pp. 2–32). Springhouse, PA: Springhouse.

Holt, S., & Robinson, T. (1979). The school nurse's assessment tool. *American Journal of Nursing, 79*, 950–953.

Leslie, G. F., & Korman, S. K. (1989). *The family in social context* (7th ed.). New York: Oxford University Press.

Nettle, C., Pavelich, J., Jones, N., Beltz, C., Laboon, P., & Pifer, P. (1993). Family as client: Using Gordon's health pattern typology. *Journal of Community Health Nursing, 10*, 53–61.

Parsons, T., & Bales, R. F. (1955). *Family socialization and interaction process*. New York: Free Press.

Pearson, A., & Vaughan, B. (1986). *Nursing models for practice*. Rockville, MD: Aspen.

Stanhope, M., & Lancaster, J. (1992). *Community health nursing: Process and practice for promoting health* (3rd ed.). St. Louis, MO: C. V. Mosby.

Toman, W. (1976). *Family constellation: Its effects on personality and social behavior* (3rd ed.). New York: Springer.

Tomm, K., & Sanders, G. (1983). Family assessment in a problem oriented record. In J. C. Hansen & B. F., Keeney (Eds.), *Diagnosis and assessment in family therapy* (pp. 101–122). London: Aspen.

von Bertalanffy, L. (1968). *General systems theory: Foundations, development, applications*. New York: George Braziller.

von Bertalanffy, L. (1972). The history and status of general systems theory. In G. Klir (Ed.), *Trends in general systems theory*. New York: John Wiley & Sons.

von Bertalanffy, L. (1974). General systems theory. In S. Arieti (Ed.), *American handbook of psychiatry* (pp. 1095–1117). New York: Basic Books.

Wegner, G. B., & Alexander, R. J. (Eds.). (1993). *Readings in family nursing*. Philadelphia: J. B. Lippincott.

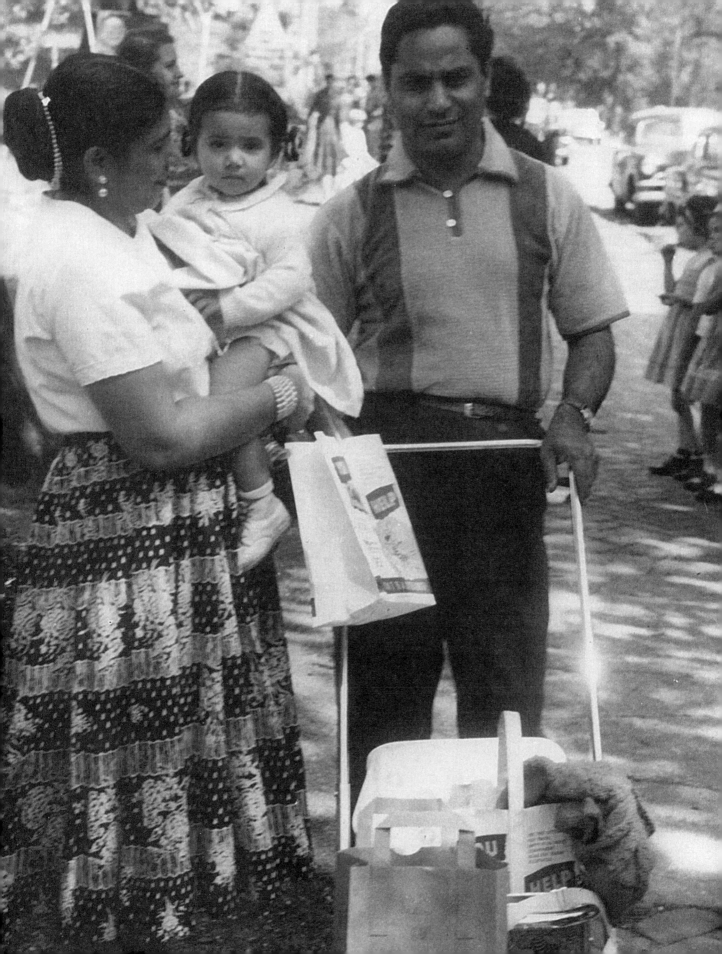

Family Health Promotion

The education of nursing students commonly focuses on illness and how nurses manage the human responses to illness. Health promotion provides nursing students with another critical element in the conceptual foundation of professional nursing practice with families.

This chapter begins with a careful description of health promotion and its historical relevance to family nursing in the United States. The discussion of family health and family health promotion will provide students with a clear understanding of these terms, their conceptual origins, and their contemporary applications. Models of both family health and family health promotion will assist the student in discriminating between them in practice.

External and internal ecosystem variables influencing family health promotion are carefully described and will add to the student's understanding of sociocultural influences on families. Students are urged to consider the influence of these factors on the roles of the family nurse identified in Chapter 1. The discussion of nursing process for family health promotion is an example of the use of health promotion as an organizing framework on which to base nursing actions with the family client. A timely discussion of the importance of health promotion to nursing practice, nursing education, family policy, and family nursing research concludes both this chapter and this section.

Before beginning the next section of this textbook, you are urged to step back and think about the material covered to this point. Consider what you have read in this section in general terms and how it has contributed to your understanding of family nursing.

Family Health Promotion

Perri J. Bomar, PhD, RN

OBJECTIVES

Upon completion of this chapter, the reader will be able to:

1. Define family health and family health promotion.
2. Understand the concept of family health promotion as distinct from but related to individual health promotion.
3. Trace the historical development of family health promotion.
4. Describe selected models of family health.
5. Explain variables influencing family health promotion.
6. Describe nursing interventions to facilitate family health promotion.
7. Examine the role of family health promotion in nursing practice, education, policy, and research.

Although the majority of health care professionals continue to focus their activities on treatment of illness in individuals and dysfunctional families, key social forces, including the wellness and self-care movement of the 1960s and 1970s, have stimulated the nursing profession to focus on health promotion for the family. In addition, the 1980 White House Conference on Families pointed to the need to target families to improve family functioning and encourage healthy family lifestyles. Each brought to light the importance of prevention and health promotion for improving the quality of family life in the United States and for reducing morbidity and mortality for individuals. Three documents from the US Department of Health and Human Services, *Promoting Health/Preventing Disease: Objectives for the Nation* (1979), *The 1990 Health Objectives for the Nation* (1980), and *Healthy People 2000* (1990), provide overall goals for the nation regarding health promotion. The objectives of the United States for the year 2000 include both health protective and disease preventive objectives.

Health protective objectives refer to reduction of unintentional injuries and improvements in occupational safety and health, environmental health, food and drug safety, and oral health. Preventive objectives are improvements in the ares of maternal and infant health, access to clinical services, and detection and treatment of diabetes and other chronic diseases; reduction and prevention of heart disease, stroke, HIV infections, and sexually transmitted diseases; prevention and treatment of cancer; increased immunization; and reduction of infectious diseases. Many state and local programs today are motivated by the desire to meet the national objectives for the year 2000. Most of the objectives will be more effectively attained if the family unit is considered along with the individual family members (Bomar, in press; Gillis, 1990; Doherty & Campbell, 1988).

For example, reducing violent and abusive behavior has implications for both individuals and the family. Family communication patterns, power issues, and decision making influence violent behavior. Negative expressions of anger by individuals and inadequate conflict resolution also will influence the likelihood of violent or abusive behaviors. Teaching individuals and families strategies to prevent abusive or violent incidents will enhance family health.

Because of the nation's emphasis on health promotion and the importance of the quality of family life in the late 1980s and the cry for a return to "family values" during the 1990s, the health professions, family scientists, sociologists, psychologists, and social workers have made considerable strides in understanding and intervening to improve the quality of family life. For example, in 1984 the National Council of Family Relations (NCFR) established a section on family health, whose members include health professionals interested in the health and illness of families across the life span. The United Nations designated 1994 as the "Year of the Family," reflecting the growing international concern for family health.

Fostering the health of the family unit as a whole and encouraging families to value health promotion and incorporate it into their lifestyle are important components of family nursing practice today. Health promotion is learned within the family, where beliefs, values, and patterns of behaviors are formed and passed along to future generations. The family is primarily responsible for providing care in health and illness, role modeling, teaching self-care and health-promoting behavior; providing care for members across the life span and during varied family transitions; and supporting each other in health-promoting activities and during acute and chronic illnesses. A major task of the family across the life span is health maintenance and health promotion for individual members and the family as a unit. The example in Box 8–1 describes a family scenario in which lifestyle changes would improve the mother's and the family's health. The role of the nurse is to help families attain, maintain, and regain the highest level of family health possible.

BOX 8-1 **Family Case Example**

The Budd Family

James (age 38 years) and Eleanor (age 36 years) have two sons Derek (age 8 years) and Dustin (age 10 years). James is a full-time engineer who teaches part-time at a community college. Eleanor has a full-time position as a professor of education and her classes are scheduled in the evenings 2 nights a week. James teaches Monday and Wednesday evenings and Eleanor teaches Tuesday and Thursday evenings. On the weekends and the other evenings the couple are either doing household chores, preparing for classes, or grading papers. Meals are usually rushed and often eaten at different times in front of the television, so that the family rarely eats meals together. While their parents are reading, working, or grading papers the boys either watch television, play video games, or do their homework. Except for family vacations and holidays, the Budds rarely spend time together enjoying each other's company. Eleanor was seen by a nurse in the family practice clinic for complaints of fatigue, lingering fluid and pain in her ears, vertigo, and nausea that has lasted 2 months. She was given antibiotics and nasal cortisone for her ear infection, after which her ear condition improved gradually. However, her complaint of extreme fatigue lingered. Laboratory tests revealed no physiological reason for the continuing fatigue. A nursing assessment of the family and Eleanor was completed using Pender's (1987) *Lifestyle Habits and Health Assessment Questionnaire* and Berkey & Hanson's (1991) *Family Systems Stressors-Strength Inventory*.

Major Family Stressors: insufficient "me" time, Eleanor's illness, decreased housekeeping standards, insufficient couple and family play time, television, inadequate time with the children, overscheduled family calendar, and lack of shared responsibility.

Family Strengths: shared religious core, respects privacy of one another, values work satisfaction, financial security, encourages individual values, affirms and supports one another, and trust between members.

Lifestyle Changes Indicated: increased individual time for parents, improved family recreation and couple time, revision of family calendar, and increased sharing of household tasks.

FAMILY HEALTH AND FAMILY HEALTH PROMOTION

The terms "family health" and "family health promotion" are not interchangeable. The term **family health** is used in referring to functional and dysfunctional families and to the biological, psychological, sociological, spiritual, and cultural aspects of family life. **Family health promotion** is directed toward achieving good family health.

Family Health

Definitions of family health have evolved from anthropological, biopsychosocial, developmental, family science, religious-cultural, and nursing paradigms, and they vary depending on their origin (Anderson & Tomlinson, 1992; Bomar, Neeley, & Palmer, in press; Doherty & Campbell, 1988; Duffy, 1988). Family scientists define a healthy family as resilient (McCub-

TABLE 8–1

TRAITS OF A HEALTHY FAMILY

Unity

Commitment

Develops a sense of trust

Teaches respect for others

Develops a sense of trust

Exhibits a sense of shared responsibility

Flexibility

Able to deal with stress

Adaptability

Sees crises as a challenge and opportunity

Open to change

Grows together in crises

Seeks help with problems

Communication

Positive Communication

Communicates and listens effectively

Fosters family table time and conversation

Shares feelings

Non-blaming

Able to compromise and disagree

Agrees to disagree

Time Together

Shares family rituals and traditions

Enjoys each other's company

Shares leisure time

Shares simple and quality time

Spiritual Well-Being

Encourages hope

Shares faith

Teaches compassion for others

Teaches ethical values

Respects the privacy of one another

Appreciation and Affection

Cares for each other

Has a sense of humor

Friendship

Respect for individuality

Has a spirit of playfulness

SOURCE: Adapted from Curran, D. (1983). *Traits of a Healthy Family.* Minneapolis, MN: Winston Press (pp. 23–24) and Olson, D. & De Frain, J. (1994). *Marriage* and the *family: Diversity* and *Strength.* Mountain View, CA: Mayfield.

bin & McCubbin, 1993) and possessing a balance of cohesion and adaptability that is facilitated by good communication (Olson, McCubbin, Barnes, Larsen, Muxen, & Wilson, 1989). Family therapy definitions often emphasize optimal family functioning and freedom from psychopathology (Bradshaw, 1988). From a developmental perspective, a healthy family is one that completes developmental tasks at the appropriate time (Duval & Miller, 1985). Taking a sociological view, Pratt (1976) described a healthy family as an "energized family"—a family that responds to the needs and interests of all its members; copes effectively with life transitions and problems; is flexible and egalitarian in the distribution of power; interacts regularly with each of its members and the community; and encompasses a health-promoting lifestyle for individual members and the family unit.

Other definitions of family health include the totality or gestalt of the family's existence and encompass the internal and external environment of the family. A holistic definition of family health encompasses all aspects of family life, including interactions and health care functions. Family health care functions include nutrition, recreation, communication, sleep and rest patterns, problem solving, sexuality, time, space, coping with stress, hygiene and safety, spirituality, illness care, health promotion, health protection, and the emotional health of family members (Bomar, 1989; Friedman, 1992). A healthy family has a sense of well-being and is free from dysfunction (Friedemann, 1989). In summary, family health is a dynamic and complex state. In a healthy family there is a sense of belonging and connectedness in family interactions, the family is flexible and adapts easily, and they work together to maintain the unit. Health is more than the absence of disease in an individual family member, or the absence of dysfunction in family dynamics; rather it is a state of family well-being.

The characteristics of a healthy family have been described by a number of authors (Curran, 1983; DeFrain & Stinnett, 1992; McCubbin & McCubbin, 1993). These characteristics include commitment to family, clear and flexible boundaries, flexible roles, resiliency, and hardiness (Bradshaw, 1988; US Department of Health and Human Services, 1990; McCubbin & McCubbin, 1993; Olson & DeFrain, 1994). The term "healthy family" is often used to denote a functional or a strong family. For example, DeFrain and Stinnett (1992) describe strong families as having commitment, appreciation, affection, positive communication, time together, spiritual well-being, and the ability to cope with stress and crisis. Table 8-1 summarizes the characteristics of health families described in the literature.

According to Anderson and Tomlinson (1992), family nurses' definitions of family health can be categorized as follows:

The *system view*, held by nursing theorists such as Berkey and Hanson (1991), Friedemann (1989), King (1983), and Neumann (1983)

The *family as the unit* of analysis (Fawcett & Whall, 1991; Gillis, 1991; Murphy, 1986; Wright & Leahey, 1984)

The holistic *biopsychosocial focus* (Bomar, 1989; Gillis, Highley, Roberts, & Martinson, 1989; Roberts, 1989; Newman, 1986; Pender, 1987).

Selected definitions of family health are shown in Box 8-2.

BOX 8-2 Selected Definitions of Family Health by Nurses

Family Health—

the family's quality of life as it is affected from a holistic perspective by such variables as nutrition, spirituality, environment, recreation, exercise, stress and coping, sexuality, health maintenance, and disease prevention (Bomar, 1994).

the health of the individual members of the family as well as the health of the family unit as whole.

the dynamic process that includes the activities a family uses to promote and protect the well-being of the family as a unit and individual members (Loveland-Cherry, 1989).

the process of expanding consciousness of the family. . . consciousness is defined as the informational capacity of the system and can be seen in the quantity and quality of interactions within the family and with the outside environment outside the family (Newman, 1983).

wellness and illness in interaction with the environment and five realms of the family experience: the interactive processes, the developmental processes, the coping processes, the integrity processes, and the health processes (Anderson & Tomlinson, 1992).

the effectiveness of family functioning. It is a dynamic balance of family maintenance, family change, family togetherness, and individuation (Friedmann, 1989).

viewed as a distinction brought forth through relationships and languaging with other human beings and continually in interaction with a unique and changing environment (Wright, Watson & Bell, 1990).

TABLE 8–2

PHASES OF THE FAMILY CYCLE OF HEALTH AND ILLNESS

Phase	Description
Family health (family health promotion and risk reduction)	The family develops and instills beliefs, values, and patterns that promote a healthy lifestyle and reduces the risk of disease or family dysfunction.
Family vulnerability and experience symptoms of illness	Members vulnerable to disease or the family unit vulnerable to dysfunction, stress, or crisis. The awareness that illness or dysfunction is present.
Family illness appraisal/sick role assumed	The meaning the family gives to the illness or situation. Also, includes initial role changes that give evidence of illness.
Contact with the health care system and diagnosis of the problem/illness	Seeking legitimating of the sick role or problem. Family acceptance of the diagnosis or solution.
Family acute response	Adjustments family make in response to an illnesses or situation. This includes making such adjustments as making arrangements in the family to care for the ill member, temporary role changes, and financial management.
Family adaptation to illness and recovery	Incorporation of the illness/event into family lifestyle while attempting to return to normalcy in family roles, structures, functions, and interactions.
Chronic adjustment/adaptation	Family makes adjustments in family roles, lifestyle, structure, functions, and interactions as it adjusts to the exacerbations and remission and treatment regimens.
Death of a member and recovery	Family adjustments and adaptations to the death of a member. This includes the period of grief and role adjustments involved in recovery to a healthy family of a different composition.

SOURCE: Adapted from Doherty, W. J. & Campbell, T. L. (1988). *Families and Health.* Newbury Park: Sage Publications, Inc. and Danielson C., Hamel-Bissel B. & Winstead-Fry, P. (1993) *Families in Health and Illness* (pp. 65–91). St. Louis: Mosby.

Anderson and Tomlinson (1992) noted ambiguity in some of the definitions of family health and suggested taking both a holistic view that incorporates wellness and illness and an ecosystems perspective. The family experience occurs in five realms: "the interactive process, the developmental processes, the coping processes, the integrity processes, and health processes of the family" (p. 61). This framework can be useful in guiding assessment, intervention, and research.

Models of Family Health

Building on Smith's (1983) models of health, Loveland-Cherry (in press) suggests that there are four views of family health:

1. The clinical model. Examined from this perspective, a family is healthy if its members are free of physical, mental, and social dysfunction.

2. The role-performance model. This view of family health is based on the view that family health is the ability of family members to perform their routine roles and achieve developmental tasks.

3. The adaptive model. In this model families are adaptive if they have the ability to change and grow, and the capacity to rebound quickly after crisis.

4. The eudiamonistic model. Professionals who use this model as their philosophy of practice focus on efforts to maximize the family's well-being and to support the entire family and individual members in reaching their highest potential (Loveland-Cherry, in press).

According to Loveland-Cherry, these family health models are useful in three ways. First, they provide frameworks for understanding the level of health a family is experiencing. Further, the models may be useful in designing interventions to assist families to maintain or regain good health or to cope with illness. Finally, the models may facilitate organization of the family nursing literature and serve as a focus for family research. There are numerous models incorporating stages of wellness and illness that explain the impact of illness on individuals and families.

The **Family Cycle of Health and Illness** of Danielson, Hamel-Bissell, and Winstead-Fry (1993) synthesizes the previous work of Doherty and McCubbin (1985) and of Coe (1970). Table 8–2 outlines this model, which depicts the dynamic movement between the phases of illness and wellness. Families do not always progress sequentially from one phase to another; some phases may be bypassed. For example, if all illness is transitory and brief (such as influenza), the family rapidly passes from a healthy state to symptom experience, the sick role, medical contact, adaptation, and then back to a health state. In transitory illness the process takes about 10 days. On the other hand, with a chronic disease the stages are longer and require more permanent family adjustments and adaptations. During each phase the family and its members engage in activities to foster family health and attain optimal levels of functioning.

Phases of the Family Health and Illness Cycle

Phase 1 in the cycle is the family health phase. During this phase the family engages in a variety of activities to improve and maintain the health of individual members and promote family functioning. For example, one health-promoting behavior is spending an evening together as a family. The second phase in the health and illness cycle is the family vulnerability and symptom experience phase, when the family perceives that its members are vulnerable and takes action to reduce the risk of illness of a member or the risk of family dysfunction. Risk reduction behaviors would include routine breast self-examination and immunizations for individuals and regularly scheduled family meetings to problem solve for family risk reduction. During this phase some families may use folk and home remedies for illnesses and consult their network for advice. If symptoms persist or adequate resources are not available, the family may then decide to make contact with a health professional. This decision initiates phase 3, assumption of the sick role and family illness appraisal. During this phase, the family accepts the sick role of the family member, evaluates potential threats or loss from the illness and their resources, and makes adjustments in family activities and the family lifestyle to accommodate the illness (Danielson et al., 1993).

In phase 4, the family consults health professionals to diagnose the illness and aid the family in understanding the illness or dysfunction. The level of family communication contributes significantly to family understanding and negotiating in this phase. After the illness is diagnosed, the family begins the fifth phase, which is called family acute response. The illness may progress to become acute or chronic, or result in death. If the ill member is cured and gives up the sick role, the family returns to phase 1, family health. If the illness continues, the family becomes a family with a chronically ill family member. Phase 6 is the period of recovery and rehabilitation in which the major tasks are relinquishment of the sick role, establishment of new patterns of family life, and return to phase 1. Long-term chronic diseases or severe disabilities bring phase 7, chronic adjustment adaptation. The family's ability to cope with the illness is influenced by their resources and their ability to adapt during crisis (McCubbin & McCubbin, 1993). After the death of a family member, the family enters phase 8, death and family reorganization, which includes the stressful processes of family grieving and reorganization of both family and extrafamilial roles and functions. After completing phase 8, the family unit returns to phase 1 of the cycle.

Family Health Promotion

Family health promotion in phase 1 of the family health and illness cycle. As with family health there is a lack of agreement on the definition of family health promotion. Bomar (in press) defines family health promotion as behaviors of the family that are undertaken to increase the family's well-being or quality of life. According to Pender (1987), family health promotion denotes family activities directed toward increasing their level of well-being and actualizing their potential. It involves the family's lifelong efforts to nurture its members, to maintain family cohesion, and to reach the family's highest potential in all aspects of health.

In the past, most of the attention of health professionals has focused on individuals and family subsystems (marital and parent-child dyads) and community health problems. There is a great need to encourage health promotion of the whole family unit since health behaviors, values, and patterns are learned within a family context. Family health promotion activities are important both during wellness and during illness of a family member. For example, if one member is ill the family may work together to provide for the physical needs of the sick person. At the same time, they must provide respite for the primary caregiver, so that this family member has time for health-promoting and health-protecting activities. An example of family health promotion is planning to have mealtimes together and to nurture the needs of all family members during an illness.

Family health promotion refers to activities families engage in to strengthen the family as a unit. The goal of these activities is to attain, retain, or regain the emotional and physical health of all family members. For example, in the Budd family in the case study (Box 8–1), health promotion can be enhanced through planning consistent family time. Family recreation and leisure time spent together promote family cohesion, unity, and bonding, and for this family participation in family time and sharing responsibilities could serve to reduce Eleanor's stress. During interactions the family may think of ways to assist each other in family maintenance.

Model for Family Health Promotion

Most models of health promotion focus on the individual. Adapting Pender's (1987) health promotion model, Loveland-Cherry (in press) suggests a family health promotion model. In this model, the probability of a family engaging in health promotion behaviors is influenced by the following factors relating to general health and specific behaviors:

General factors
   Family systems patterns
   Demographics
   Biological characteristics

Health-related factors
    Family health socialization patterns
    Family definition of health
    Perceived family health status
Behavior-specific factors
    Perceived barriers to health-promoting behavior
    Perceived benefits to health-promoting behavior
    Prior related behavior
    Family norms
    Intersystem support for behavior
    Situational influences
    Internal and family cues

A lay model for family health promotion is offered by Paul Pearsall (1990) in his book *Power of the Family: Strength, Comfort and Healing*. He encourages families to use their inner resources to strengthen, comfort, and heal family relationships. The major focus is on lifelong family unity and caring, using 10 strategies that he calls the "RXs" (Table 8–3). Nurses could encourage families to work together and use these strategies to promote health in family life.

In the past decade, family health promotion has received considerable emphasis in nursing and related fields. However, reports on the effectiveness of family-focused health

TABLE 8–3

PRESCRIPTIONS FOR A HEALTHY FAMILY

Families are encouraged to consider the following strategies to promote family health:

Family Rituals are the receptive behaviors or activities between two or more family members that occur with regularity in the day-to-day activities of daily living. Examples are a hug when a member leaves or returns, saying grace at meals, bedtime stories for children and so forth. Rituals provide security and attachment to oneness (unity) of the family system.

Family Rhythms means learning to do things together. This is a calm moving together in harmony during the family activities of daily living.

Family Reason is being reasonable during irrational times. Is there fairness and effort on everyone's part to reduce conflict? Recognition that one is a family is created not by being an actor but rather by interaction with others.

Family Remembrance is keeping of the family heritage, respect for family history and learning from the conflicts of members of the previous generation.

Family Resilience is the process of staying together through the stresses of life, to tolerate and grow as a unit with family spirit.

Family Resonance is to make good family vibes. It is a sense of the family as a unit of energy rather than a group of individuals. Family members are free to self-actualize as well as work together for family unity.

Family Reconciliation is the process of getting back together again after conflict. This includes always forgiving, tolerating, loving no matter what the family problem. Not allowing anything to destroy the family because unforgiveness leads to a life of regret.

Family Reverence is protecting the dignity of the family unit by concern for "us." Having a pride and respect for the uniqueness of the family unit and an "enduring commitment to the eternal unity of the family."

Family Revival is quick recovery from family conflicts, arguments, and feuds.

Family Reunion is the process of recollecting the family for the purpose of celebrating life together, maintaining family cohesion, comforting one another, learning from each other, and loving.

SOURCE: Pearsall, P. (1990). *The power of the family: strength, comfort, and healing.* New York: Doubleday.

promotion interventions are limited. In a study of parents' health-promoting lifestyles 6 months after contracting with a family nurse to make one change in the family lifestyle patterns, Bomar (1991) noted significant changes in lifestyles. There is a need for more research on the effectiveness of interventions to promote family health.

ECOSYSTEM FACTORS INFLUENCING FAMILY HEALTH PROMOTION

Family health promotion is the by-product of interactions with both external ecosystems and internal family processes. External ecosystem factors include such things as the national economy, family and health policy, societal and cultural norms, media, and environmental hazards (noise, air, soil, crowding, and chemicals). Internal factors include family type, family lifestyle patterns, family processes, the personalities of family members, power structure, family role models, coping strategies and processes, resilience, and culture.

External Factors Influencing Family Health Promotion

National Economy

The national economy directly affects the family's economic health; that is, the availability of jobs to meet the family's basic and health promotion needs directly affects the quality of a family's lifestyle. In addition, the availability of goods and services (food, clothing, shelter, medical care, insurance, transportation, and recreation) is basic to survival. In the past, the primary targets for health promotion programs were the workplace, some schools, and the middle class. Emphasis was placed on preventing heart disease by cessation of smoking, improved nutrition, and moderate exercise. Until the mid-1980s little attention was given to the health of minorities, people of low income, and the elderly (US Department of Health and Human Services, 1985).

Family Economic Resources

When a family has economic health, they have the resources needed for family health promotion. Adequate family income contributes to emotional well-being and supplies resources for family recreation and leisure. Socioeconomic class is an important ingredient in family health promotion. Middle- and upper-class families are more likely than poor families to engage in health-promoting and preventive activities. The cost of buying recreational and exercise equipment and apparel or paying for recreational activities is often beyond the means of low-income families. The activities of low-income families are often directed toward meeting basic needs — providing for food, shelter, and safety, and curing acute illness, rather than prevention or health promotion. Achieving better health for vulnerable and poor families in adverse family circumstances should be a goal for health professionals.

Family Policies

The United States does not have a national family policy. Historically, policy has focused on individuals rather than families, and even though there was a White House Conference on Families in 1980, there are still only a few policies specific to families. Debates on family policies are often highly politicized, and there is great disagreement about the need to provide family housing, universal access to health care, intergenerational supports, and consideration for family diversity (Wisensale, 1993).

Health Policies

Health policies at state, county, and city levels also affect the quality of family health. Local communities provide water and monitor its quality, maintain sanitation, develop and maintain parks for recreation, and provide health services to low-income and elderly families. Such local services enhance the health of individuals and enhance family health. At the state level services include assistance with medical care through Medicaid, the maintenance of state recreational areas and parks, health promotion and prevention programs, and economic assistance for low-income families. At the federal level, policies and fiscal support are needed to improve the quality of family health; in particular there is a need for (1) primary care for individuals across the life span, (2) child care policy, (3) more national parks and recreation areas, (4) agencies that monitor and develop legislation and implement health policies, (5) economic support for vulnerable families, and (6) research on families and family health. Many of the objectives in *Healthy People 2000* are couched in terms of individuals; however, many of these objectives can only be attained by changing family health lifestyles. Because of the number of different government agencies involved in health care and family issues, there is a need for collaboration among these policy-making bodies in a nation of diverse individuals and families.

Environment

Family nurses need to be aware of environmental issues that affect health. According to Wiley (1989), the family living environment (visible and invisible) is crucial. The family and its members are exposed to both occupational and nonoccupational hazards. Because not all environmental hazards are consistently monitored, it is crucial to teach families to prevent and remove environmental hazards.

Media

Another influence on family health is the visual and print media. Many advertisements advocate consumption of foods high in sugar, salt, and fat; alcoholic beverages; and the use of tobacco products. Health promotion advertisements have generally targeted the middle class, who are more health conscious than the vulnerable and underserved, who are often the targets for alcohol and tobacco advertising campaigns.

Science and Technology

Advances in science and technology have increased the life span of Americans, decreased the length of hospital stays, and contributed to our understanding of how to prevent, reduce, and treat disease. There are now many valuable sources of information on health promotion for families and individuals. At the same time, however, the development of more effective medications and advanced medical equipment (such as respirators, ventilators, electronic intravenous pumps, and smaller kidney dialysis machines) has greatly increased the feasibility of home health care for chronically ill family members of all ages. Families are often the caregivers for ill members, and they provide the majority of care to older adults. Often, the well-being of the family and caregivers is compromised, beginning with phase 3 of the Family Health and Illness Cycle and continuing to the end of phase 8 (from the sick role and family appraisal to the chronic illness phase or death and reorganization phase).

Internal Factors Influencing Family Health Promotion

Factors within the family that influence health promotion activities include:

Family developmental, for example, childbearing, school age launching, or retirement

Family type, for example, vulnerable, secure, durable, or regenerative (McCubbin & McCubbin, 1993)

Family structure, for example, single, nuclear, multigenerational, or dual career

Family process, for example, communication skills and patterns (Miller et al, 1988), social support networks (Roth, in press), family roles and role models (Friedman, 1992), vertical diffusion, and cultural health practices, values, and beliefs

Family lifestyle, for example, leisure, recreation, and exercising (McCown, 1994); eating patterns and rituals (James, 1994); sleep patterns (Kick, 1994); expressions of sexuality (Heinrich, in press); stress management and coping strategies (McCubbin & McCubbin, 1993); hygienic practices; illness behaviors, rituals and routines; and religious beliefs and practices.

Family Type and Development

Families who are flexible and able to adjust to change are more likely to be involved in health-promoting activities. Vulnerable families are often coping with a pileup of stressors and unable to focus on activities to enhance health. When families experience transitions, changes in their health-promoting lifestyles are often required. Thus, when a family member becomes ill, the health-promoting activities of the caretakers are generally curtailed. The stage of family development and the accomplishment of development tasks also significantly influence a family's ability to be healthy. For example, in the case study in Box 8-1, Eleanor's ability to reach her potential is influenced by the fact that her children are of school age and that she and her husband are a dual-career couple.

Family Structure

Families in the 1990s are quite different from the families of the 1970s. Family structures are more diverse; there are more dual-career/dual-earner families, blended families, and single-parent families. Vulnerable families have also increased — single-parent teen families, homeless families, low-income families, low-income single-parent teen families, migrant families, and low-income older adults. Health promotion for these different families presents different challenges. For example, a single working parent may have little parent-child time, experience role stress, and have poor lifestyle patterns (Hanson, 1986; Loveland-Cherry, 1986). Low-income families may focus less on health promotion but more on basic needs of obtaining shelter, adequate food, and health care.

Family Processes

Family processes are continual actions or series of changes that take place in the family experience. Essential family processes of a healthy family are functional communication and family interaction, which are both necessary to parenting and sharing of affection. Through both verbal and nonverbal communication, parents teach behaviors, share feelings and values, and make decisions about family health practices. It is through communication that families adapt to transitions and develop cohesiveness (Olson et al, 1989).

Culture

The influences of culture on family beliefs, attitudes, lifestyle patterns, and health behaviors are discussed in Chapter 4. Often, different cultures define and value health, health promotion, and disease prevention differently. For example, in some cultures family recreation is viewed as a waste of time and relaxation for stress management is considered laziness. Clients may not respond to the family nurse's suggestions for health promotion because they conflict with their health beliefs and values. Hence, it is crucial to assess the family culture and health beliefs before suggesting changes in health behavior.

Family Lifestyle Patterns

Lifestyle patterns affect family health. For example, when family members and the family as a whole engage often in leisure activities, recreation, and exercise, they are better able to cope with day-to-day problems (Curran, 1983). In addition, time together often promotes family closeness. In families with children, parents teach health practices and beliefs to children. Moreover, healthy lifestyle practices such as good eating habits, good sleep patterns, proper hygiene, and positive approaches to stress management are passed from one generation to another. Also, when one family member initiates a health behavior change, other family members often make a change too. For example, when an individual family member changes eating patterns, perhaps by going on a diet, other family members often change their eating pattern. Moreno (1975) calls this process "**vertical diffusion**."

Role Models

Family members provide both negative and positive role models. For example, smoking, use of drugs and alcohol, poor nutrition, and inactivity are often intergenerational patterns (Crooks, Iammarino, & Weinberg, 1987; Loveland-Cherry, 1986). Stress management, exercise, and communication are learned from parents, siblings, and extended family members such as grandparents (Duffy, 1986). Health professionals can promote positive family role modeling by health teaching in the community, the churches, and the workplace.

Religion

Another factor that influences family health promotion is religion. In a review of the research on religion and family health, Thomas and Cornwall (1990) note that research suggests that there is significant positive relationship between religion and marital well-being and satisfaction. In a study of 225 families in California on a nine-item religiousness scale, family religiousness was positively related to general well-being and social relations (Ranson, Fisher, & Terry, 1992). Further, in a study of the health of 42 single-parent families, Hanson (1986) found a significant positive relationship between religiousness and a child's mental and physical health. Curran (1983) has also reported that religion is a significant factor in family health.

Religion may be a positive force in family life because it: (1) is a source of social support and belonging; (2) encourages family togetherness through family activities and recreation; (3) provides a sense of meaning in family life and life; (4) promotes love, hope, faith, trust, forgiveness, forbearance, goodness, self-control, morality, justice, and peace; (5) encourages the use of divine assistance during times of family stress and crisis; and (6) teaches reverence for family life (Abbott, Berry, & Meredith, 1990; Curran, 1983; Brigman, 1992; Warner, in press). The social support of religion and the clergy is particularly helpful during family transitions such as weddings, baptisms, confirmations or Bar Mitzvahs, and at times of loss such as death, divorce, and so on (Warner, in press). Many churches have support groups for single parents, stepfamilies, single adults, the bereaved, widows and widowers, the unemployed, and parents of young children. For example, to meet the spiritual needs of a congregation of over 2000 members, the Rancho Bernardo Presbyterian Community Church in San Diego, California, has pastors for a family life ministry, healing ministries (emotional healing), youth and single adults, and a senior ministry.

In order to provide holistic care, the nurse needs to assess a family's spiritual health, support the family's spiritual beliefs, assist families to meet their spiritual needs, provide spiritual resources for family transitions and lifestyle changes, and assist families to find meaning in their circumstances (Carson, 1989; Warner, 1994; Brigman, 1992). Such activity is validated by findings that a family is spiritually strengthened by togetherness, making the family a priority, honor and respect for each family member, support of the needs of **individuation**, commitment to the family, daily prayer, dedication and renewal, honesty, and integrity (Friedemann, 1989; Warner, 1994).

THE NURSING PROCESS FOR FAMILY HEALTH PROMOTION

Family nurses have a crucial role in facilitating health promotion within the family context across the life span. Enhancing the well-being of the family is essential during periods of wellness, as well as during illness, recovery, and stress. A primary goal of nursing care for families is empowering the family to work together to attain and maintain family health. The family nursing process includes family assessment, contracting and goal setting, intervention and health teaching, evaluation, and follow-up.

According to Pender (1987) there are four phases in the nurse-client relationship: the initial phase, the transition phase, the working phase, and the step-down and follow-up phase. During the initial contact phase, the nurse identifies the need for health care. This is followed by the transition phase, when the client decides whether to continue the nurse-client relationship. Commitment to do so may be demonstrated by signing a contract. In the working phase, the energies of both the nurse and client are expended to meet the stated goals — a process requiring that the nurse and client collaboratively devise a plan for reaching these goals; that the client and nurse meet periodically to review progress; and that the nurse provide feedback and reinforcement. This periodic review process requires commitment on the part of both the nurse and family. A final evaluation of progress and provisions for follow-up comprise the terminal phase of the nurse-client relationship.

When working with families in the realm of health promotion, the nurse often makes assumptions about families and self-responsibility for their health. According to Bomar (in press), the following assumptions are a useful guide for family health promotion and nursing practice:

1. Families are ultimately responsible for their own health.

2. Families have the capacity to change in constructive as well as destructive directions.

3. Families have a right to health information in order to make informed decisions about behaviors and lifestyle choices.

4. The health-seeking process occurs in the context of interpersonal and social relationships.

5. Families will only employ health behaviors that they find relevant and compatible with their family lifestyle and structure.

6. Families have the potential for improvement in their health, and this can be enhanced by a nurse who is caring.

Family health promotion needs and interventions, which differ for each family, will be influenced by the nurse's assumptions.

Assessment

The purpose of assessment is to determine a family's health status by thorough examination of family interaction, development, coping, health processes, and integrity (Anderson & Tomlinson, 1992). As explained in Chapter 2, the models that nurses use to assess family health vary. A holistic nursing model for family health promotion includes structural and functional, health promotion, and health protection components of the family system.

Assessment helps the nurse to identify family strengths that foster health promotion and stressors that impede health promotion. It also assists the nurse to identify areas for intervention. Such interventions may include promotion of family integrity, maintenance of family process, exercise promotion, environmental management, mutual goal setting, and parent education (Iowa Intervention Project, 1992). The assessment of the Budd Family (Box 8-1) provides an example in which there are many areas for growth in health promotion and lifestyle.

Family Contracting

Contracting with a family to change or initiate an activity to strengthen family health increases the likelihood of attaining desired goals (Hill & Smith, 1990; Gray, 1994; Pender, 1987). A **contract** is based on a set of goals mutually agreed on by a health care provider and an individual or family (Hill & Smith, 1990; Steiger & Lipson, 1985). It may be oral or written. There are three types of contracts. The first is a nurse/client contract, which is an agreement between the nurse and client (family) to work together to attain goals that are determined by the client. The second type is called a contingency contract. This type of contract includes the process of setting a goal and identifying costs and rewards of goal attainment with a health professional or other support person (Steckle, 1982). The purpose of the contingency contract is to reinforce the behaviors needed to reach a goal. The third type of contract is the self-care contract. The client develops this type of contract independently of a health professional. The contract is between two individuals for the purpose of improving a health behavior.

Contracts are useful for making lifestyle changes, reframing attitudes, and modifying unhealthy interaction patterns. They are most effective when the components are negotiated and signed by all family members. The disadvantages of contracts are that they are time-consuming to develop and that they require commitment by the health professional and all family members involved. In addition, periodic re-evaluation and renegotiation may be necessary.

The health of the Budd family (Box 8-1) might be improved by contracting to work as a family on such activities as increasing family time and recreation, providing personal time for Eleanor, sharing household tasks, and revising the family calendar. The family could be advised to contract as a unit to reduce each of the identified stressors. There are few reports on the success rate of family contracting. However, Swain and Steckle (1981) reported improvement in health promoting behaviors in clients with hypertension, diabetes, and arthritis who followed their contracts. Detailed discussions of contracting can be found in Hill and Smith's (1990) *Self-Care Nursing Promoting Health* and Pender's (1987) *Nurses and Family Health Promotion*. These authors also suggest strategies to facilitate attaining, regaining, or maintaining a health-promoting lifestyle.

Nursing Interventions in Family Health Promotion

In the working phase, the family and the nurse collaborate to make changes in the family's lifestyle that will enhance the family's health. The nurse collaborates with the family and provides information, encouragement, and strategies to help the family make lifestyle changes. This process is termed empowerment.

Empowerment is the process of providing people information and resources to help them attain their goals. A family's goal may be to reframe a situation, strengthen behaviors that enhance coping with stress or crisis, or incorporate health-promoting activities in family behavior patterns. A family whose member is dying of AIDS can be empowered by teaching them how to cope with feelings of isolation and how to obtain resources and social support in the family and the community. The primary emphasis in family empowerment is on involvement of the family in goal setting and planning, and not on having the nurse do this for the family (Gray, 1994).

Often, contemporary families focus on individual family members and the family unit seems to be forgotten. For example, the Budd family spent little time together as a family. The parents provided food, shelter, safety, health care, and education for their family, but there was little time for family bonding and closeness. Antibiotics cured Eleanor's inner ear infection; however, getting rid of her extreme fatigue might require changes involving the entire family. After an assessment of the Budd family's strengths and stressors, nursing interventions might include: (1) evaluation of the family and individual calendars and schedules, (2) discussion of strategies to provide rest and personal time for James and Eleanor, (3) discussion of the significance of family togetherness, and (4) encouragement to plan for more couple time and parental time with each of their sons.

A key role of nurses in health promotion for families is encouraging them to value their "oneness," to appreciate family togetherness (Bradshaw, 1990; Friedemann, 1989), and to plan activities to foster their unity. One way to enhance family bonding among the Budds would be to share meals together when possible. Because Eleanor has extreme fatigue, other family members could help with meal preparation. This would give them an opportunity to be together, enhance communication, and reduce role strain for Eleanor. This family could also negotiate a family contract for weekly scheduled family time. Each member would make that family time a priority and let no other activity interfere with it. The nurse could help by consulting local newspapers, family magazines, and community agencies for activities that might interest the entire family.

During their life course, families will inevitably experience crises and stress. The family resilience, unity, and resources will influence how they cope with crisis and stress (McCubbin & McCubbin, 1993; Pearsall, 1990). The goal of the family nurse is to facilitate family adaptation by suggesting strategies to promote family resilience, reduce the pileup of stressors, make use of resources, and negotiate necessary changes to enhance the family's rebound from stressful events or crises. The nurse can teach families to anticipate life changes, make the necessary adjustments in family routines, evaluate roles and relationships, and cognitively reframe events. For example, in military families changes occur in family decision-making, roles, responsibilities, communication patterns, and power when the military member is deployed. Anticipatory guidance by health professionals could help military families plan to maintain communication, anticipate economic changes, maintain the household, and parent the children long distance.

Families may need help in meeting both the needs of the family as a whole and individual needs. In order to find a balance, each family member should have time alone to develop a sense of self and to focus on spiritual growth. Friedemann calls this "individuation." The family also needs to plan "family time," when the sense of belonging and "oneness" or "togetherness" can be experienced. Healthy families have both kinds of time (Olson & DeFrain, 1994; Friedemann, 1989).

Families may need to be reminded of the importance of togetherness, a sense of which can help them cope with life stressors and crises more effectively. Family unity often improves as a result of family celebrations, rituals, and routine family activities. Instruments such as the Family Times and Routines Inventory (McCubbin & McCubbin, 1993) can help the professional to identify family routines and the APGAR (Smilkstein, 1978) can be used to determine the level of family satisfaction.

Confluence

Confluence, or the process of combining activities to promote togetherness, fosters family unity and closeness (Friedemann, 1989). The use of confluence by the Budd family (Box 8–1) would give them more time for family interaction and reduce the work load for Eleanor. For example, James and Eleanor could work side by side doing household chores on Saturday, everyone could alternate in assisting Eleanor with meal preparation and clean up, the boys could do their homework in the same room while their parents graded papers, and everyone could be assigned a task so that they could work together to complete the weekend household upkeep. Pearsall (1990) suggests that family togetherness is fostered by planning to routinely eat most meals as a unit, having regularly scheduled family time, and going to bed and waking up at the same time.

Strategies to Intervene in Family Health Promotion

Once the nurse and family have identified family strengths and areas for growth or change, the family should prioritize their goals. The commitment of all family members to achieving a goal is crucial to the family's success in reaching it. Goal attainment can be encouraged by negotiating contracts, which often include agreements to change family interaction patterns, behaviors, or lifestyle patterns. The nurse can help to negotiate and implement contracts and can also serve as health teacher, resource finder, and evaluator of the family's health promotion plan, Pender (1987) provides in-depth information on developing a plans for health protection and promotion.

An example of an activity to promote family unity is an African-American family's desire to start an annual celebration of Kwanza (Mgeni, 1992). To be successful, the specifics of rituals, time, supplies, and activities must be learned and negotiated by each family member. The primary role of the nurse is health teaching about the goal and strategies to reach this goal, including information about community resources. The family's primary activity is to agree on family system changes and to evaluate their progress. Periodic discussions are needed to determine the effectiveness of the activities.

Areas in which the nurse can provide family support, anticipatory guidance, family education, and family enrichment include:

Coping with family transitions (such as births, acute and/or chronic illnesses, separations, launching children, divorce, death, and retirement)
Family and individual dietary patterns
Family and individual recreation and exercise
Family sexuality
Family sleep and rest patterns
Family environmental practices
Socialization and rearing of children
Risk reduction and socialization in health care practices (prevention and promotion)

Encouraging a balance between togetherness and individuation

Providing for family systems and household maintenance

Encouraging family spirituality (Bomar, in press; Friedman, 1992; Friedemann, 1989; Warner, in press)

Although beginning family nurses may not be skilled in all these areas, they can seek out community resources (family recreation, or classes on parenting, communication, or understanding family dynamics) for well families.

Family needs and nursing interventions will differ with different family structures and at different times in the family life course. For example, in a nuclear family, health promotion includes promotion of a healthy marriage. In such a family, the family nurse can suggest that the family:

Make the marriage a priority

Communicate regularly

Practice encouragement

Schedule meetings about family maintenance and couple issues

Set up rules for negotiations and conflict resolution

Plan regularly for activities to have fun (Carlson, Sperry, & Dinkmeyer, 1992, p. 86).

A major force in the development of a healthy family is commitment to family unity and shared negotiation of family goals. An important aspect of family nursing practice is provision of anticipatory guidance to adult family members to help them understand and value individual, dyad, parent-child, and family development issues and transitions.

Health Teaching and Anticipatory Guidance

Nurses working with well families can teach family awareness, encourage family enrichment, and provide information on community agencies that are resources for strengthening and enriching families. One example of a community resource is a family wellness program founded in 1980 in San Jose, California (Doub & Scott, 1992). A class in the program, called "Survival Skills for Healthy Families," is taught to families in schools, churches, community centers, and hospitals, and also is a component of drug, alcohol, and spouse and child abuse prevention programs. A contract can be made with the family to attend or find out more about such a program. The family nurse should be able to provide families with information about available community resources. In some cases, the nurse may need to call or visit and observe an agency in action to determine its appropriateness.

The beginning family nurse is prepared to intervene by teaching about healthy processes (basic nutrition, exercise routines, hygiene, preventive health practice, and awareness of family). Basic teaching strategies are suggested by Redman (1993). Advanced family nursing interventions such as family life education, family enrichment, and marriage enrichment are more appropriate for graduate nurses, family life educators, marriage and family counselors, and therapists.

Some communities have family enrichment programs for well families, and recently "ministers of health" have been appointed in churches, parishes, and synagogues. In the early 1980s, a national multidisciplinary organization called the Health Ministries Association was formed with the goal of promoting a healthy body, mind, and spirit for all persons in religious congregations. Members include pastors, health educators, health professionals, and concerned congregation members. With the development of such health ministries many nurses are assuming positions as parish nurses, in which they combine nursing care with spiritual counseling from a holistic perspective (Mikulencak, 1992). In 1990 three universities had graduate specialty degrees in parish nursing (Chandler, 1992), and there is now a National Parish Nurse Resource Center.

Activities of a health ministry program often include:

Education on health promotion, wellness, disease prevention, and other topics for families and individuals across the life span

Coordination of volunteers to provide social and network support to members with lifestyle and health problems

Personal counseling

Monitoring and screening for health promotion, disease prevention, and treatment of chronic diseases

Parenting and fatherhood classes

Service as a health resource and referral agent

Support groups for single parents, older adults, and remarried families

Promotion of the integration of faith and health

The address of the Parish Nurse Resource Center is in the Resources List (Appendix A).

Many communities provide resources such as couple communication workshops, family retreats, family magazines, parenting classes for young and adolescent families, support for stepfamilies, lesbian and gay support groups, and so forth. A list of selected family agencies and resources appears in Appendix A.

Preparation for Termination

As the individual or family approaches their goal, the nurse sees the client less frequently. Pender (1987) calls this the step-down phase. During this phase the family takes on more responsibility for planned activities and becomes more self-reliant in problem solving and evaluating their progress toward goals.

Evaluation and Follow-Up

The follow-up phase (Pender, 1987) is the last phase of nursing intervention. During this phase, the progress of the client/family toward the health promotion goals is reviewed, and if the goals are not met, other options are discussed and planned. After the desired change has been incorporated into the family lifestyle, the nurse discontinues family appointments; however, an opportunity is provided for families to follow up with the nurse by appointments, calls, or periodic visits. The family is taught how to contract as a family and is provided with resources for other areas of family health promotion and protection.

HEALTH PROMOTION AND FAMILY NURSING

As resources change in the 1990s and individuals and families are encouraged to assume more responsibility for their care, supporting families in the area of health promotion will be very important. Major tasks of nursing with families are to use the nursing process in partnership with families, to help families find ways to achieve their lifestyle and health care goals, to illuminate the importance of family health promotion, to serve as a family advocate, and to be an expert in family health promotion matters. The goals is for families to attain, maintain, or regain the highest possible level of family health. The following discussion concerns the importance of health promotion to the future of family nursing.

Nursing Practice

In the next decade, the settings where nurses encounter families will change. There is a continuing shift in health care from the hospital to community settings, so that nurses will have more direct interactions with families in ambulatory health care settings and homes. A comprehensive family assessment may facilitate the development of a holistic health plan for those who are ill; and because more ill family members will receive care in their homes, the impact on family wellness will also need evaluation. In addition, strategies will be needed to provide health promotion and health protection for individual members and the entire family in community-based as well as inpatient settings. Basic and advanced roles of family nurses are listed in Table 8-4.

At all stages of the family health and illness cycle, the goal is to return the family as a whole to their highest health potential. In community settings such as churches and work sites, the nurse can provide programs for family health promotion. Selected topics include parenting from infancy to old age; role changes during family and individual transitions such as retirement, birth of a new baby, bereavement, and so forth; and coping with individual and family stressors. Single-parent and blended families often need anticipatory guidance, family enrichment activities, and parent and stepparenting education. The nurse can encourage all family members to monitor their family for its unity, strengths, and a sense of belonging.

TABLE 8-4

ROLES OF THE FAMILY HEALTH NURSE IN FAMILY HEALTH PROMOTION

Beginning Family Nursing Roles

Health teacher

Counselor

Facilitator

Caregiver

Collaborator

Advocate

Role model

Advanced Family Nursing Practice Roles

Case manager

Clinical specialist

Family consultant

Family advocate

Leader in family health matters

Researcher

Supervisor

Health planner

Theory developer

SOURCE: Adapted from Bomar, P., McNeeley, G., & Palmer, I. (1989). Family health nursing: History and role. In P. Bomar (Ed.) *Nurses and Family Health Promotion: Concepts, assessment and interventions.* (pp. 1–12). Philadelphia: WB Saunders.

In any setting, nurses can advocate for families by writing and voting on family issues, supporting a philosophy of practice that encourages family nursing, volunteering in community activities for families, and supporting family programs.

Nursing Education

There is little standardization of family content in schools of nursing in the United States (Hanson, Heims, & Julian, 1992; Hanson & Heims, 1992). In addition to traditional content on family theoretical frameworks, illness, stress and coping, and crisis, curricula at the undergraduate and graduate level should include content on family health promotion. At the present time, however, few students are prepared in family health promotion. The emphasis in most curricula is on acute and chronic physical illness, psychosocial problems, and community nursing; the primary focus is on the individual in the context of the family. Limited attention is paid to groups of families in the community or to well families.

If nurses are to be a part of the efforts to meet the national health goals for the year 2000, undergraduate and graduate curricula in schools of nursing will need to include content on the family as the unit of care and on family health promotion and disease prevention. Schools of nursing will need to find or create innovative sites for clinical practice where students can provide nursing care to well families. Such sites might include a nursing clinic in a low-income housing project, a senior center, or a family exercise center; practice with a parish nurse; work site classes; or a school or nursing clinic.

Family Policy

The document *Healthy People 2000*, which incorporates 22 specific goals, and the current emphasis on comprehensive health care for all citizens will help to shape local, state, and national policies geared toward improving family health. The passage of the 1993 Family Leave Policy marked a beginning in the effort to implement policies to improve the quality of family health. In order to reach the 22 goals for the nation by the year 2000, families must be empowered to assume more responsibilities in the realm of health promotion and disease prevention for family members. Family issues most frequently reviewed by policy makers include marriage, divorce, family violence, abortion, child care, child health care, and family health insurance coverage. Based on an in-depth review of the literature, Zimmerman (1992) concluded that the well-being of individuals and families is better in states where the government meets the needs of the citizens through policies to improve the quality of life. According to Wisensale (1993), family health policy should include (1) a national family policy agenda, (2) universal access to health care, (3) housing for low- and middle-income families, (4) intergenerational family issues, and (5) work and family issues; further, policy should reflect the diversity in family structure (pp. 249–250). The family nurse needs to be aware of policies advancing family health throughout the family life course and should support them. Nurses can support family policy legislation by keeping informed about issues, voting, communicating with policy makers, giving expert testimony, maintaining membership in and supporting professional nursing organizations, and financially supporting the political advocacy activities of health professional organizations.

Family Nursing Research

Research on family health promotion is beginning to be carried out (Duffy, 1988). The creation of the National Institute of Nursing Research (NINR) in 1993 has provided a focus for family nursing research. The NINR's agenda for nursing research includes developing and testing community-based programs to promote family health using nursing models, and assessing the effectiveness of nursing interventions for families during the chronic illness of a family member (National Institute of Nursing (NINR) Outreach, Fall, 1993). Although in the past most family research was actually research on individuals in the family context, the research agenda set by NINR will provide significant knowledge about approaches to improving the quality of family life.

SUMMARY   As resources change in the 1990s and as individuals and families are encouraged to assume more responsibility for their health care, supporting families will be an important task for the nurses who treat them. The major tasks are to use the nursing process in partnership with families, help families find ways to achieve their lifestyle and health care goals, illuminate the importance of family health promotion, serve as a family advocate, and be an expert in family health promotion. The goal is to assist families to attain, maintain, or regain the highest possible level of family health.

STUDY QUESTIONS

1. Many factors help determine whether a family is involved in health promotion. Which of the following factors may influence promotion of a family's health?
   a. Type of family
   b. Quality of family interaction
   c. Developmental level of family
   d. Quality of family housing
   e. All of the above

The Jones family has four members: Tyrone, the father, age 39 years; Marcia, the mother, age 30 years; Barbara, age 8 years; and James, age 15 years. James has hemophilia and has AIDS, which he contracted from a blood transfusion about 3 years ago. He began to show symptoms a year ago, was prescribed an experimental drug, and is currently asymptomatic. He attends high school daily but tires easily. The parents come in to the HIV clinic with James for a routine checkup. They say that he does not have much to say and stays in his room a lot after school; in fact all the family members stay in their own rooms most of the time. Meals are usually eaten separately. James says he eats dinner in his room most evenings and complains about feeling lonely and avoided. The parents, in turn, feel that James is avoiding them at meals.

2. What stage of the Family Health and Illness Cycle is this family experiencing?
   a. The vulnerability and symptom experience cycle
   b. The health phase
   c. Chronic adjustment/adaptation phase
   d. Rehabilitation

3. Family process influences how a family adapts to a family health issue. Which of the following processes would be most helpful in improving the quality of this family's life?
   a. Communicating as a family about how each feels about James' health

   b. Ignoring the problem; it will take care of itself
   c. Insisting that James eat with the family
   d. Understanding that each one is grieving and deciding not to worry about it

4. Which of the following best describes key traits of a healthy family that this family does *not* appear to have?
   a. Experiences happiness, is financially secure, takes vacations
   b. Resilience, spends time together, and communicates positively
   c. Resilience, united in coping with AIDS,

spends time together

d. Flexibility, sense of humor, communicates positively

5. Internal family factors possibly influencing the level of this family's well-being are:
   a. James' disease
   b. Reaction of peers to AIDS
   c. Fear of the family of AIDS
   d. Lack of exercise of members
   e. a and b only

6. To empower this family to resolve the crisis so that James does not feel alone and the rest

of the family does not feel avoided, the nurse would:

a. Tell them exactly what to do to resolve the issue

b. Teach them ways to communicate and problem solve

c. Encourage development of a family contract to spend time together as a family

d. Allow them to work the issue out by themselves

e. b and c

REFERENCES

Abbott, D. A., Berry, M., & Meredith, W. H. (1990). Religious belief and practice: A potential asset in helping families. *Family Relations, 39*, 443–448.

American Nurses' Association. (1980). *Nursing: A social policy statement.* (ANA Publication No. NP-63-35M).

Anderson, K. H., & Tomlinson, P. S. (1992). The family health system as an emerging paradigmatic view for nursing. *Image: Journal of Nursing Scholarship, 24*, 57–63.

Berkey, K. M., & Hanson, S. M. H. (1991). *Pocket guide to family assessment and intervention.* St. Louis, MO: C. V. Mosby.

Bomar, P. J. (Ed.). (1989). *Nurses and family health promotion: Concepts, assessment, and intervention.* Philadelphia: W. B. Saunders.

Bomar, P. J. (1991) Health-promoting lifestyles of childbearing parents. *Proceedings Second International Family Nursing Conference.* Oregon Health Sciences University School of Nursing: Portland, Oregon.

Bomar, P. J., Neeley, G., & Palmer, I. S. (in press). Family health nursing: History and role. In P. J. Bomar (Ed.), *Nurses and family health promotion: Concepts, assessment and intervention* (2nd ed.). Philadelphia: W. B. Saunders.

Bradshaw, J. (1988). *Bradshaw on the family.* Deerfield Beach, FL: Heath Communications.

Brigman, K. (1992). Religion and family strengths: Implications for mental health professionals. *Topics in Family Psychology and Counseling, 1*, 39–52.

Burr, W. R., Day, R. D., & Bahr, K. S. (1993). *Family science.* Pacific Grove, CA: Brooks/Cole.

Carlson, J., Sperry, L., & Dinkmeyer, D. (1992). Marriage maintenance: How to stay healthy. *Topics in Family Psychology and Counseling, 1*, 84–90.

Carson, V. (1989). *Spiritual dimensions of nursing practice.* Philadelphia: W. B. Saunders.

Chandler, R. (1991, June 19). Nurses — Ministers of Health. *Los Angeles Times,* Al.

Coe, R. (1970). *Sociology of medicine.* New York: McGraw-Hill.

Crooks, C., Iammarino, N., & Weinberg, A. (1987). The family's role in health promotion. *Health Values, 2,* 7–12.

Curran, D. (1983). *Traits of a healthy family.* Minneapolis, MN: Winston Press.

Danielson, C. B., Hamel-Bissel, B., & Winstead-Fry, P. (1993). *Families in health and illness.* St. Louis, MO: Mosby.

DeFrain, J., & Stinnet, N. (1992). Building on the inherent strengths of families: A positive approach for family psychologists and counselors. *Topics in Family Psychology and Counseling, 1*, 15–26.

Doherty, W., & Campbell, T. (1988). *Families and health.* Newbury Park, CA: Sage Publications.

Doherty, W., & McCubbin, H. I. (1985). Families and health care: An emerging arena of theory, research, and clinical interventions. *Family Relations, 34*, 5–10.

Doub, G., & Scott, V. (1992). Family wellness: An enrichment model for teaching skills that build healthy families. *Topics in Family Psychology and Counseling, 1*, 72–83.

Duffy, M. E. (1986). Primary prevention behaviors: The female-headed, one-parent family. *Research in Nursing and Health, 9*, 115–122.

Duffy, M. E. (1988). Health promotion in the family: Current findings and directives for nursing research. *Journal of Advanced Nursing, 13*, 109–117.

Duval, E. M., & Miller, B. C. (1985). *Marriage and family development* (6th ed.). New York: Harper & Row.

Friedemann, M. L. (1989). Closing the gap between grand theory and mental health practice with families: Part 1. The framework of systematic organization for nursing of families and family members. *Archives of Psychiatric Nursing, 3*, 10–19.

Friedman, M. M. (1986). *Family nursing theory and assessment* (2nd ed.) Norwalk, CT: Appleton & Lange.

Friedman, M. M. (1992). *Family nursing theory and assessment* (3rd ed.) Norwalk, CT: Appleton & Lange.

Gillis, C. (1991). Family nursing research, theory, and practice. *Image: Journal of Nursing Scholarship, 22,* 19–22.

Gillis, C. L., & Davis, L. L. (1992). Family nursing research: Precepts from paragons and peccadilloes. *Journal of Advanced Nursing, 17,* 28–33.

Gillis, C. L., Highley, B. L., Roberts, B. M., & Martinson, I. M. (1989). *Toward a science in family nursing.* Reading, MA: Addison-Wesley.

Gray, R. (1994). Family self-care. In P. J. Bomar (Ed.), *Nurses and family health promotion: Concepts, assessment, and intervention* (2nd ed.). Philadelphia: W. B. Saunders.

Hanson, S. M. H. (1986). Healthy single parent families. *Family Relations, 35,* 125–132.

Hanson, S. M. H., & Heims, M. (1992). Family nursing curricula in U.S. schools of nursing. *Journal of Nursing Education, 31,* 303–308.

Hanson, S. M. H., Heims, M., & Julian, D. (1992). Education for family health care professionals: Nursing as a paradigm. *Family Relations, 41,* 4952.

Heinrich, K. (in press). Family sexuality. In P. J. Bomar (Ed.), *Nurses and family health promotion: Concepts assessment, and intervention* (2nd ed.) Philadelphia: W. B. Saunders.

Hill, L. & Smith, N. (1990). *Self-care nursing promoting health.* Englewood Cliffs, NJ: Prentice-Hall.

Hoffer, J. (1994). Family communication. In P. J. Bomar (Ed.), *Nurses and family health promotion: Concepts, assessment, and intervention* (2nd ed.). Philadelphia: W. B. Saunders.

Iowa Intervention Project. McClosky, J. C., & Bulechek, G. M. (Eds.) (1992). *Nursing interventions classification (NIC).* St. Louis, MO: Mosby Year Book.

James, K. (1994). Family nutrition. In P. J. Bomar (Eds.), *Nurses and family health promotion: Concepts, assessment, and intervention* (2nd ed.). Philadelphia: W. B. Saunders.

Kick, E. (1994). Sleep and the family. In P. J. Bomar (Ed.), *Nurses and family health promotion: Concepts, assessment, and intervention* (2nd ed.). Philadelphia: W. B. Saunders.

King, I. M. (1983) King's theory of nursing. In I. W. Clements & F. B. Roberts (Eds.), *Family health: A theoretical approach to nursing care* (pp. 177–188). New York: John Wiley & Sons.

Labun, E. (1988). Spiritual care: An element in nursing care planning. *Journal of Advanced Nursing, 13,* 314–320.

Loveland-Cherry, C. J. (1986). Personal health practices of single parent and two parent families. *Family Relations, 35,* 133–139.

Loveland-Cherry, C. J. (in press). Family health promotion and protection. In P. J. Bomar (Ed.), *Nurses and family health promotion: Concepts, assessment, and interventions* (2nd Ed.). Philadelphia: W. B. Saunders.

McCown, D. (in press). Family recreation and exercise. In P. J. Bomar (Ed.), *Nurses and family health promotion: Concepts, assessment, and intervention* (2nd ed.) Philadelphia: W. B. Saunders.

McCubbin, M. A., & McCubbin, H. I. (1993). Families coping with illness: The resilience model of family stress adjustment and adaptation. In C. B. Danielson, Hamel-Bissel, B., & Winstead-Frye, P. (Eds.), *Families in health and illness* (pp. 21–63). St. Louis, MO: Mosby.

Melson, G. F. (1980). *Family and environment: An eco-systems perspective.* Minneapolis, MN: Burgess.

Mgeni, Y. (1992, December 17), Kwanza holidays celebrate black principles, unity. *Minneapolis Star Tribune,* p. 4.

Mikulencak, M. (1992). The satisfying role of parish nursing. *The American Nurse,* 10.

Miller, S., Miller, P., Nunnally, D., & Wackman, D. (1991). *Talking and listening together.* Littleton, CO: Interpersonal Communication Programs.

Mischke, K. B., & Hanson, S. M. H. (in press). Family health assessment and intervention. In P. J. Bomar (Ed.), *Nurses in family health promotion: Concepts, assessment, and interventions* (2nd ed.). Philadelphia: W. B. Saunders.

Moreno, P. R. (1975). Vertical diffusion effects within black and Mexican-American families participating in the Florida parent education model. *Dissertation Abstracts International, 36,* 1358.

Murphy, S. (1986). Family study and family science. *Image: Journal of Nursing Scholarship, 18,* 170–174.

Neuman, B. (1983). Family intervention using the Betty Neuman health-care system model. In I. W. Clements & F. B. Roberts (Eds.), *Family health: A theoretical approach to nursing care* (pp. 239–254) New York: John Wiley & Sons.

Newman, M. A. (1986). *Health as expanding consciousness.* St. Louis, MO: C. V. Mosby.

Nursing Outreach (Fall, 1993). Bethesda, MD: National Institute of Nursing Research.

Olson, D. H., & DeFrain, J. (1994). *Marriage and the family: Diversity and strengths.* Mountain View, CA: Mayfield.

Olson, D. H., McCubbin, H. I., Barnes, H., Larsen, A., Muxen, M., & Wilson, M. (1989). *Families: What makes them work* (2nd ed.). Beverly Hills, CA: Sage Publications.

Pearsall, P. (1990). *The power of the family: Strength, comfort, and healing.* New York: Doubleday.

Pender, N. J. (1987). *Health promotion in nursing practice* (2nd ed.). Norwalk, CT: Appleton & Lange.

Pratt, L. (1976). *Family structure and effective health behavior and the energized family.* Boston: Houghton

Mifflin.

Ranson, D. D., Fisher, L., & Terry, H. E. (1992). The California Family Health Project: II. Family world view and adult health. *Family Process, 31*, 251–267.

Redman, B. (1993). *The process of patient education* (7th ed.) St. Louis, MO: C. V. Mosby.

Roth, P. (in press). Family social support. In P. J. Bomar (Ed.), *Nurses and family health promotion: Concepts, assessment, and intervention* (2nd ed.). Philadelphia: W. B. Saunders.

Steckle, S. (1982). *Patient contracting.* Norwalk, CT: Appleton-Century-Crofts.

Steiger, N. J., & Lipson, J. G. (1985). *Self-care nursing: Theory and practice.* Bowie, MD: Brady.

Smilkstein, G. (1978). The family APGAR: A proposal for a family function test and its use by physicians. *Family Practice, 6*, 1231–1239.

Smith, J. (1983). *The idea of health: Implications for the nursing profession.* New York: Teachers College Press.

Swain, M. S., & Steckle, S. (1981). Contracting with patients to improve compliance. *Hospitals, 51*, 81–84.

Thomas, D. L., & Cornwall, M. (1990). Religion and family in the 1980s: Discovery and development. *Journal of Marriage and the Family, 52*, 983–992.

US Department of Health and Human Services. (1979). *Promoting health/preventing disease: Objective for the nation.* Washington, DC: US Government Printing Office.

US Department of Health and Human Services. (1985). *Report of the secretary's task force on black and minority health.* Washington, DC: US Government Printing Office.

US Department of Health and Human Services. (1986). *The 1990 health objectives: A midcourse review.* Rockville, MD: Office of Disease and Health Promotion, Public Health Service.

US Department of Health and Human Services. (1990). *Healthy people 2000: National health promotion and disease prevention objectives* (DHHS Publication No. PHS 91-50213). Washington, DC: US Government Printing Office.

Warner, C. G. (1994). Religion and family health. In P. J. Bomar (Ed.), *Nurses and family health promotion: Concepts, assessment, and interventions* (2nd ed.). Philadelphia: W. B. Saunders.

Whall, A. L., & Fawcett, J. (1991). The family as a focal phenomenon in nursing. In A. L. Whall & J. Fawcett (Eds.), *Family theory development in nursing: State of the science and art* (pp. 7–29). Philadelphia: F. A. Davis.

White House Conference on Families. (1980). *Listening to America's families: Action for the 1980s.* Washington, DC: US Government Printing Office.

Wiley, D. (1989). Environment and family health. In P. J. Bomar, (Ed.), *Nurses and family health promotion: Concepts, assessment, and intervention* (pp. 293–219). Philadelphia: W. B. Saunders.

Wisensale, S. K. (1993). State and federal initiatives in family policy. In T. H. Brubaker (Ed.), *Family relations: Challenges for the future* (pp. 229–250). Newbury Park, CA: Sage Publications.

Wright, L., Watson, W., & Bell, J. (1990). The family nursing unit: A unique integration of research, education and clinical practice. In J. Bell, W. Watson, & L. Wright (Eds.), *The cutting edge of family nursing.* Calgary, Alberta: Family Nursing Unit Publications.

Wright, L., & Leahey, M. (1984). *Nurses and families: A guide to interviewing families.* Philadelphia: F. A. Davis.

Zimmermann, S. L. (1992). *Family policies and family well-being.* Newbury Park, CA: Sage Publications.

BIBLIOGRAPHY

Curran, D. (1989). *Working with parents: Delores Curran's guide to successful parent group.* Circle Pines, MN: American Guidance Services.

Department of Family and Community Medicine. (1992). *Developing healthy families: A resource list.* Toronto, Ontario: Working with Families Institute.

Mace, D. (1983). *Prevention in family services: Approaches to family wellness.* Beverly Hills, CA: Sage Publications.

Miller, S., et al. (1988). *Connecting with self and others.* Littleton, CO: Interpersonal Communication Programs.

U N I T

II

Family Nursing Practice

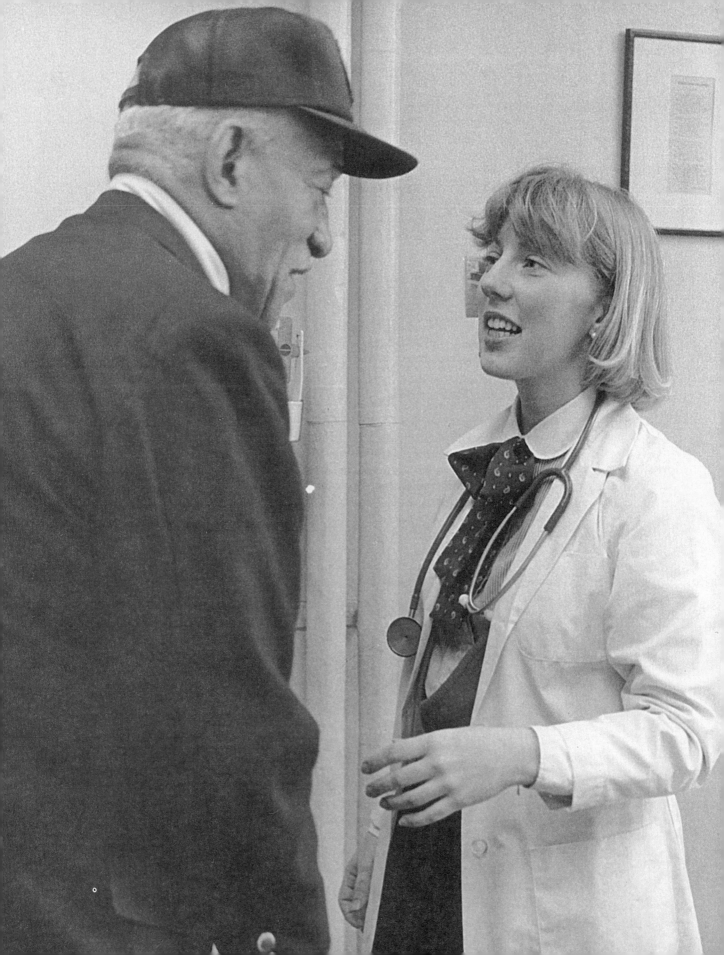

Family Nursing Across Settings

This short chapter sets the stage for the clinical chapters that follow in Unit II, Family Nursing Practice. It begins with a discussion of the philosophy of family nursing and the roles that nurses play as a result of that philosophy in a variety of practice settings and continues with an examination of the constraints of health care settings that influence family nursing practice, such as location and accessibility, cost, and agency policies.

A clinical example aptly reflects family nursing practice in a school nurse setting. The description of the application of the nursing process with a pregnant adolescent demonstrates sensitivity to the family and underscores the importance of the family to this young woman's circumstances.

Another clinical vignette provides the reader with an entirely different perspective, demonstrating the different roles of family nurses in occupational health, clinical nursing, acute institutional care, community health, and home care. In all of these practice areas the philosophy of family nursing guides the care provided to the family client.

In stressing the importance of the family nurse role in various practice settings and in conveying the challenge for the nurse of identifying roles appropriate to the setting, this chapter provides a perspective for the chapters that follow.

CHAPTER 9

Family Nursing and Health Care Settings

Doris Julian, RN, EdD ■ *Karen B. Mischke, PhD, OGNP/WHCNP, CFLE*

OUTLINE   CONTEXT OF FAMILY NURSING

CASE STUDY: FAMILY NURSING IN A SCHOOL SETTING
  Family Nursing Roles of the School Nurse

CASE STUDY: FAMILY NURSING ROLES IN MULTIPLE SETTINGS

OBJECTIVES   *Upon completion of this chapter, the reader will be able to:*

1. Develop a personal definition of family nursing.
2. Identify characteristics of health care settings that can influence the delivery of family nursing care.
3. Identify characteristics of specific nursing positions that can influence the delivery of family nursing care.
4. Describe family nursing roles that can be adapted to a variety of settings.

Family nursing can occur in any setting — the home, the hospital, a clinic, the office of a family nurse practitioner, or a rehabilitation unit. Opportunities for the practice of family nursing are everywhere. Given the diversity of settings in which nurses practice, it is important to be open to opportunities to practice family nursing, since the physical and social environment of health care settings can both determine the resources available to families and influence the practice of family nursing.

Gilliss, Highley, Roberts, and Martinson (1989) comment that although family nursing can be provided in all settings, adaptations may be needed in traditional settings to ensure inclusion of the family. These adaptations include modifications in the role of the nurse. Bomar (in press; Bomar, McNeeley, & Palmer, 1989) proposes a variety of roles for family nurses: (1) client (family) advocate, (2) collaborator, (3) consultant, (4) coordinator, (5) facilitator, (6) family health educator, (7) leader, (8) primary caregiver, (9) researcher, (10) role model, (11) supervisor and health planner, and (12) theory developer.

Figure 9–1 depicts the broader environment or context of family nursing.

CONTEXT OF FAMILY NURSING

Family nursing is viewed here as intertwined with the family and the health care setting. The broader environment for family nursing reflects the culture, politics, historical time, and socioeconomic condition. The environment may be defined in terms of (1) urban or rural location; (2) population density; (3) geographic or topographic features; (4) climate; and (5) industrial and economic conditions. Environmental characteristics have a significant influence on the interaction of family, family nursing, and the health care setting (Henson, Sirles, & Sloan, 1984).

The element of historical time depicted in Figure 9–1 needs to be emphasized, for this is a major aspect of context that is often taken for granted. Events do not occur in a historical vacuum, and health practices are always influenced by local, national, and world responses to contemporaneous occurrences. Historical time may be characterized by war or peace, depression or prosperity, the presence or absence of natural disasters, rapid or minimal technological changes (as in transportation or communication), and ecological changes.

In the first example below, family nursing care is provided by a school nurse serving students attending a rural high school. The nursing services provided originate in a single setting. The second example involves multiple health professionals located in a variety of care settings: employee health facility, outpatient clinic, doctor's office, community hospital, and employee's home. Each example concludes with a discussion of the relationship of the setting to family-centered nursing care.

Case Study: Family Nursing Roles in a School Setting

Kim is 16 years old and a junior in the only high school in a community of 24,000 people. The nearest metropolitan area is approximately 2 hours away. Until this school year, Kim's school performance was characterized by steady attendance and active participation in classes and school activities. At the midpoint of her junior year, her social science teacher linked her frequent absences with her unusual pallor and tendency to sleep or withdraw during class and suggested she make an appointment with the school nurse.

During the initial appointment, the school nurse collected data on her overall health with special attention to physiological, emotional, and developmental

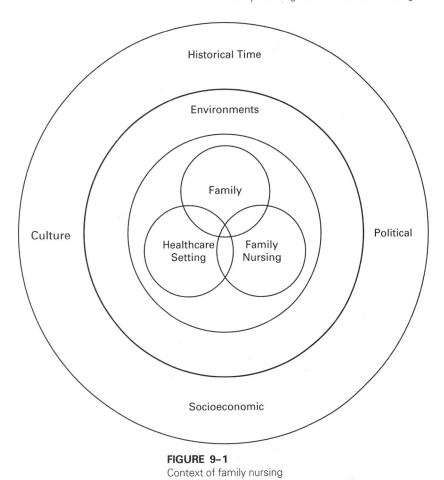

FIGURE 9–1
Context of family nursing

issues. Kim said that she had been sexually active for 5 months and had missed one menstrual period. She wondered if she could be pregnant because she had never used any method of birth control. Kim also described using alcohol, smoking cigarettes, and using cocaine during the summer. The family history revealed that she was an only child whose parents had recently separated. Her father contributed about $300 a month to her support and her mother had a part-time job as a waitress. Kim said she missed her father very much.

The school nurse used this initial visit as an opportunity to assess Kim's perception of a potential pregnancy and what this might mean to her and to those she identified as family. Confidentiality and genuine caring guided this beginning assessment. Kim was provided information on the purchase and use of a pregnancy kit and given an appointment to return the following week. Upon return, Kim told the school nurse that the pregnancy test was positive. With this information the school nurse began to assess Kim's perceptions of the physical, emotional, and social resources available to her, including family, friends, health care providers, health insurance, education, and transportation. A third visit was then scheduled for the following week. At this visit the school nurse explored Kim's knowledge and views about pregnancy, her relationship with the father of the baby, and her interactions with the primary parent, her mother.

Weekly or bimonthly appointments were then scheduled between Kim and the school nurse. They afforded the school nurse an opportunity to take a family-centered nursing approach, based on her knowledge that the health situation affecting Kim would influence the family as well. The nuclear family at the outset consisted of Kim and her recently separated parents. Kim lived with her mother and her father lived close by. The influence of the father of the unborn child on the family was yet to be determined.

Discussion The setting presented in this example is a school-based health office run by a school nurse responsible for providing on-call health services to high school students. The school nurse's responsibilities, in addition to this school, include a high school in an adjacent community and four elementary schools. Each school is allocated a specific day and time each week for regular nursing services. A beeper/telephone arrangement allowed the school nurse to respond to or coordinate emergency health care among the various settings.

Providing family-centered care is a challenge for this nurse, given the constraints of time, travel, and the availability of clients and family members. The nurse must offer family care within the boundaries of the social, cultural, and health values of the family, and the resources available in the community. Major issues for consideration include: (1) establishing a relationship between the school nurse and the client family members living in the community; (2) implementing family nursing care plans based on shared goals of the family and health care provider; and (3) coordinating social, economic, and health resources available in the community.

Family Nursing Roles of the School Nurse

The school nurse can take a variety of caregiving roles in providing family-centered nursing care. These are illustrated with references to the preceding case study:

1. *Advocacy* involves supporting Kim's right to make informed choices about her potential pregnancy (Kim stated her wish to keep the child if she were pregnant) and her future education, parenthood, and work plans. The realities of motherhood are often misunderstood by individuals in this developmental stage. Therefore, the school nurse, in essence, must become a positive reframer for Kim. The nurse does this by communicating the positive and the not-so-positive aspects of the situation. To the individual who views teenage pregnancy in a solely negative manner, the school nurse can point out that this experience, although unplanned, will serve as an ongoing challenge. It will require Kim to use the strengths she already possesses, expand others now lying dormant, and develop still others. Kim may doubt her ability to cope with a pregnancy when she thinks about what this entails—her own health care needs and those of her unborn child. Her inner questioning may focus on issues surrounding prenatal needs, school attendance and telling significant others, or on what she has heard or read about; for example, the stigma of being an unmarried pregnant teenager, the issues of poverty, and the unending demands placed on a parent by an infant. Kim might wonder if she will be able to handle a pregnancy and raise a healthy baby. The advocacy provided by the school nurse is essential when Kim faces these times of inner questioning.

2. As *educator/teacher* the school nurse can offer appropriate information to Kim and her mother (if she chooses to have her mother present) about what constitutes a healthy pregnancy and what Kim needs to know in order to plan for a healthy pregnancy. This needs to be done in an atmosphere that is conducive to learning. The establishment of trust must take place between the nurse as teacher and Kim as learner. Also, Kim's readiness to learn and her cognitive interest are vital elements in the learning milieu. If Kim is highly anxious, fearful, or overwhelmed, she will be unable to hear what the school nurse has to share. A good time for the nurse to do in-depth teaching is when Kim is experiencing periods of inner questioning and is seeking answers; that is, when Kim is in a listening mode and the nurse sees a beginning in readiness to problem solve.

   The school nurse must also assess whether Kim is motivated to follow a healthy prenatal course. Motivation cannot be imposed on Kim; however, the school nurse can influence whether Kim becomes motivated by describing attainable goals and the rationale behind them, for example, preventing nausea and excessive weight gain, ensuring adequate nutrition and rest, preventing fetal distress imposed by drugs and alcohol, and so on. Since motivation comes from within, Kim needs specific objectives to reach for and the means by which to reach them. Objectives devised by the school nurse and Kim must be precise and concrete and must contain elements that can be evaluated, since motivation cannot occur in the abstract.

3. As *resource facilitator* the school nurse can explore the financial and peer group resources available to Kim and her family. In particular, she can (1) assist Kim in locating an appropriate health care professional for prenatal care, and (2) assist Kim's mother in finding and using a support group for newly divorced women. If they lack emotional and social support from family, friends, and health professionals, both Kim and her mother may believe that "they must do it all on their own." Pregnancy and divorce are two overwhelming life events and should not be faced alone. Adequate resources exist for pregnant unmarried teenagers and for women in marital transition. Examples include schools and public or private agencies offering education and group support. These resources accept individuals where they are in their life's journey and provide them with information and opportunities to practice problem solving in a safe environment.

4. As *counselor* the school nurse can establish a therapeutic, trusting relationship with Kim. She should promote friendly negotiations between Kim's father and mother to encourage a supportive relationship with their daughter. Kim's changing physical, social, emotional, and financial status must be dealt with. The parents, who have known Kim the longest, can provide the calm and security that Kim needs. Parental love and approval of her as a person are important aspects of Kim's self-acceptance. The nurse counselor may also include a session with the young father of the baby and a clarification of what his future relationship to Kim and his unborn child may be.

5. As *health promoter* the school nurse provides health care information to Kim and her family. Prevention of illness and health maintenance should be encouraged and supported, and the mechanisms by which this can be facilitated need to be identified. Health promotion activities applicable to Kim can be expanded to include other high school students as well, in after-school sessions.

SUMMARY

This discussion describes approaches to family-centered care by a nurse who, in a school setting, responded to the needs of one teenager and her family. The school setting also provides opportunities for discussing health promotion with other teenagers attending the school and for involving the families of these young people. The nurse plays a variety of roles in providing family-centered care. These roles will be further explored in the next example, which illustrates how family nursing care is carried out in multiple settings.

Case Study: Family Nursing Roles in Multiple Settings

Fred, aged 58 years, was employed in an electronics plant located 10 miles outside a metropolitan area. He lived with his wife, Anna, in a suburban housing development a few miles from his work. Their children, Fred, Jr. and Nancy, were each married and living in a nearby state. Fred had health insurance through his company and was also required to have an annual physical examination by the plant's occupational health nurse.

During his annual examination, Fred mentioned to the nurse that his wife had observed a pigmented mole on his upper back. It was not painful and he was not concerned but he would like to reassure his wife. The nurse completed a thorough history and examined all skin areas. Information was provided on the potential significance of skin lesions and options for follow-up. Referral to a dermatologist was proposed after Fred consulted with his primary health care provider.

During the visit to his physician, Fred, accompanied by his wife, had a brief contact with the office nurse. This nurse, in addition to noting changes in height, weight, and blood pressure from his last visit, had an opportunity to assess Fred and Anna's response to the change in skin pigmentation. She helped them to recognize that their concerns were not trivial and encouraged them to ask specific questions.

Their subsequent visit to a dermatologist's office introduced them to a nurse who had specialized in the field of dermatology. She consulted with the family about what to expect during the office visit, including the possibility of a biopsy, and let them know she would be available during the entire visit. Her brief exit interview alerted her to family concerns about health implications of this condition.

Additional health care visits for this family took them through a variety of settings. Fred's mole was diagnosed as multiple myeloma with multiple metastases. Over an extended period of time, he required surgical procedures with hospitals stays. Visits to his physician and the occupational health nurse provided ongoing monitoring. Fred and Anna recognized the long-term nature of his health condition and, due to his deteriorating physical health, decided on early retirement for Fred when he reached the age of 62 years. His physician made a referral to a community health agency to provide Fred and Anna with home-based care as needed.

The community health nurse made additional referrals to rehabilitative services for useful adaptations to the home environment. Anna was provided with ongoing counseling to assist her in exploring and planning her own life goals. Both Fred and Anna were encouraged to maintain communication with their son and daughter.

Fred's health continued to gradually deteriorate, and as additional problems appeared and respiratory and kidney failure became imminent, he and Anna conferred with their community health nurse. A referral was made to the local hospice center and to a nurse assigned to provide hospice services in the home. These services continued until his death.

Discussion   The multiple settings presented in this example represent a cross-section of health care resources used by one individual over a period of years. The opportunity for family nursing care exists in varying degrees in each of these settings (Pluth, 1993). The roles undertaken by nurses in these various settings overlapped with one another. They seemed to ebb and flow based on Fred's current health needs. For example, the nurse in the industrial setting was an employee advocate, health educator, and resource facilitator. The nurse in the clinical setting assumed the additional roles of mediator and health promoter in providing family-centered care. The roles of the office and hospital nurses encompassed primary care, patient and family education, and coordination of health care (Conkling, 1989).

The first setting in this case example was an electronics plant with on-site health care provided by an occupational health nurse. In this setting the nurse was attentive to family concerns expressed by the client and provided case finding, that is, early identification, education, and referral. The second setting was a physician's office, where the nurse offered family-focused counseling and supportive education. Hospital settings became a frequent part of Fred's health care. In this setting nurses had opportunities to interact with Fred's wife and other family members. In addition to providing physical care, these hospital nurses played a key role in interpreting Fred's responses to treatment, offering relevant education, and encouraging use of additional hospital resources such as nutrition, physical therapy, and chaplain services.

As Fred's disease progressed, the family needed assessment and teaching. Fred wanted to go home and family members were willing to care for him, provided proper support was available. The nurse responsible for discharge planning arranged for at-home support services.

At-home care was provided by a community health nurse. Such a setting was ideal for a family nursing approach because the nurse could interact with family members in their own environment. The enactment of multiple roles was possible, as well as direct care and monitoring of Fred's health condition by the nurse, Fred's wife, and other family members. When hospice care in the home was elected by Fred and his wife rather than care in a hospice center the community health nurse's role changed to one of consultation. The hospice nurse provided home care with particular attention to family needs for grief counseling and preparation for the changing roles of all family members. Thus the nurse also paid attention to the family's existing social, emotional, and physical resources and elicited others the family deemed important, that is, legal, spiritual, and financial resources (Donnelly, 1993).

SUMMARY   Fred's case illustrates the opportunities for family nursing care in the workplace, the physician's office, the hospital, and the home. Other settings could well have been a part of this individual's health care history. Outpatient clinics with a general or specialty focus and emergency rooms are examples of other potential service settings.

CONCLUSION

Each setting provided both constraints and challenges for the nurse in offering a family approach to care (Ferrell & O'Neil-Page, 1990). Each nurse had the opportunity to assess both the work situation and the patient and family needs. This assessment provided the basis for selecting one or more professional roles to enhance patient and family care. Roles discussed in this section included: educator, counselor, case manager, direct caregiver, and resource referral person. The major goal of all of these nursing approaches was recognition of the importance of the family in the care of the individual and continuity of services (Harter, Grossman, Swanke, 1989; Pluth, 1993).

STUDY QUESTIONS

1. Identify four health care settings in which family nursing could be practiced.

2. What are the distinguishing characteristics of family nursing?

3. Identify two possible roles that might be undertaken by a family nurse as required by the setting. Define these roles.

4. What are the distinguishing characteristics of the environment that will influence the delivery of family nursing?

5. What are some issues that nurses in any health care setting need to consider in offering family nursing care?

REFERENCES

Bomar, P. (in press). Family health nursing: History and role. In P. Bomar (Ed.), *Nurses and family health promotion: Concepts, assessment and interventions.* Philadelphia: W. B. Saunders.

Bomar, P., McNeeley, G., & Palmer, I. (1989). Family health nursing: History and role. In P. Bomar (Ed.), *Nurses and family health promotion: Concepts, assessment and interventions* (pp. 1–12). Baltimore: Williams & Wilkins.

Bozett, F. W., & Fields, M. (1984). *The role of the nurse in providing family health care.* Unpublished manuscript, University of Oklahoma School of Nursing, Oklahoma City.

Conkling, V. K. (1989). Continuity of care issues for cancer patients and families. *Cancer, 64*(Suppl.), 290–301.

Detmer, S. (1986). The future of health care delivery systems and settings. *Journal of Professional Nursing, 2,* 20–38.

Donnelly, G. F. (1993). Chronicity: Concept and reality. *Holistic Nursing Practice, 8,* 1–7.

Ferrell, B. R., & O'Neil-Page, E. (1990). Continuity of care. In S. L. Groenwald, M. H. Frogge, M. Goodman, & C. H. Yarbro (Eds.), *Cancer nursing: Principles and practice* (2nd ed., pp. 1078–1088). Boston: Jones & Bartlett.

Friedman, M.M. (1992). *Family nursing: Theory and assessment* (3rd ed.). Norwalk, CT: Appleton & Lange.

Gilliss, C. L., Highley, B. L., Roberts, B. M., & Martinson, I. M. (1989). What is family nursing? In C. Gilliss (Ed.), *Toward a science of family nursing* (pp. 64–73). Reading, MA: Addison-Wesley.

Harter, E., Grossman, L. K., & Swanke, E. (1989). Networking to implement affective health care. *Maternal Child Nursing, 14,* 387–392.

Henson, C. S., Sirles, A., & Sloan, R. (1984). The community health nurse as family nurse practitioner. In M. Stanhope & J. Lancaster (Eds.), *Community health nursing: Process and practice for promoting health* (pp. 762–779). St. Louis, MO: C. V. Mosby.

Pluth, N. (1993). Continuity of cancer care for patients and families through health care systems. In P. C. Buchsel & C. H. Yarbro (Eds.), *Oncology nursing in the ambulatory setting: Issues and models of care* (pp. 49–70). Boston: Jones & Bartlett.

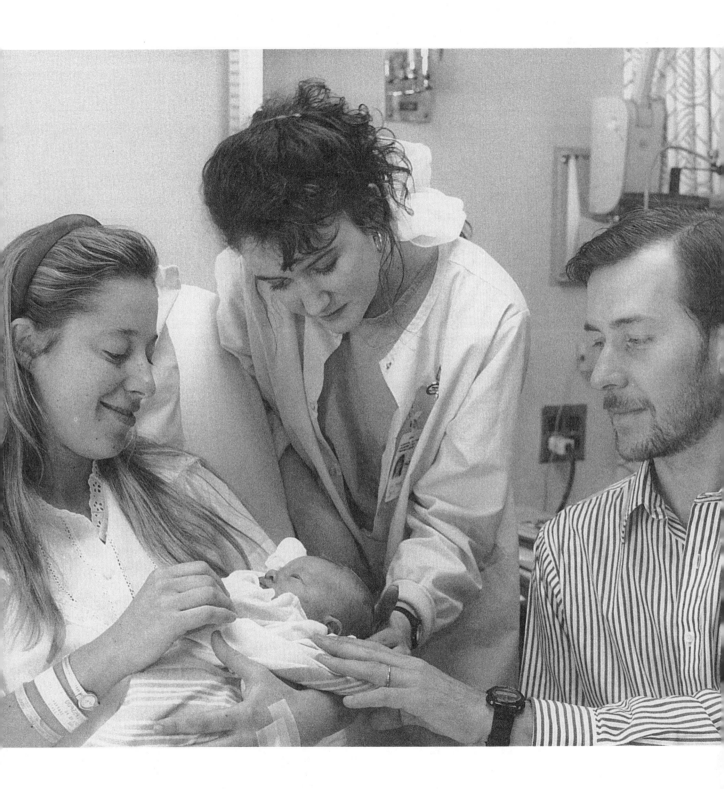

Family Nursing with Childbearing Families

This chapter explains the difference between childbearing nursing and maternity nursing. After a brief history of childbearing family nursing, it describes the theoretical foundations of family nursing with childbearing families and provides the reader with clear examples of the use of theory in practice. The discussion will further the students' understanding of the material in Chapter 2, Theoretical and Research Foundations of Family Nursing, by providing relevant examples.

Family resources such as coping skills, social support, and health care attitudes and practices affect individual members' experiences during childbearing. The authors describe in detail mechanisms that can be used by family nurses to assist childbearing families in developing their resources and improving their health during reproductive and childbearing experiences. The development of these resources and skills in families is the focus of family nursing assessment and interventions for both healthy and high-risk childbearing situations.

This chapter focuses on health promotion activities with childbearing families and how to facilitate parenting so that the student can learn about the actual practice of nursing with childbearing families. Finally, the clinical case study examines the various roles of the professional nurse in the context of the transitions experienced by a childbearing family.

CHAPTER 10

Family Nursing with Childbearing Families

Louise Kelly Martell, RN, PhD ■ *Margaret A. Imle, RN, PhD*

OBJECTIVES *Upon completion of this chapter, the reader will be able to:*
1. Differentiate between childbearing family nursing and maternity nursing.
2. Discuss the history of childbearing family nursing.
3. Apply structural-functional, family systems, and developmental theories to the nursing care of childbearing families.
4. Analyze the impact on family health of developmental tasks of the childbearing stage in the family life cycle.
5. Use the developmental tasks of the childbearing family stage to guide family health promotion.
6. Determine when childbearing families should be referred to other family health care providers.
7. Analyze how threats to childbearing health affect family health.
8. Discuss nursing care for families with threats to health during childbearing.
9. Describe the implications of childbearing family nursing for education, research, and policy development.

WHAT IS CHILDBEARING FAMILY NURSING

Today, as awareness grows about the impact of reproductive events on all family members and vice versa, increasing numbers of health care providers for women are including families in their care. Consequently, family nursing concepts are being integrated more into traditional care of women.

Family nursing with childbearing families covers the period prior to conception, pregnancy, labor, birth, and the postpartum period. Childbearing family nursing traditionally begins when families are considering whether to start having children, and continues until parents have achieved a degree of comfort in their roles and have ceased adding babies to their families. It often expands to include family planning and sexuality. Decisions and changes surrounding the bearing of children vary for families and depend on cultural and psychological needs, as well as social customs, so that the beginning and end point of the reproductive years may be different for different families.

Childbearing family nursing is not synonymous with maternity nursing. Rather, it focuses on the family as the unit of care and the family as context for the care of the individual members, with a concentration on health and wellness rather than disease and illness.

Family functioning, family structure, and life events have been shown to be related to pregnancy outcomes (Ramsey, Abell, & Baker, 1986). For example, women living with spouses or family members were more likely to have healthy, full-term babies than women living alone. Women living with families who were sources of stress, rather than protectors from stress, however, had smaller babies. Mercer and Ferketich (1990) found that hospitalization during pregnancy was stressful to women and their partners, and that negative (or stressful) life events during pregnancy had a negative impact on family functioning.

In childbearing family nursing, the nurse uses family concepts and theories as part of assessment, diagnosis, planning, interventions, and evaluation. In particular, family nursing process addresses relationships, the essence of families. Thus, while childbearing family nursing practice incorporates the traditional components of nursing such as direct physical care, patient teaching, and referral to other health care providers, these components are oriented to the entire childbearing family.

HISTORY OF CHILDBEARING FAMILY NURSING

Before there were professional nurses in the United States, during the late nineteenth century, caregivers during childbearing were primarily midwives, or female neighbors, friends, servants, and relatives, and most caregiving was done in the home during the birth and postpartum period. Care extended not only to the birth process, but also included maintaining the household, tending to the new baby and the other children, and providing postpartum physical care. Family roles, including those related to childbearing, were fixed by gender, and men were not usually involved with any part of the childbearing process.

With the industrialization of the United States, many families moved to urban areas and household size diminished. The traditional networks of women were not always available, and mothers needed to replace the care previously provided in the home. At the same time, with the development of anesthesia and surgical obstetrics, care for childbirth shifted from networks of women to male physicians. Nevertheless, even with the rise of physician-attended births in the late nineteenth and early twentieth centuries, many middle-class women still gave birth at home (Leavitt, 1986; Wertz & Wertz, 1989).

During the first third of this century, physicians began to centralize their services in hospitals and the hospital became the place for labor, birth, and early postpartum recovery. Although more and more middle-class families in the twentieth century had hospital births tended by physicians, many working-class urban families continued to have babies at home with the traditional female care providers. One impetus for the development of public health nursing was concern for the health of these urban mothers and babies. The early public health nurses were the predecessors of childbearing family nurses. When those early public health nurses made home visits to new mothers, they often turned their attention to the other family members. For example, while on a home visit, a nurse might discover that the unemployed father of the family had suffered a job-related illness and that the other children were undernourished. Realizing that the health needs of all the family members were intertwined, early public health nurses made families, not individuals, their clients. Their concern for families laid the foundation for maternity care reforms such as the family planning movement and prenatal and postnatal home visits.

From the 1930s through the "Baby Boom" of the 1950s, there was a dramatic shift of births to hospitals, and family involvement in childbearing diminished (Leavitt, 1986). Women were heavily sedated and anesthetized for labor and birth. Births became "deliveries," which were more similar to surgery than a life event. Because of concerns about infection control, family members and other companions were forbidden to be with a woman in labor. Young children were barred from visiting their mothers during the postpartum period. Babies were segregated in nurseries and brought out to their mothers only for brief feeding sessions. The contribution of nurses was to ensure smooth operation of the postpartum wards and nurseries through the imposition of routine and orderliness. Nursing care was inflexible. Despite these conditions, families tolerated the control of childbearing by physicians and nurses because of the prevailing belief that hospital births were safer for mothers and babies.

Not all families were satisfied with the hospital experience for childbearing, however. In the late 1950s and 1960s, some women and a few physicians began to question the need for heavy sedation and analgesia during childbirth and embraced "natural childbirth," a movement that was taking place in Europe and the Soviet Union. A feature of "natural childbirth" was the close relationship between the laboring woman and a supportive person serving as a coach. In the United States, husbands assumed the supportive role for women who chose "natural childbirth" (Wertz & Wertz, 1989).

In the 1970s, many families decided they wanted more involvement by fathers not only in labor and birth but throughout childbearing experiences, and families went to classes to prepare them for the birth experience. In many parts of the country, prospective parents sought out physicians and hospitals that would meet their expectations, and control over childbearing began to shift from health care professionals to families.

Nurses responded in different ways to this shift in the role of families in childbearing. Some were skeptical about the changes families demanded. Others were enthusiastic about increased family participation; they conducted childbirth classes, taught parents to be assertive with their physicians, and lobbied hospital policy makers to allow fathers in delivery rooms. In line with these changes, many hospital-based childbearing nurses began to consider themselves mother-baby nurses rather than nursery or postpartum nurses, and labor and delivery nurses often collaborated with family members to help women cope with the discomforts of labor.

In early research conducted by Klaus and Kennel (1976) on mother-infant bonding, contact between a mother and her baby soon after birth appeared to have a positive impact on their relationship. This finding served as the impetus for the growth of **family-centered care** (American College of Obstetricians and Gynecologists, 1978). Today, the maintenance or promotion of family contact throughout the birth experience is a hallmark of childbearing care. Many hospitals have relabeled their obstetrical services, using names such as "Family Birth Center" to convey the importance of family members in childbearing health care.

In the future, family-centered care may not be possible for many childbearing families because diminished resources of time and personnel may make it difficult for hospital nurses to do more than meet basic needs of patients. Most nurses address some of the needs of family members, but their practice may not yet encompass the family as a unit (Jordan, 1994). A study of history shows, however, that the partnership of families and nurses in the childbearing experience is constantly evolving.

THEORIES TO GUIDE CHILDBEARING FAMILY NURSING

A number of theories have contributed to nurses' understanding of how families grow, develop, function, and change during childbearing. These include structural-functional theory, family systems theory, and developmental theory. Certain well-known theoretical approaches help nurses predict normal, common occurrences for the family during the childbearing portion of the family life cycle. These theories can guide family nurses in making more complete assessments and planning interventions that fit the predictable consequences of childbearing.

Structural-Functional Theory

Structural-functional theory, described in a previous chapter of this book, is applicable to childbearing. The functions of reproduction and the socialization of children are of particular importance to the childbearing family. Closely related to these functions are the expression of affection, family coping, health care, economic support, and provision for basic needs, all of which are important to childbearing family nursing. Successful achievement of many family functions depends on how well a family meets the basic needs for food, shelter, and clothing, and census data on childbearing outcomes show a strong relationship among socioeconomic status, access to prenatal care, and childbearing outcomes (Johnson, 1986; Mercer, 1989; Ramsey, et al., 1986); that is, families who do not have adequate economic resources may not be able to obtain prenatal care, and consequently are at greater risk for poor perinatal outcomes.

Family structure has several aspects—power, roles, values, and communication (Friedman, 1992)—and many of the activities of expectant parents are oriented toward changes in family power and roles as they take on the functions of reproduction and the socialization of children. Family communication and values influence these changes in power and roles that are required to accommodate the new family member.

The power structure of a family, when balanced so as to maintain the status quo, may be relatively comfortable for a family until a time of change. With the first child, however, the balance of power within the family shifts. The power that is often associated with resources such as money may decrease for an expectant or new mother if her income decreases or stops during childbearing; and as her money-related power decreases, that of her partner may increase. Knowledge, another resource valued during new experiences, also may affect the power balance within a family. The parent with the most knowledge and experience in the care of infants and children may have the most power in making decisions about the children's care. Typically, mothers tend to have this informational power. Other sources of power in childbearing families may be rooted in the family's values.

Structurally, family roles are challenged when a baby is added to the family. These roles are influenced by the social class, culture, economic status, and values of a family. When couples have their first child, family roles tend to become more traditional. Even the most untraditional families experience pressure to conform to more traditional expectations, and role behaviors tend to become more separated when people become parents. Open communication and flexible expectations about roles and power facilitate the changes needed in families during childbearing.

Using structural-functional theory, childbearing family nurses can assess the family power structure, roles, family communication patterns, and how their values affect the way a family takes on reproduction and the socialization of children. Interventions based on structural-functional theory can be designed to help family members become aware that their values and communication patterns influence their power and role structures, which will change with the birth of a child. For example, the nurse can help the members of a middle-class family who value egalitarian power and role structures discuss their expectations about family roles on a day-to-day basis when a first baby is born.

It is important that family nurses become aware of their own personal family structures and how they affect the way they assess and intervene with an expectant family. When nurses and families have different family values, their expressions of family power and role structures may also differ.

Family Systems Theory

Another theory useful for childbearing family nursing is family systems theory, which focuses on both family process and outcomes. The central idea of family systems theory is that a family functions or adapts in such a way as to maintain **homeostasis**. Because a family is considered an open system, it is affected by exchanges with its environment. The degree of openness is regulated by the family boundaries, which may impede or facilitate interaction with social systems outside the family (Broderick, 1993; Mercer, 1989). The interdependence of individuals within a family contributes to a family's ability to adapt and maintain homeostasis, even when the family is experiencing stress and strains from both inside and outside. When a family encounters **stress,** the family engages its coping resources to meet these stressors and attempts to return to a state of homeostasis. The ability to adapt depends on the family's ability to use feedback, from the external environment and within the family itself, to mold the behavior of the family system and its components.

Becoming parents or adding a child brings many stressors that challenge family homeostasis. As disequilibrium occurs, adjustments are needed and new roles must be learned. Families with greater flexibility about role expectations and behaviors tend to weather these periods of disequilibrium with less discomfort. The greater the flexibility of family members and the more they are able to engage in various family roles, the more effective will be the family's response to the stressors associated with childbearing.

Family systems theory can be used to describe changes in the family that occur in response to changes in individual family members and family subsystems (Miller & Winstead-Fry, 1982). As subsystems are created or modified by pregnancy and childbirth, there is a sense of disequilibrium until a family adapts to its new member. For example, changes in the marital partner subsystem occur in response to development of the mother-fetus or parent-child subsystems.

With the transition to parenthood, the family system is enlarged. Not only do the extended families of childbearing couples also have to adjust in order to maintain homeostasis, but, in most families, contact and exchange of help across generations increase with the advent of parenthood and grandparenting (Belsky & Rovine, 1984). Intergenerational family patterns and conflicts sometimes exacerbate the disequilibrium accompanying childbearing. Past patterns of family relationships may be recalled by parents and grandparents and contribute to disagreement and a sense of unresolved conflict. During pregnancy, expectant parents are likely to consider and evaluate how they were raised by their own parents; some fear that they will repeat their parents' mistakes, while others consciously decide to use their parents' methods themselves (Imle, 1983, 1989).

Research by Tilden (1983) and by Norbeck and Tilden (1983) on **social support**, stress, and disequilibrium in childbearing women suggests that external stressors are an important source of disequilibrium in pregnant women, and that nurses should assess the effect of stress on family homeostasis. Family systems theory is especially useful because it takes into account the needs of a family as it struggles to return to stability or homeostasis during the upheavals and changes brought about by childbearing. Using family systems theory, childbearing family nurses assess the family system, including its various subsystems, intergenerational patterns, boundaries, exchange of energy and resources with the environment, and the way the family copes with change and stress. Nursing interventions guided by this theory focus on adaptation and coping with the change inherent in childbearing. For example, a nurse may bring up the topic of intergenerational patterns and conflicts if the expectant parents do not discuss it spontaneously and the nurse has had cues from the family that this is an area of concern.

Childbearing family nurses can also use systems theory to determine if a family will be amenable to family nursing care. With the changes inherent in childbearing, the **permeability of family boundaries** increases and families become more open to influences from the environment—both positive and negative. Families that can transcend their usual boundaries to obtain assistance in times of change can benefit, and their openness can allow health care providers, particularly family nurses, to assist in health promotion. In fact, families may be becoming more receptive to health teaching than in former times.

Families who have closed, nonpermeable boundaries typically reject influences from the environment and, as a result, may be less open to the assistance provided by family nurses and may not get the help they need. Very closed or enmeshed families do not allow stress or energy to diffuse out from the family and are thus at greater risk for poor childbearing outcomes than are more open families (Ramsey et al., 1986).

Developmental Theories

Family development theories are particularly useful for childbearing family nursing, especially when a birth is the first one for a family. Developmental theories focus on predictable changes and growth that occur during individuals' and families' lives. Changes come in stages during which upheaval occurs and adjustments are made. What occurs during these stages is generally referred to as developmental tasks. Stages of upheaval are followed by periods of relative stability. Two developmental models are the Family Life Cycle Theory of Duvall (Duvall & Miller, 1986), described in Chapter 2 and further elaborated here, and the theory of family transitions proposed by Cowan (1991).

Family Life Cycle Theory

Duvall's Family Life Cycle Theory describes family tasks and processes in different stages. In this theory, the family childbearing stage is defined as the period from the beginning of the first pregnancy until the oldest child reaches 18 months of age. During this stage, families have the following nine **developmental tasks:**

1. Arranging space (territory) for a child
2. Financing childbearing and childrearing
3. Assuming mutual responsibility for child care and nurturing
4. Facilitating role learning of family members
5. Adjusting to changed communication patterns in the family to accommodate a newborn and young child
6. Planning for subsequent children
7. Realigning intergenerational patterns
8. Maintaining family members' motivation and morale
9. Establishing family rituals and routines

Some of these tasks reoccur as other children are added during a family's life cycle, while other tasks are more salient for first children.

Transition Concepts

Cowan's (1991) model of the transition to parenthood may be considered a developmental model because parenthood represents normal, predictable change in a family. This transition model includes process and structure. Process involves the dynamic mechanisms of route, both internal and external, and the level of **adaptation** as the family makes a transition to parenthood; structure refers to linkages among the parts of the family system. These linking structures are roles, relationships, and self.

A period of disequilibrium is inevitable as the family moves from one state to another. The transition to parenthood has been defined as a long-term process that results in reorganization of both inner life and external behavior (Cowan, 1991). Reorganization occurs in three phases: first comes disbelief in the reality of the change; second, there is frustration over not being able to cope in the old ways; third, the family accommodates as they claim their new identity as parents and learn new role expectations consistent with being parents.

These two developmental theories can guide childbearing family nurses in assessing family achievement of developmental tasks and assessment of roles and relationships, as well as a parent's internal sense of self.

ECLECTIC USE OF THEORIES FOR CHILDBEARING FAMILY NURSING

None of the theories described above is entirely satisfactory for guiding childbearing family nursing. Family systems theory emphasizes the need to maintain balance and counteract change; but with childbearing, change is inevitable and may be in conflict with homeostasis—considered in some perspectives the goal of a family system. Family developmental theory is rooted in change but it is not applicable to many contemporary families, such as blended or single-parent families, because it was based on the typical experiences of traditional, mainstream American families in the 1950s. Transition may imply a negative response to a new situation, which may not be the case with childbearing. However, the idea that transition is both normal and potentially unsettling can help nurses to accurately assess and manage the impact of predictable and unpredictable events during childbearing.

The following ideas derived from these three theories are especially useful for childbearing family nursing:

- Childbearing is a transition but not necessarily a crisis.
- Changes occur in a family during the **childbearing cycle**.
- Change in one member or one aspect of a childbearing family induces changes in other members and aspects of a family.
- Family structures and functions must change for adaptation to be possible.
- Developmental tasks for pregnancy and childbearing are predictable and lead to new ways of functioning for individuals and families.
- Families are usually more open to influences from the environment during the childbearing cycle.
- Environmental influences such as social support and family nursing can have a positive impact on a childbearing family.

This eclectic approach, using all three theories, can guide assessment, diagnosis, planning, intervention, and evaluation of family nursing with regard to both health promotion and threats to the health of the childbearing family.

HEALTH PROMOTION FOR THE CHILDBEARING FAMILY

Nurses come into contact with members of childbearing families in the offices of health care providers, in clinics, classes, hospitals, homes, and other community settings. While nurses typically may have only mothers or infants as identified patients, the health promotion actions of family nurses are directed toward the entire family. Because families are systems, nursing care directed toward individual members will affect other family members. Likewise, nursing care directed toward an entire family will affect individual members.

The developmental tasks of the childbearing family that are listed in the theory of the family life cycle (Duvall & Miller, 1986) can be used to guide health promotion. This theory is helpful because it addresses the pattern of adaptation to parenthood that is typical for many families in Western cultures. Even families of different configurations and from other cultural backgrounds undergo developmental processes during childbearing. The developmental tasks listed previously, with appropriate nursing actions, are discussed below.

Arranging Space (Territory) for a Child

Typically, during the third trimester of pregnancy, families make material and space preparations for their babies. Often families move to a new residence during pregnancy or the first year after birth to obtain more space, or they modify their living quarters and furnishings to accommodate a new baby.

Family nurses are not involved in arranging or providing space for childbearing families; however, families' concerns about space are of interest to family nurses. By simply asking during the third trimester about living space and physical preparation for the baby, nurses can assess whether these are being taken care of. If a family has not made physical preparations for the baby, the nurse should investigate the reasons. Busy families may inadvertently delay preparations. Nurses' inquiries about space and physical preparations for the baby may prompt such parents to arrange space. Lack of spatial preparation, however, may have other causes. Families who fear or have experienced perinatal loss often delay preparations. These families may fear that their baby will not live and they do not wish to go through the heartbreak of dismantling a nursery that will not be used. Nurses can help these families explore and manage their fears about survival of the baby. Lack of spatial preparation may be due to the fact that the parents have not accepted the reality of the coming baby, perhaps because of stress, which has diverted their attention. Stressors affecting childbearing families need to be recognized and dealt with promptly. A further difficulty may be inadequate, unsafe housing and homelessness, which may be real threats to the safety of some childbearing families. Nurses should refer such families to appropriate resources, such as rent subsidy programs, in order to obtain safer housing or for further investigation of their living situations.

Financing Childbearing and Childrearing

Childbearing family nurses recognize the importance of financing childbearing. For example, health care providers may not accept patients who are not insured or cannot pay for obstetrical services. The nurse's role is to help families seek out needed resources such as nutrition programs and prenatal clinics that fit with the financial resources of the childbearing family. A less obvious but equally important role is to help families overcome nonfinancial barriers to needed care. Such barriers to prenatal care often include lack of transportation and child care, hours of service that conflict with family employment, and cultural insensitivity of health care providers.

For most present-day families, childbearing will result both in additional expenses and lower family income, because most employed women will miss some work during childbearing. Even with legislation to protect women from loss of jobs during childbearing, maintaining previous earnings and opportunities for advancement may be difficult to realize for women returning to work after childbirth. This can be extremely stressful for mothers without partners who provide the sole income to their families.

Families cope with threats to their income in a variety of ways. It is not uncommon for new and expectant fathers to work more hours than average or to change jobs, which may be a source of more anxiety and stress for the family. Women tend to alter their employment situation to make it more compatible with life with a new baby. Families may fall back onto savings or alter their lifestyle to make up the loss of income.

Child care should be considered long before families need this service. Last-minute scrambling to obtain safe and adequate child care can be extremely stressful for families and often results in less than satisfactory arrangements for both parents and babies. Nurses can direct families to information resources to help them choose safe and appropriate child care and encourage them to make such arrangements well in advance of need.

Assuming Mutual Responsibility for Child Care and Nurturing

Besides additional expenses, the care and nurturing of infants bring sleep disruptions, demands on time and energy, additional household tasks, and personal discomfort for caretakers. Most people would not consider these aspects of parenting pleasant. Why, then, do adults voluntarily assume responsibility for a helpless infant? Explanations range from the biological drive to reproduce, the expectation of producing a new generation, or fulfillment of personal expectations, to social desirability and acceptance. The affectional bond or attachment that develops between parents and their children may be one of the driving forces for engaging in infant care and nurturing, even under difficult circumstances.

Interventions to promote parent-infant attachment are well described in recent maternity texts (Bobak & Jensen, 1993; May & Mahlmeister, 1994; Olds, London, & Ladewig, 1992) and in the human development and nursing literature. Promotion of family integrity, feeding management, and identification of those at risk for poor attachment are particularly important for family nurses, whose goal is to enhance nurturing among all family members.

Promotion of Family Integrity

Throughout the childbearing cycle, nurses can assist families to understand and respond to the impact of a new baby on existing children. No matter what age siblings are, the addition of a new baby will affect the position, role, and power of other children, which is stressful for both parents and children. Nurses can emphasize the positive aspects of adding a family member by focusing on sibling "relationships" rather than "rivalry." Parents may need help to recognize that *all* the children, not just the new baby, have needs. Some parents may be concerned about whether they have "enough" energy, time, and love for additional children. Practical ideas for time and task management can alleviate some of their concerns.

Once a baby has been born, opportunities for children to visit their mother and new sibling in childbearing health settings can enhance the development of sibling relationships. Nurses can make the older children feel special by expressing warmth and hospitality to them, recognizing their new role as "big brother" or "big sister," and having age-appropriate toys, furnishings, and educational materials available. Family nurses can also use sibling visitation as an opportunity to explain to parents the older children's expected or unexpected behavior in an inpatient setting. For example, crying by a 2-year-old child may be the child's way of expressing stress in response to a strange environment rather than rejection of the new baby. Although parents may want to discourage children's visits because of crying, the nurse can use these visits to discuss the needs of children in adapting to the new sibling, including ongoing contact with their mothers.

In some settings, children may be present at birth. What is important for children at the time of birth, whether they are present or not, is that they are cared for and supported by a responsible adult whom they trust. During pregnancy, the nurse should remind parents to consider the logistics of caring for other children at the time of birth and during the mother's hospital stay.

All family members experience upheaval during the first few days to weeks that a new baby is in the home. Nurses need to remind parents to be realistic in their expectations for themselves, each other, and their children. Such realistic expectations help families plan ahead to identify appropriate support resources, such as help with household chores.

Feeding Management

Feeding tends to be synonymous with love and nurturing, and success in feeding their babies induces feelings of competence in mothers and love toward their babies. Feeding is such a powerful reinforcement of love and attachment that some fathers have expressed envy of their partners' ability to breast-feed (Jordan, 1986).

Even though breast-feeding is recommended for infants, nurses must recognize that a family's comfort with the method of infant feeding is as crucial for the physical, emotional, and social well-being of an infant as the food itself. Regardless of the choice of feeding method, nurses' instructions need to emphasize the development of the relationship between infant and parent through feeding. Being held during feeding enhances social development whether a baby is breast-fed or bottle-fed. Parents should take the time during feedings to enjoy interaction with their babies.

Nurses can promote paternal-infant attachment by encouraging breast-feeding women to involve fathers in the feeding experience. For example, the father can comfort the baby while the mother is getting ready to nurse, or burp the baby during and after feedings. Another way to involve the father in feeding is to have him feed the baby an occasional bottle of expressed breast milk. Early involvement of fathers in feeding is especially beneficial later when infants are being weaned or mothers are preparing to return to work.

Risk Identification

Risk identification involves identifying families and individuals who are likely to have difficulty with attachment. The difficulty may be related to the health of either parents or the infant, or to the parents' ability to carry out their role as parents.

Extreme stress, health-risk factors, and illness can interfere with the parent-newborn contact needed for the development of **attachment**. Stressful conditions that pull parents' energies and attention away from their newborns can also be detrimental to attachment. Family nurses can be instrumental in assuring contact between families and supportive networks in these situations. In extremely stressful family situations, such as chemical dependency or severe postpartum depression, childbearing family nurses may refer families for appropriate therapy.

In a family where a parent has suffered abuse, neglect, or abandonment there is risk for poor attachment. Nurses need to help such families gain a perspective on the poor parenting they experienced and make them aware that they can choose not to repeat these behaviors with their own children, as well as to convey to these families a sense of caring and concern, which may have been missing in their own childhood. In addition, the family nurse can also help parents develop new skills in caregiving and interacting with their babies, such as soothing a fussy baby. In these situations family nurses often work with social workers, psychotherapists, and developmental specialists to help the parents care for and nurture their children.

Nurses often identify families at risk for poor attachment through observing parent behaviors. Behaviors that could cause concern include verbal expressions of dissatisfaction with the baby, comparisons of the baby and disliked family members, failure to respond to the infant's crying, lack of spontaneity in touching the baby, and stiffness or discomfort in holding the baby after the first week. Isolated incidences of these behaviors are probably not detrimental to attachment. What is important are trends and patterns of behaviors; that is, whether the parent-infant relationship is progressing positively. Love for and enjoyment of children grow over time. If the parents' enjoyment of the baby as a unique individual and commitment to the baby are not progressing, the family needs continuing support, education, role modeling, encouragement, and realistic appraisal. Childbearing family nurses may need to refer families who do not demonstrate these behaviors to other professionals who can provide intensive interventions.

FACILITATING ROLE LEARNING OF FAMILY MEMBERS

Learning roles is particularly important for the childbearing family. For many couples, taking on the role of parents is a dramatic shift in their lives. Difficulty with adaptation to parenthood may be related to the stress of learning new roles as well as to role conflicts. Role learning involves having expectations about the role, developing the ability to assume the role, and taking on the role.

Expectations About the Parent Role

Expectations about parent roles are part of the stress new parents experience during the transition to parenthood. Mothers compare their actual experiences with their expectations, and those whose actual experience was disappointing regarding their relationship with their spouse, physical well-being, maternal competence, and maternal satisfaction have had more difficulty adjusting to parenthood (Imle, 1989; Kalmuss, Davidson, & Cushman, 1992). Expectations about the partner's role also influence the transition to parenthood. For example, men have often been regarded as helpmates, supports, and bystanders during childbearing rather than as parents. If women are regarded as the "real" parents, men are not encouraged to grasp the reality of fatherhood. These expectations can keep men from believing that they have the knowledge, support, or skills to become involved parents.

In the United States, societal expectations of the parent role, especially motherhood, are unrealistic and may set up parents who feel inadequate (Jordan, 1990). The myth of motherhood is supported by the media, which are full of images of new mothers clad in luxurious lace while they feed glowing, contented babies in immaculate houses. The reality of early motherhood is that prepregnancy clothes do not fit, babies periodically become demanding malcontents, and houses are messy because family members are too exhausted to clean. Nursing and medical textbooks reinforce the myth of motherhood by implying that 6 weeks after birth, when healing of the reproductive system is complete, women are ready to resume all their activities. In reality, it takes longer for women to resume their roles. A recent study of 110 postpartum women showed that at 6 months after birth virtually no woman had regained full functioning (Tulman, Fawcett, Groblewski, & Silverman, 1990). Incongruence between the ideal and the reality of the parent role may result in frustration, turmoil, and loss of confidence. Unrealistic expectations about being parents and about children's development are often present in angry, abusive families (Johnson, 1986).

The nurse can help parents discuss and face their ideals and bridge the gap between idealized and actual roles. One way to start is to have expectant parents, before their baby's birth, describe what they think being parents will be like. From their responses family nurses can assess their expectations and begin to educate parents about the realities of parenting. For example, nurses can help expectant parents see themselves in very real situations — with interrupted sleep and little free time. Nurses must present a realistic but balanced view of parenthood; having parents shift from a totally positive view to an entirely negative one may not help them carry out the parent role. Encouraging contact with new parents who are in the process of assuming the role may be more effective than any descriptions of parenting a nurse can give.

Family nurses can also help pregnant couples explore their attitudes and expectations about the role of their partners. For instance, a woman may not realize that she is placing her mate in a role subordinate to her as the primary parent or "expert." Nurses can encourage expectant women to bring their mates into their experience by sharing their physical sensations and the emotions of being pregnant. Many men need to be encouraged to think about how they expect to enact their role as fathers. Being relegated to a subordinate role can be discouraging and ultimately may result in the man's becoming less involved in parenting. If women expect their mates to be fully involved parents, they need to provide opportunities for partners to become skilled infant caregivers. For example, when her mate assumes infant care responsibilities, a woman should not rush in to correct her mate's "mistakes" such as a loose diaper or a shirt on backwards.

Developing Abilities for the Parent Role

Family nurses in all childbearing care settings teach parenting skills. The content and process of teaching these skills are well delineated in textbooks (Bobak & Jensen, 1993; May & Mahlmeister, 1994; Olds, London, & Ladewig, 1992) and other sources of information on expectant parent education (Nichols, 1993; Peterson & Peterson, 1993; Starn, 1993).

Expectant mothers and fathers develop parenting abilities and skills through their own childhood experiences and through contact with other parents, friends, family members, and health care providers. Consequently, when planning educational strategies for parents, nurses must consider expectant parents' past experiences and the range and diversity of their information sources.

The role of a parent is a dynamic one because children's needs change as they develop. Fortunately, parents' skills grow and change along with their children. Family nurses can continue to help families develop the abilities they need for the parent role beyond the childbearing stage.

Taking on the Role of Parent

Taking on the parent role requires not only learning to perform caretaking tasks but also developing the feelings associated with parenting and the ability to solve problems associated with being a parent. Family nurses can assist parents in taking on the parental role by praising parents in their early efforts and modeling the feelings associated with the role. Specific behaviors to model include displaying warmth toward the baby and expressing pleasure over care of the baby.

As parents take on their roles, they begin, through problem solving, to modify these roles to suit their own life situations and needs (Drayden & Imle, 1991). As parents meet their baby's needs more consistently and successfully under a variety of conditions, their positive feelings about being parents grow. Nurses can help families discuss how to perform parenting tasks in their own environment with their own equipment. This problem-solving process can be enhanced by helping parents associate their baby's behavior with its meaning. For example, a baby may be crying because of hunger and not to annoy his or her parents. While helping parents empathize with their baby, nurses should also help them understand what is developmentally appropriate behavior for their baby so that they do not misinterpret the infant's behavior. If parents are becoming skilled caregivers with warmth, concern, and affection for their babies in their own environments, then they are clearly taking on the parent role.

Parents who experience frustration in taking on the parent role tend to evaluate themselves negatively. Intensive work with these parents to help them develop empathy for their baby and understand the parent problem-solving process is necessary. If new parents do not display warmth and affection toward the baby, a family nurse should be concerned. These parents may need interventions to help them develop attachment.

Adjusting to Changed Communication Patterns in the Family to Accommodate a Newborn and Young Child

As parents and infant learn to interpret and respond to each others' communication cues, they develop effective communication patterns. However, infant cues may be so subtle that parents may not notice them until the nurse points them out. Because of differences in temperament, different infants respond in different ways, which may make it difficult for parents to interpret cues. Many babies respond to being held by cuddling and nuzzling, but others respond by back arching and stiffening. Parents may interpret the latter as rejecting and unloving responses, and these negative interpretations may adversely affect the parent-infant relationship. Family nurses can help by educating parents about different infant temperaments so that they can interpret their baby's unique style of communication. A useful tool to help parents learn about their infant's interactive behavior is the Brazelton Neonatal Behavioral Assessment Scale (BNBAS). By observing the baby's assessment parents can learn about the interaction style of their infant. Learning to perform the BNBAS involves extensive training; however, for the family nurse involved with parent-infant interaction issues, learning the BNBAS is definitely worthwhile.

Communication between parents changes with the transition to parenthood. During the years of childbearing many men and women devote considerable time to career development. The time demands of work often affect the couple's communication adversely (Belsky, Perry-Jenkins, & Crouter, 1985), yet parenthood requires effective communication between the parents. One effective expectant parent communication program focuses on information, skills, and support (P.L. Jordan, personal communication with the author, 1993). The information component teaches effective communication strategies. The skills component includes supervised discussions using the communication strategies that have been taught. The coach for the supervised discussion of parenting also provides support.

Planning for Subsequent Children

Some families with their first baby have definite, mutually agreed-upon plans for additional children, while others have definitely decided not to have more children. Families who have definite plans primarily need information about family planning options so they can carry out their plans.

Often, family nurses encounter couples who are uncertain about having more children. In these situations the nurse can help the family clarify its values and decision making. However, when discussing childbearing decisions, family nurses must consider the power structure and locus of decision making in the family. Mutuality in decision making implies that both persons have equal power and status, which is rarely the case. It would be counterproductive for a nurse not to consider the male partner in a family with a male-dominated power structure. In such a family the women may acquiesce in her husband's decisions even when she does not agree with him.

Realigning Intergenerational Patterns

The first baby adds a new generation in the family lineage and carries the family into the future. During the first pregnancy, expectant parents change from being the children of their own parents to becoming parents themselves (Bennet, Wolin, & McAvity, 1988). As they see themselves approaching the status held by their own mothers and fathers, they begin to redefine themselves, to consider themselves as parents as well as adults (Imle, 1989). For many parents, with parenthood comes prestige and sense of their own power as they see themselves becoming more like their parents.

When the expected baby is the first grandchild, the parents of the expectant parents also experience a change in status and become grandparents (Hagestad & Lang, 1986). Nurses working with pregnant women can promote the development of grandparent-parent relationships in several ways (Martell, 1990a). Many women will talk spontaneously about their mothers, but the nurse can encourage discussion with a simple question such as, "Tell me about how things are going between you and your mother." From the pregnant woman's response, the nurse can assess the quality of the relationship and, where appropriate, consider interventions. For example, the nurse might suggest that the pregnant woman ask her mother to tell her about her own pregnancy and birth experiences. Sharing these experiences can enhance the sense of continuity. If conflict exists, family nurses can help by teaching pregnant women some simple communication strategies to open discussion with their mothers and help resolve conflict.

Potential areas of conflict between generations include infant feeding methods, dealing with crying babies, and other aspects of childrearing. Current recommendations for infant care and feeding may not be the same as what grandparents did with their children. Consequently, new parents may receive conflicting information. If conflicts persist or if, out of sheer exhaustion, new parents take outmoded or unwanted advice, they can become resentful and intergenerational bonds can break down. Even with the change in their status, new parents may find it stressful to confront their parents on an adult-to-adult level, especially when their parents genuinely want to be helpful. Nurses can suggest tactful ways for expectant parents to confront their own parents who have outmoded advice and information. Ideally, conflict can be prevented through information sharing and open discussion about what would be helpful prior to the arrival of the baby. Nurses can educate new grandparents about current recommendations by helping them compare their experiences with present-day practices, giving them tours of hospital facilities, and providing up-to-date reading materials (Starn, 1993).

Reliance on health care professionals for childbearing and childrearing guidance is primarily a middle-class phenomenon; for other socioeconomic and cultural groups, health care professionals may not be as esteemed as the older women in families on matters relating to childbearing. In these situations, nurses may feel frustrated when new parents accept the advice of other family members, such as their own mothers, rather than the recommendations of health care providers. Such a reaction should not be allowed to interfere with the nurse's primary goal of enhancing family function.

Maintaining Family Members' Motivation and Morale

The care, feeding, and comforting of infants demand time, energy, and resources. Moreover, women may be fatigued for months from the physical exertion and blood loss of birth, compounded by the demands of infant care, and some women have little chance to be well rested before they are expected to return to their jobs (Killien, 1993). In addition, maternal exhaustion can contribute to postpartum depression, which is detrimental to families (Martell, 1990b).

Family nurses can help family members to maintain motivation and morale and to avoid becoming overwhelmed by the transition to parenthood. Before new mothers are discharged from the hospital, both parents need to know about ways to promote rest and sleep. For example, helping a new mother with comfort measures for a sore perineum or uterine cramps makes it easier to rest and improves morale. Families need to be realistic about infant sleep patterns; typically, babies will need night-time feedings for several months, no matter how parents modify the timing and content of the feedings. Time-honored ways to promote rest while a baby needs night-time feedings are to alternate who responds to the baby and to feed the baby in the parents' bed. Infant crying seems to be more irritating if parents are fatigued, and it can exacerbate sleep loss and fatigue. Thus helping parents to cope with crying can help family morale: being able to soothe a fussy baby can boost the confidence of new parents and allow them to get additional sleep.

In present-day American families, the postpartum period can be lonely. Many young families live in communities far distant from their extended families. They may have recently moved into a new neighborhood and not had a chance to establish friendships or community affiliations. Family nurses need to counsel families realistically about the duration of postpartum recovery and how isolated they may feel during this time. Expectant parents should be encouraged to ask their support networks for help with meals and household tasks after the birth. Frequently, new parents can find such support from childbirth education groups and colleagues at work. It is also helpful to connect with other new parents. When young families find that their parenting experiences are similar to those of others, their morale tends to improve. Morale is also boosted by nurses and other health professionals who give realistic and positive feedback. Often new parents want to appear self-sufficient and are reluctant to accept offers of help; they may be vague about their needs. In such cases, nurses can help them to articulate their needs and accept help.

The demands of early parenting tend to draw mothers and fathers away from the couple relationship. Couples may feel that the baby has interfered in their relationship and can feel that they are each being ignored by the other as the baby, with immediate and continuing demands, becomes the primary focus of each parent. A mother, especially, can feel torn between her baby and her partner. The impact of a baby on a relationship may be distressing for couples who have invested much of their interest and energy in their relationship as a couple.

Couples need to be aware of potential changes in their sexual relationship with the arrival of a baby. Sensitive family nurses can counsel couples about changes in sexuality after birth and assist them to develop mutually satisfying sexual expression. Often couples need to be encouraged to take time for themselves apart from the baby. The actual separation from the baby is not as important in itself as the fact that it allows parents to interact with each other and enjoy each other's company outside of the parenting role. This can be done even in very brief periods of conversation and physical closeness when the baby is asleep.

Most parents also need companionship and interests beyond the family. Family nurses need to recognize these needs, and help families maintain their adult interests and friendships.

Establishing Family Rituals and Routines

Rituals develop as children come into a family, and these become part of the uniqueness and identity of a family. Family rituals include bedtime and bathing routines, baby's special possessions such as a treasured blanket, and nicknames for body functions. When families are disrupted or separated during childbearing, nurses can help them deal with stress by encouraging them to carry out their usual routines and establish new rituals related to their babies.

THREATS TO HEALTH DURING CHILDBEARING

For the majority of families, childbearing is a physically healthy experience. For some families, however, health is threatened during childbearing and the childbearing experience becomes an illness experience. In such cases, concern for the physical health of the mother and fetus tends to outweigh other aspects of pregnancy, and rather than eagerly anticipating the birth and baby, family members are dominated by fear and apprehension. Moreover, the family developmental tasks are disrupted as they focus attention on the health of the mother and survival of the baby. The following case study of a family with a preterm birth is used to illustrate the impact of threats to health on childbearing families.

Case Study: The Johnsons: A Family with a Preterm Birth

Tom and Mary Johnson's first child, Jenny, was born at full term. Mary had no health problems during the pregnancy. At that time the Johnsons lived in a large city in the western part of the United States, near their parents, siblings, and childhood friends.

Two years later the Johnsons moved to a small town 500 miles away from their friends and families, to find better professional opportunities for Tom and more affordable housing. A month after the move, they discovered that Mary was about 3 months pregnant. Mary decided to postpone seeking employment as a secretary until after the birth and concentrate on fixing up the older two-story house they had bought.

Unexpectedly, Mary had problems with this pregnancy. At 27 weeks, her obstetrician diagnosed gestational diabetes and she had to modify her diet to keep her blood glucose level under control. At 29 weeks she began to have preterm labor. To stop the contractions, her physician insisted that Mary stay on bed rest around the clock, except for a very brief daily shower and use of the bathroom. Tom had to take over meal preparation, house cleaning, and bathing and dressing Jenny. He also arranged the living room so Mary could lie on the couch and Jenny could play near her mother while he was at work. Because he had no accumulated vacation or sick time, Tom could not take off time from his job to help Mary and take care of Jenny without sacrificing pay.

Mary found it difficult to follow her diet and stay on bed rest. She was frustrated because she had to stop her house renovation project, and Tom's cooking and housecleaning were not up to her standards. She was tempted to run the vacuum cleaner, wash dishes, and eat sweets while Tom was at work. The medication to suppress contractions made her so anxious and tremulous that she could not amuse herself with crafts and sewing. She was lonely for her mother and friends, 500 miles away; she longed for companionship but found herself complaining and nagging Tom when he was home. Jenny frequently had tantrums because she could not play outside with her mother, and began to have lapses in toilet training.

At 32 weeks of pregnancy, Mary's membranes ruptured, and her physician sent her to a perinatal center 100 miles away from home because it had better facilities to care for preterm babies. Jenny went with her parents to the perinatal center to wait until one of her grandmothers could come and take care of her. Jason was born 28 hours after the Johnsons arrived at the hospital.

Mary had an uncomplicated recovery and was discharged from the perinatal center within 24 hours after she gave birth. Jason, the new baby, remained at the perinatal center in the special care nursery until he was mature and stable enough to go home 4 weeks later.

Impact of Threats to Health on the Childbearing Family Even though problems of gestational diabetes and preterm labor are often managed at home, these threats to childbearing health are disruptive for the family. Other family members must assume household and family tasks so that the expectant mother can stay on her prescribed regimen. As the description of the Johnson family shows, shifting these tasks may be stressful and affect the family's functioning. Expectant fathers, especially, find that *all* their time and energy are consumed by employment and household tasks that previously were shared, or done solely by their partners. Children's lives change when their mother is confined to bed. Toddlers do not understand why their mothers cannot pick them up or run after them. The resulting frustration for children can manifest itself in behavior changes such as Jenny's tantrums and lapses in toilet training. The demands of families, on the other hand, may make bed rest a stressful experience for women. Certainly Mary's anxiety was in part a response to feeling unable to handle family demands, and her nagging and complaining were probably expressions of her anxiety. Because of their frustration and the burdens of family tasks, women may not fully comply with the regimens necessary to control threats to health.

The at-risk pregnancy is stressful in terms of the family's financial and other resources. Loss of income may result from time away from work, and medical expenses rise due to the need for increased care, including possible neonatal intensive care. Personal expenses may also increase if there is need for changes in diet, medications, alterations in transportation, and help with household tasks. The cost in terms of family energy and emotional responses cannot be measured as easily, but their impact is evident in a situation like Tom's, where the demands of household management are added to those of a new job.

Because of the unpredictable nature of high-risk childbearing, planning for the future becomes more difficult. The family may have to cope with sudden hospitalization, and if there are other small children in the home, they may become extremely anxious about their mother's sudden departure if they have not been prepared for it, especially if they are unable to comprehend what is going on.

High-risk childbearing is especially stressful when a family has a limited social network to assume family tasks such as meal preparation, child care, and household maintenance. Mary's premature labor occurred before the Johnsons had developed a social network in their new community. Had they had a supportive network, some of the burden of household management may have been eliminated. With adequate support Mary may not have felt so lonely and perhaps someone could have taken Jenny out to play. In other families, both parents' jobs may be affected by unpredictability. With a pending preterm birth, for example, parents, especially employed women, may not be able to accurately determine when to begin a parental leave or when it will end.

Transfer to a distant perinatal center is not uncommon for families in remote rural areas. Such transfers can separate family members for days or months and make it difficult to maintain established relationships. In Tom and Mary's case, being with their new son Jason was difficult because each visit required a 200-mile round trip, Tom had a full-time job, and Mary cared for Jenny during the day. Even if logistical problems are solved and a family can be together, coping with even the basic tasks of living is a challenge in these high-tech settings. For instance, a family may not know where to stay, how to find reasonably priced meals, or even where to park the car.

Interventions for health promotion need to be modified for the family with a high-risk pregnancy. For example, a family nurse managing Mary's care for preterm labor would see that the prescribed regimen of bed rest was disrupting family morale and plans to arrange space for the new baby, that Tom was suffering role overload, and that the mother-child relationship between Mary and Jenny was strained. Lacking a local social network, the Johnsons had little exchange with outsiders and consequently, stress could not diffuse out from this family. A family nurse might help a family identiify and use resources, such as home health agencies and parents' groups, in the community for assistance with household management and morale. The nurse could help Tom and Mary discuss the frustration of Mary's bed rest and diet changes and Tom's role overload and how these stressors were affecting their relationship. Information about the impact of change on a 2-year-old child could help Tom and Mary understand and better manage Jenny's behavior. When Jason needed to remain at the perinatal center, a neonatal nurse with a family focus would recognize the impact of having a preterm baby in a regional neonatal intensive care unit on development of attachment to the baby, role learning, and family morale. Interventions for the Johnson family would include creating ways for them to have contact with

Jason, through telephone updates of his condition and photographs, even when they could not be physically with him, allowing them to do normal infant care tasks for Jason when they visited him, and encouraging them to develop a support system with other parents of intensive care infants.

In situations of threat, the coping strategies of families may be inadequate or even exhausted in the face of extreme stress. Before an at-risk pregnancy, many young families have never had to face situations of threats to health, drain of financial resources, or separation from loved ones. In these situations family nurses can help childbearing families develop appropriate coping strategies. The family's coping strategies can be further compromised by the fact that families under stress often have unrealistic perceptions of their situation. Nurses can help them realistically appraise threats to health, and identify their strengths and resources for coping. Strengths include the ways they have coped with stressful situations in the past; resources include available helpful persons, financial assistance, and informational sources. Finally, nurses can assist families in the longer term by teaching them to problem solve and develop new resources and strategies for healthy, effective coping.

IMPLICATIONS FOR EDUCATION, RESEARCH, AND POLICY

Family nursing with childbearing families has developed in part in response to the increasing emphasis in nursing education on families as the client or the context for nursing care. With the shift of health care into nonacute care settings and homes, education about family nursing will become even more important for childbearing health care.

Research on family nursing interventions and outcomes needs to increase. Evaluation of the effectiveness of family nursing interventions is especially critical when health care costs are under close scrutiny and third-party payers need to be convinced that family nursing interventions result in improved outcomes for childbearing and that they are cost-effective.

The incorporation of the word "family" in the names of many health care institutions may make nurses complacent about the state of family nursing practice in their settings. Serious examination of institutional policies can help nurses determine whether the word "family" is part of a catchy title for marketing purposes or betokens a strong influence on philosophy, policies, and nursing standards. Nurses also need to be aware of the impact of social policies on childbearing families. One example is family leave for childbirth, which can profoundly affect the health and development of childbearing families.

SUMMARY   Childbearing family nursing is not synonymous with maternity nursing. Family nurses care for all members of the childbearing family and focus on families who are healthy, as well as those who experience threats to health during the childbearing cycle. While childbearing family nursing is not yet universally practiced in health care settings, it is evolving through education, research, and policy development. Various family theories help family nurses organize nursing assessments, plan interventions, and evaluate the outcomes of nursing care with childbearing families. Through its impact on adaptation to parenthood, family nursing can make a major difference in family health during the childbearing phase of the family life cycle.

STUDY QUESTIONS

1. Early predecessors of childbearing family nurses were:
   a. Childbirth educators
   b. Nurse midwives
   c. Nursery nurses
   d. Public health nurses

2. Family roles, values, communication, and power are components of which of the following theories?
   a. Family life cycle development
   b. Family systems
   c. Structural-functional
   d. Transition

3. Currently the best theory to guide childbearing family nursing is:
   a. Family systems
   b. Structural-functional
   c. Transition
   d. None of the above

4. Families with closed boundaries are often not accessible to nursing interventions because:
   a. These families do not have children
   b. These are unstable families
   c. Family members do not interact with each other
   d. These families reject influences from the outside environment

5. Childbearing family nurses may ask about a family's space arrangement for an expected baby to assess whether the family:
   a. Is meeting its basic needs
   b. Is accepting the reality of the expected baby
   c. Has fears about the survival of the baby
   d. All of the above

6. Priority in research related to childbearing families is on:
   a. The effectiveness of family nursing interventions
   b. Development of theories that describe childbearing families
   c. The importance of immediate contact between newborn babies and their parents
   d. How the baby boom of the 1950s influenced present-day childbearing family nursing.

7. Discuss ways that childbearing family nurses can enhance an expectant father's role as a parent.

8. A new mother and her mother do not agree on how to handle a newborn's persistent crying. Discuss nursing actions that would help them resolve their differences.

9. Write a care plan to help the Johnson family develop a relationship with Jason while he is in the special care nursery.

REFERENCES

American College of Obstetricians and Gynecologists (ACOG) and the Interprofessional Task Force on Health Care of Women and Children. (1978). *Joint statement on the development of family centered maternity/newborn care in hospitals.* Chicago: ACOG.

Belsky, J., Perry-Jenkins, M., & Crouter, A. C. (1985). The work-family interface and marital change across the transition to parenthood. *Journal of Family Issues, 6,* 205–220.

Belsky, J., & Rovine, M. (1984). Social network contact, family support, and the transition to parenthood. *Journal of Marriage and the Family, 46,* 455–462.

Bennet, L. A., Wolin, S. J., & McAvity, K. T. (1988). Family identity, ritual and myth: A cultural perspective on life cycle transition. In C. J. Falico (Ed.), *Family transitions* (pp. 211–234). New York: Guilford Press.

Bobak, I. M., & Jensen, M. D. (1993). *Maternity and gynecologic care: The nurse and the family.* St. Louis, MO: C. V. Mosby.

Broderick, C. B. (1993). *Understanding family process.* Newbury Park, CA: Sage Publications.

Cowan, P. A. (1991). The individual and family life transitions: A proposal for a new definition. In P. A. Cowan & M. Hetherington (Eds.), *Family transitions* (pp. 3–30). Hillsdale, NJ: Laurence Erlbaum.

Drayden, T., & Imle, M. (1991, May). *First-time parents' perspectives of family care needs during the postpartum period of transition to parenthood.* Paper presented at the Second International Family Nursing Conference. Portland, OR.

Duvall, E. M., & Miller, B. C. (1986). *Marriage and family development.* New York: Harper & Row.

Friedman, M. M. (1992). *Family nursing: Theory and practice* (3rd ed.). Norwalk, CT: Appleton & Lange.

Hagestad, G. O., & Lang, M. E. (1986). The transition to grandparenthood. *Journal of Family Issues, 7,* 115–130.

Imle, M. A. (1983). *Indices to measure concerns of expectant parents in transition to parenthood.* Unpublished doctoral dissertation, University of Arizona, Tucson.

Imle, M. A. (1989). *Adjustment to parenthood: Model and scale development: Final report (1984–1988).* (USDH Grant #5R23NU01181). Washington, DC: PHS Division of Nursing.

Johnson, S. H. (1986). Role theory strategies. In S. H. Johnson (Ed.), *Nursing assessments and strategies for the family at risk: High-risk parenting.* Philadelphia: J. B. Lippincott.

Jordan, P. L. (1986). Breastfeeding as a risk factor for fathers. *Journal of Obstetric, Gynecologic, and Neonatal Nursing, 15,* 94–97.

Jordan, P (1990). Laboring for relevance. *Nursing Research, 13,* 11–16.

Jordan, P. L. (1994). *Family centered maternity care: Fact or fiction.* Manuscript submitted for publication.

Kalmuss, D., Davidson, A., & Cushman, L. (1992). Parenting expectations, experiences, and adjustment to parenthood: A test of the violated expectations framework. *Journal of Marriage and the Family, 54,* 516–526.

Killien, M. G. (1993). Returning to work after childbirth: Considerations for health policy. *Nursing Outlook, 41,* 73–78.

Klaus, M. H., & Kennel, J. H. (1976). *Maternal-infant bonding.* St. Louis, MO: C. V. Mosby.

Leavitt, J. W. (1986). *Brought to bed: Childbearing in America 1750–1950.* New York: Oxford University Press.

Martell, L. K. (1990a). The mother-daughter relationship during daughter's first pregnancy: The transition experience. *Holistic Nursing Practice, 4*(3), 47–55.

Martell, L. K. (1990b). Postpartum depression: A family problem. *Maternal-Child Nursing, 15,* 90–93.

May, K. A., and Mahlmeister, L. R. (1994). *Maternal and neonatal nursing: Family centered care.* Philadelphia: J. B. Lippincott.

Mercer, R. T. (1989). Theoretical perspectives on family. In C. L. Gilliss, B. L. Highley, B. M. Roberts, & I. M. Martinson (Eds.), *Toward a science of family nursing* (pp. 9–36). Menlo Park, CA: Addison-Wesley.

Mercer, R. T., & Ferketich, S. L. (1990). Predictors of family functioning eight weeks following birth. *Nursing Research, 39,* 76–82.

Miller, S. R., & Winstead-Fry, P. (1982). *Family systems theory in nursing practice.* Reston, VA: Reston Publishing.

Nichols, F. H. (Ed.). (1993). Perinatal education. *Clinical Issues in Perinatal and Women's Health Nursing, 4,* 1–159.

Norbeck, J., & Tilden, V. P. (1983). Life stress, social support and emotional disequilibrium in complications of pregnancy: A prospective multivariate study. *Journal of Health and Social Behavior, 24,* 30–46.

Olds, S. B., London, M. L., & Ladewig, P. W. (1992). *Maternal-newborn nursing: A family centered approach.* Redwood City, CA: Addison-Wesley.

Peterson, K. J., & Peterson, F. L. (1993). Family-centered perinatal education. *Clinical Issues in Perinatal and Women's Health Nursing, 4,* 1–4.

Ramsey, C. N., Abell, T. D., & Baker, L. C. (1986). The relationship between family functioning, life events, family structure, and the outcome of pregnancy. *Journal of Family Practice, 22,* 521–527.

Starn, J. (1993). Strengthening family systems. *Clinical Issues in Perinatal and Women's Health Care Nursing, 4,* 35–43.

Tilden, V. P. (1983). The relation of life stress and social support to emotional disequilibrium during pregnancy. *Research in Nursing and Health, 6,* 167–174.

Tulman, L., Fawcett, J., Groblewski, L., & Silverman, L. (1990). Changes in functional status after childbirth. *Nursing Research, 39,* 70–75.

Wertz, R. W., & Wertz, D. C. (1989). *Lying-in: A history of childbirth in America.* New Haven, CT: Yale University Press.

BIBLIOGRAPHY

Aguilera, D. C., & Messick, J. M. (1974). *Crisis intervention: Theory and methodology.* St. Louis, MO: C. V. Mosby.

Ainsworth, M. D. S. (1973). The development of infant-mother attachment. In B. M. Caldwell & H. N. Riccuiuti (Eds.), *Review of infant research* (Vol. 3). Chicago: University of Chicago Press.

Brazelton, T. B. (1989). *The earliest relationship: Parents, infants, and the drama of early attachment.* Reading, MA: Addison-Wesley.

Carter, E., & McGoldrick, M. (1980). *The family life cycle: A framework for family therapy.* New York: Gardner Press.

Cowan, C. P., & Cowan, P. A. (1992). *When partners become parents: The big life change for couples.* New York: Basic Books.

Imle, M. A. (1990). Third trimester concerns of expectant parents in transition to parenthood. *Holistic Nursing Practice, 4(3),* 25 – 36.

Johnson, S. H. (1986). *Nursing assessments and strategies for the family at risk: High-risk parenting.* Philadelphia: J. B. Lippincott.

Mercer, R. T. (1990). *Parents at risk.* New York: Springer.

Mercer, R. T., Nichols, E. S., & Doyle, G. C. (1989). *Transition in a woman's life: Major life events in developmental context.* New York: Springer.

Shewin, L. N. (1987). *Psychosocial dimensions of the pregnant family.* New York: Springer.

Spero, D. (1993). Sibling preparation classes. *Clinical Issues in Perinatal and Women's Health Care Nursing, 4,* 122 – 131.

Sumner, G. (1990). *Keys to caregiving.* Seattle: NCAST Publications.

Walker, L. O. (1992). *Parent-infant nursing science: Paradigms, phenomena, methods.* Philadelphia: F. A. Davis.

Whall, A. L., & Fawcett, J. (1991). *Family theory development in nursing: State of the science and art.* Philadelphia: F. A. Davis.

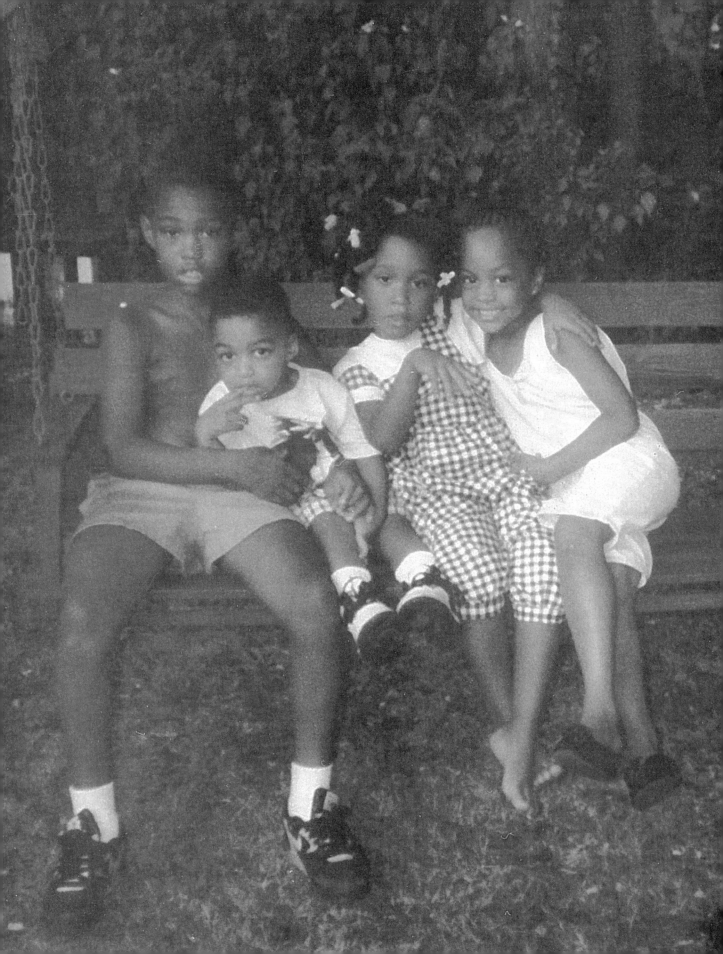

Family Child Health Nursing

Family nurses focus on the relationship of family life to children's health and illness, and they assist families to achieve well-being. This chapter describes the practice of family child health nursing. It begins by examining the history of family-centered care and then describes the Family Interaction Model, using examples to illustrate the connection between theory and practice.

Through family-centered care, nurses facilitate family life and the development of family members to their fullest potential. Using the Family Interaction Model, this chapter explains how nurses can take a comprehensive and collaborative approach to families, incorporating relevant components of family life and interaction, family development and transitions, and family health and illness.

Health promotion in family child nursing is examined and the importance of grandparents, day care, and after-school facilities to child health is explored. The chapter goes on to provide a detailed description of the use of the Family Interaction Model to screen for potentially harmful situations, to instruct families about health issues, and to help families cope with acute illness, chronic illness, and life-threatening conditions.

After completing this chapter students may find it helpful to think about their own family child nursing experiences or those they have read about and consider how the information contained in this chapter might have been used in those situations.

CHAPTER 11

Family Child Health Nursing

Vivian Gedaly-Duff, RN, DNSc ■ *Marsha L. Heims, RN, EdD*

OBJECTIVES   *Upon completion of this chapter, the reader will be able to:*

1. Define and describe family child health nursing.
2. Describe the major features of the Family Interaction Model.
3. Formulate family career-based nursing actions for the family child health nurse.
4. Describe how family child health nurses screen various types of families in transition for health-related issues.
5. Formulate nursing intervention strategies for families with children based on the transitions experienced during patterns of health and illness.
6. Formulate health outcomes for a child and/or family with children during the family career.
7. Formulate health outcomes for a child and/or family experiencing a health transition during an acute illness, a chronic illness, and a life-threatening illness.
8. Describe the influences of social and legal policies and standards of practice and care on family child health nursing.

A major task of **families** is to nurture children to become healthy, responsible, and creative adults. Parents, as primary caretakers of their children, are charged with keeping them healthy as well as caring for them during illness. Yet most mothers and fathers have little formal education for parenting and must rely on memories of their childhood experience in their families of origin. In fact, most parents learn the role "on the job" during the process of raising their own children.

Family child health nurses help families promote health, prevent disease, and cope with illness. The importance of family life for children's health and illness is often invisible, because families' everyday routines are commonplace and lie below the level of conscious awareness. However, family nurses assume that family life influences the promotion of health and the experience of illness in children.

Families are groups with unique features, including specific family memories and intergenerational relationships; family rules and routines; family aspirations and achievements; and ethnic or cultural patterns (Burr, Herrin, Day, Beutler, & Leigh, 1988).

Healthy outcomes for children — for example, achievement of three times their birth weight at 1 year of age, or successful completion of high school by adolescents with juvenile diabetes — are partially attributable to the intangible, invisible daily interactions among family members. Family features related to illness are often not discussed, but they are evident in daily activities. Nurses, in collaboration with families, examine how the unique features of the family influence health.

Family child health nursing focuses on the relationships between family life and children's health. It is applied to families in two ways: nurses care for children within the context of their families, and they care for children by treating their families as units. In both approaches, families affect children's health, while children's health affects their families.

This chapter provides a brief history of family-centered care of children and then presents a family interactional model that can be used to guide nursing practice with families with children in health promotion, acute illness, chronic illness, and life-threatening illness situations.

HISTORY OF FAMILY-CENTERED CARE OF CHILDREN

Consideration of the role of the family in the health care of children is not new. In a history of the 125-year existence of Great Ormond Street Hospital for Sick Children in London, Besser (1977) reports that Drs. Armstrong and West disagreed about the need to separate children from their families to treat disease. Armstrong, who opened the first Dispensary for the Infant Poor in 1769, argued that taking a sick child from its parent would break its heart and said that the "air" of a crowded open room was contaminated. The poor survival rates of children in institutions supported this view. The Foundling Hospital in London admitted 14,934 infants between 1756 and 1760, but only 4400 lived to enter apprenticeships (Besser, 1977). In opposition, West, who founded Britain's Great Ormond Street Hospital in 1852, was convinced that a hospital was essential for promoting children's health because of his visits to families in "homes" that were dark, cold hovels (Besser, 1977).

Nurses' have always worked with families with children (Schultz & Meleis, 1988). Lillian Wald (1904), the founder of public health or community nursing, described a 2-year-old child ill with pneumonia:

> . . . Baby was found on a feather bed covered with feather pillows, with a temperature of 105°F. The nurse explained to the mother the desirability of cooler bedding and taught her

how to arrange the crib properly. The front room was reserved for the sick baby and the mother was taught how to give the medicines, how to sponge the baby, and how to keep a record of the treatment. She devoted herself to the sick child, while her sister came to take care of the house and the two other children. The child's fever ran on for 4 days, and at the end subsided and the baby recovered (p. 605).

The following description (Faville, 1925) shows a nurse working with the whole family. It tells of a nurse's visit to a child's home after sending home a note explaining that the child had a communicable disease and could not return to school without a note from the doctor.

The visiting nurse walked with Tony and Mike up the alley to their home. . . . The mother could read no English and so had attached small importance to the printed slip of paper brought from school. Two more children, Mary and the baby, were found to be scratching vigorously, and the father was sick in bed with a bad cold. "All the time, he cough," the mother explained. "Now hot, now cold." "Did he spit blood?" "Yes, last week." The Italian doctor had been in and said that the man must go to the country at once. "But how can we? No place to go; no money and I must stay here to get Jimmie off to work each night;" Jimmie being the pale-faced boy of 17 who was eating his supper preparatory to going on night shift at the mill (p. 14).

As these vignettes illustrate, nurses have always worked to improve the health of children and their families.

An area of family child health care that is of interest to nurses involves the effects of hospitalizing children to treat disease. Hospitalized children suffer from a lack of family nurturance. During and after World War II, Burlingham and Freud's work (1942) and Spitz's study (1945) demonstrated the effects of separating infants and children from their families during institutionalization. Goslin (1978), after reviewing the literature on hospitalization, concluded that young children (particularly infants older than 6 months and children under 4 years) demonstrated, in sequence, protest, despair, and detachment when separated from their families.

Nurse clinicians (Wood, 1988) and researchers (Godfrey, 1965; Mahaffy, 1965; Miles, Carter, Riddle, Hennessey, & Eberly, 1989) have examined ways to reduce the negative effects of hospitalization on children and families, and this research has led to policies of open visiting for all family members, parent rooming-in, family preparation for procedures, consistent nursing care, and therapeutic hospital play (Thompson, 1986). Nurses in particular can reduce the stress of hospitalization for children, demystify for siblings what their sisters or brothers are experiencing, educate parents and grandparents concerning the child's disease, and support the family as a unit during hospitalization.

In past decades American families hospitalized their children for illness care. Today, there is a blurring of the division between hospital and home care for ill children (Feetham, 1986). Infants and children may be hospitalized for hours as in day-surgery, for months as in neonatal intensive care units, or repeatedly for chronic disease. In each of these cases, the families ultimately care for their children during illness. When a child is hospitalized, families have the desire to participate but often feel left out of the decision making concerning their children's health needs. They are also often unprepared for the burden of daily illness care at home (Harrison, 1993; Shelton, Jeppson, & Johnson, 1987). "Family-centered care" has emerged in response to the increasing family responsibilities for health care.

Family-centered care involves collaboration by families, nurses, and other health professionals to deliver health care to children and families (Lash & Wertlieb, 1993). The principles of family-centered care include (1) recognizing that families are "the constant" in children's lives, while personnel in the health care system fluctuate; (2) openly sharing information about alternative treatments, ethical concerns, and uncertainties about health care treatments; (3) forming partnerships between families and health professionals to decide what is important for the families; (4) respecting the racial, ethnic, cultural, and socioeconomic diversity of families and their ways of coping; and (5) supporting and strengthening families' abilities to grow and develop. For example, families that live with the everyday routine of a child's chronic disease not only know the pattern of the disease, drugs, and other medical treatments, but also know the responses of their child and family member to these factors. Many times health professionals fail to recognize the expertise that families acquire as they care for their own children (Ferraro & Longo, 1985).

As a result of their ongoing involvement, families learn that health professionals base decisions on theory, research, and clinical experience but do not know exactly how a particular child will respond until after their interventions are completed (Paget, 1982). Families acknowledge the uncertainty that surrounds their child's disease, but they want to be informed partners of the health team in decision making. In an American society that respects family diversity, a health team that includes the family is preferable to a hierarchical team with physicians at the top, nurses in between, and families at the bottom. Family-centered care brings attention back to the importance of families in health care.

FAMILY INTERACTION MODEL

Family child health nurses need a theoretical model that can describe, explain, predict, and prescribe nursing care (Dickoff, James, & Wiedenbach, 1968) and address diverse family situations. Nurses work with families when they are healthy and ill; they know some families for a short time and with others have ongoing relationships; they see families in homes, clinics, and hospitals. To be useful, a model for nurses caring for families with children must be applicable to all these situations. The **Family Interaction Model** uses the concepts of **family career**, **individual development**, and **patterns of health/disease/illness** to guide nursing practice of families with children (Gedaly-Duff, 1990a, 1990b).

The Family Interaction Model is derived from **symbolic interaction theory** and developmental theory. Symbolic interactionists suggest that families influence individuals' learning of meanings and gestures through societal and family interactions. That is to say, both adults and children learn the meanings of and respond to events through their daily interactions with family members.

When two people join together to begin a new family, their interactions create new meanings of health and illness. Much of the time the daily nature of family activities makes meanings implicit rather than explicit. When nurses understand that families and family members have unique perceptions and meanings for a health or illness situation, they can help families redefine a situation if necessary, and create a shared family meaning for the situation. For example, a child diagnosed with sickle-cell anemia may be labeled by the family as a "son with a handicapping, painful disease." The nurse would work with the family to redefine the situation to "a son who can grow and develop but who lives with an episodic, painful condition."

The **developmental perspective** suggests that families and individuals change over time. Families who consist of adults and children experience various developmental stages simultaneously among their members, and they progress through a series of family developmental stages. Conflict is expected because of differences in the needs of individuals and the family. By comparing their observations of particular families to expected family and individual developmental stages, nurses can plan appropriate care.

The Family Interaction Model, which is based on the insights of social interactionist George Herbert Mead (1934), assumes that (1) meanings and responses to health, disease, and illness are created through interactions among family members and between the family and society, and (2) families' meanings and responses are partially influenced by family and individual development (Fig. 11-1). Not only do families shape their members, but members shape their families (Turk & Kerns, 1985).

The Family Interaction Model has three concepts that guide nursing care: (1) family career, which is the experience of family life over time; (2) individual development, which is the expected changes in humans associated with growth and development; and (3) patterns of health, disease, and illness, which are expected behaviors in these health situations. Knowledge of these three concepts can introduce nurses to an understanding of the effects of health and illness on family interactions.

Family Career

Family career is the dynamic process of change that occurs during the life span of the unique group called the family. American families are diverse, as can be seen from the fact that single, divorced and remarried, and homosexual parents are caring for children. The notion of family career includes the diverse paths that unfold during their family lives.

Family career represents the family like a motion picture showing family growth and development over time. By contrast, the family life cycle representation is more like a series of snapshots of family stages with their various expected roles and tasks. The family career consists of family life that changes predictably over time and moves through devel-

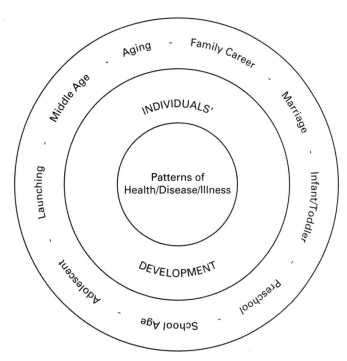

FIGURE 11-1
Family interaction model.

opmental stages such as establishing a family, raising and launching children, and experiencing the death of a parent figure (Turk & Kerns, 1985, p. 3). It requires reorganizing family roles and tasks as families progress through different stages of development and situational events (J. Aldous, personal communication, April 11, 1994; White, 1991).

These predictable changes, however, do not necessarily occur in a linear fashion. For example, childbirth may occur in middle to late adulthood, rather than in early adulthood; or a person may marry into a family with an adolescent and experience parenthood, but not the parenthood of young children. New research is describing additional family career stages and developmental tasks in such nontraditional groupings as single-parent, divorced, and remarried families. The concept of family career is useful because it reminds us that families are dynamic (Table 11 – 1). Nurses working with childrearing families need to examine family career, the stage of family development, and transition events that affect health.

Family Stages

Duvall's eight stages of family development describe expected changes in families who are raising children. The typical family career starts with marriage without children, then come childbearing, preschool children, school children, adolescents, the launching of young adults (first child gone to last child leaving home), middle age of parents (empty nest to retirement), and aging of family members (retirement to death of both parents) (Duvall & Miller, 1985). **Family stages** help nurses anticipate the family reorganization necessary to accommodate the growth and development of its members. For example,

TABLE 11–1

FAMILY CAREER: STAGES, TASKS, AND TRANSITIONS

Period	Family Stage	Family Tasks	Family Transitions
Early Adulthood	Families without children Families with infants Families with preschoolers	Provide economic resources that secure shelter, food, and clothing	Transitions or times of change are expected in families
Middle Adulthood	Families with school-age children Families with adolescents	Develop emotionally healthy individuals who manage crises and experience achievement	Families reorganize predictably when children grow Families reorganize when unpredictable changes occur in personal relationships, role and status, environment, physical and mental capabilities, and there is loss of possesions
Late Adulthood	Launching children Middle-aged families Aging families	Assure each member's socialization as a member of society in school, work, spiritual, and community life Give birth, adopt a child, or contribute to next generation Promote health and care for members experiencing injury, disease, and illness	Family routines change at transition points Family rituals acknowledge and celebrate family transition points

families with school-aged children expect them to be able to take care of their own hygiene, whereas families with infants expect to do all the hygiene care.

Across all family stages, there are basic **family tasks** that are essential to survival and continuity (Duvall & Miller, 1985): (1) to secure shelter, food, and clothing; (2) to develop emotionally healthy individuals who can manage crisis and experience nonmonetary achievement; (3) to assure each individual's socialization in school, work, spiritual, and community life; (4) to give birth, to adopt a child, or to contribute to the next generation; and (5) to promote the health of its members and to care for them during illness. The intangible services that families provide to individuals and society are evident in these basic family tasks. Families nurture human potential through building family and individual competencies (Andrews, Bubolz, & Paolucci, 1980). The aim of the nurse is to help childrearing families develop appropriate ways to carry out the tasks necessary to prevent illness or disease, and to promote or restore health.

Family Transitions

Family careers include both developmental and situational transitions. **Family transitions** are events that signal a reorganization of family roles and tasks. Developmental transitions are predictable changes that occur in an expected time line congruent with movement through the eight family stages. Thus, family members expect and learn to interact differently as children grow. Sometimes families may not make the transition to an expected family stage, a scenario often seen in families raising handicapped children. Families whose children are not capable of independent living cannot launch all their children.

Five types of situational transitions that require family reorganization are changes in personal relationships, roles and status, the environment, physical and mental capabilities, and the loss of possessions (Rankin, 1989). Such changes are embodied in the following examples: changes in personal relationships occur when a new baby or stepchild is integrated into the family group, or when one becomes a new stepparent after divorce and remarriage; changes in roles and status happen when an only child becomes a sibling after the family adopts a new child; changes in the familiar environment occur when working parents move to a new job and family members encounter a new house, school, friends, and community. Even greater changes occur when families immigrate to a new country, learn a new language and a new culture, and perhaps have to work at a lower-status job. Changes in physical and mental capabilities—for example, an illness that incapacitates a working parent—may shift caregiving activities to other members of the family. A natural disaster may destroy family possessions and heirlooms and alter family structures and ways of interacting.

Family transitions may follow expected or unexpected time lines. Increased independence is expected in children as they grow older, but children are not expected to die before their parents. Nurses screen families for transition events because transitions, both developmental and situational, are signals to nurses that families may be at risk for health problems.

Individual Development

Families with children are complex groups of adults and children. Because no one perspective explains humans adequately, nurses consider multiple dimensions of human development. Some family developmental stages are related to the growth of individual members and the differing needs of maturing human beings. Table 11–2 is a schematic representation of human development. It is not all-inclusive but highlights some stages of

TABLE 11–2

SOCIAL-EMOTIONAL, COGNITIVE, AND PHYSICAL MATURATIONAL DIMENSIONS OF INDIVIDUAL DEVELOPMENT

Period	Age	Social-Emotional Stages	Radius of Significant Relations	Stage-Sensitive Family Development Tasks	Human Needs	Values Orientation
Infancy	Birth	Trust vs. mistrust (I am what I am given.)			Physiological: air, food, and shelter	
	3 mo		Primary parent	Having, adjusting to, and encouraging the development of infants Establishing a satisfying home for both parents and infant(s)		Undifferentiated
	6 mo 9 mo					
	1 yr	Autonomy vs. shame or doubt (I am what I "will.")	Parental persons		Safety/security	
Preschool- Age Period	2 yr					
	3 yr	Initiative vs. guilt (I am what I imagine I can be.)	Basic family	Adapting to the critical needs and interests of preschool children in stimulating, growth-promoting ways Coping with energy depletion and lack of privacy as parents	Belonging, rootedness, family, friends	Punishment and obediance
School- Age Period	4 yr					
	5 yr					
	6 yr	Industry vs. inferiority (I am what I learn.)	Neighborhood school	Fitting into the community of school-age families in constructive ways	Esteem: self-respect, self-esteem	

Cognitive Stages of Development	Developmental Landmarks	Physical Maturation	Developmental Steps (Lines)	Developmental Problems
Sensory-Motor Infants move from neonatal reflex level of complete self-world undifferentiation to relatively coherent organization of sensory-motor actions. They learn that certain actions have specific effects upon the environment. Minimal symbolic activity is involved. Recognition of the constancy of external objects and primitive internal representation of the world begins.	Gazes at complete patterns Social smile (2 mo) 180° visual pursuit (2 mo) Reaches for objects (4 mo) Rolls over (5 mo) Raking grasp (7 mo) Crude purposeful release (9 mo) Inferior pincer grasp Walks unassisted (10–14 mo) Words: 3–4 (13 mo) Builds tower of 2 cubes (15 mo) Scribbles with crayon (18 mo) Words: 10 (18 mo) Builds tower of 5–6 cubes (21 mo) Uses 3-word sentences (30 mo) Names 6 body parts (30 mo) Uses appropriate personal pronouns, i.e., I, you, me (30 mo)	**Rapid (Skeletal)** Transitory reflexes present (3 mo) (i.e., moro, sucking, grasp, tonic neck reflex) Muscle constitutes 25% total body weight Birth weight doubles (6 mo) Eruption of deciduous central incisors (5–10 mo) Birth weight triples (1 yr) Anterior fontanel closes (10–14 mo) Transitory reflexes disappear (10 mo) Eruption of deciduous first molars (11–18 mo) Babinski reflex extinguished (18 mo) Bowel and bladder nerves myelinated (18 mo) Increase in lymphoid tissue	Anticipation of feeding Symbiosis (4–18 mo) Stranger anxiety (6–10 mo) Separation anxiety (8–24 mo) Self-feeding Oppositional behavior Messiness Exploratory behavior Parallel play Pleasure in looking at or being looked at Beginning self-concept Orderliness Disgust Curiosity Masturbation Cooperative play Fantasy play Imaginary companions	Birth defects Feeding disorders: colic, regurgitation, vomiting, failure to thrive, marasmus, feeding refusal, atopic eczema Stranger anxiety Physiologic failure to thrive Sleep disturbances: resistance or response to over-stimulation Extreme separation anxiety Pica Teeth grinding Poisonings Temper tantrums, negativism Toilet training disturbances: constipation, diarrhea Excessive feeding Bedtime and toilet rituals Speech disorders: delayed, elective mutism, stuttering Physical injuries: falls Nightmares, night terrors Extreme separation anxiety Excessive thumb sucking Phobias and marked fears
Preoperational Thought (prelogical) Children make their first relatively unorganized and fumbling attempts to come to grips with the new and strange world of symbols. Thinking tends to be egocentric and intuitive. Conclusions are based on what they feel or what they would like to believe.	Rides tricycle (36 mo) Copies circle (36 mo) Matches 4 colors (36 mo) Talks of self and others (42 mo) Takes turns (42 mo) Tandem walks (42 mo) Uses 4-word sentences (48 mo) Copies cross (48 mo) Throws ball overhand (48 mo) Copies square (54 mo) Copies triangle (60 mo) Prints name Rides two-wheel bike Copies diamond	**Slower (Skeletal)** Weight gain 2 kg per year (12–36 mo) **Rapid (Skeletal)** Weight gain 2 kg per year (4–6 yr) Eruption of permanent teeth (5.5–8 yr) Body image solidifying	Task completion Rivalry with parents of same sex Games and rules Problem solving Achievement Voluntary hygiene	Developmental deviations: lags and accelerations in motor, sensory, and affective development Food rituals and fads Sleep walking School phobias Developmental deviations: lags and accelerations in cognitive functions, psychosexual, and integrative development Self-destructive behaviors Enuresis, soiling, and excessive masturbation Physical injuries: fractures

Continued

TABLE 11–2

SOCIAL-EMOTIONAL, COGNITIVE, AND PHYSICAL MATURATIONAL DIMENSIONS OF INDIVIDUAL DEVELOPMENT *(Continued)*

Period	Age	Social-Emotional Stages	Radius of Significant Relations	Stage-Sensitive Family Development Tasks	Human Needs	Values Orientation
School-Age Period	7 yr			Encouraging children's education achievement		Instrumental exchange: "If you scratch my back, I'll scratch yours."
	8 yr					
	9 yr					
	10 yr					
	11 yr	Identify vs. identity diffusion (I know who I am.)	Peer in-groups and out-groups Adult models of leadership	Balancing freedom with responsibility as teenagers mature and emancipate themselves Establishing postparental interests and careers as growing parents		
Adolescence	12 yr					
	13 yr					
	14 yr					
	15 yr					Conventional Law and order: "They mean well."
	16 yr					
	17 yr 18 yr					
Early Adulthood		Intimacy vs. isolation	Partners in friendship, sex, competition	Releasing young adults into work, military service, college, marriage, and so on with appropriate rituals and assistance Maintaining a supportive home base		Principled social contract
Middle Adulthood		Generativity vs. self-absorption or stagnation	Divided labor and shared household	Refocusing on the marriage relationship Maintaining kin ties with older and younger generations	Self-actualization: doing what one is capable of	
Late Adulthood		Integrity vs. despair, disgust	"Humankind" "My kind"	Coping with bereavement and living alone Closing the family home in adapting to aging Adjusting to retirement		Universal ethical principles

Adapted from D. Prugh (1983) in *The Psychological Aspects of Pediatrics*, Philadelphia: Lea & Febiger.
R. Murray Thomas (1992) in *Comparing Theories of Child Development* (pp. 166–167, 501), Belmont CA: Wadsworth.
E.M. Duvall and B.C. Miller (1985) in *Marriage and Family Development* (6th ed.) (p. 62), New York: Harper and Collins.

Cognitive Stages of Development	Developmental Landmarks	Physical Maturation	Developmental Steps (Lines)	Developmental Problems
Concrete Operational Thought Conceptual organization takes on stability and coherence. Children begin to seem rational and well organized in their adaptation. The fairly stable and orderly conceptual framework is systematically brought to bear on the world of objects around them. Physical quantities, such as weight and volume, are now viewed as constant despite changes in shape and size.	Simple opposite analogies Names days of week Repeats 5 digits forward Can define brave and nonsense Knows seasons of the year Able to rhyme Repeats 4 digits in reverse Understands pity, grief, surprise Knows where sun sets Can define nitrogen, microscope	**Slowest (Skeletal)** Weight gain 2–4 kg per year (7–11 yr) Uterus begins to grow Budding of nipples in girls Increased vascularity of penis and scrotum Pubic hair appears in girls Menarche (9–16 yr) **Spurt (Skeletal)** (Girls 1.5 yrs ahead) Pubic hair appears in boys Rapid growth of testes and penis Axillary hair starts Down on upper lip appears	Competes with partners Hobbies Ritualistic play Rational attitudes about food Companionship Invests in community leaders, teachers, impersonal ideals	Learning problems Psychophysiologic disorders Personality disorders: compulsive, anxious, overly dependent, oppositional, overly inhibited, overly independent, isolated and mistrustful personality, tension discharge disorders, and sexual deviations
Formal Operational Thought People can now deal effectively not only with the reality before them, but also with the world of the abstract and the world of possibility ("as if"). Cognition is of the adult type. Adolescents use deductive reasoning and have the ability to evaluate the logic and quality of their own thinking. Their increased abstract power provides them with the capacity to deal with laws and principles. Although egocentrism is still evident at times, important idealistic attitudes are developing in the late adolescent and young adult.	Knows why oil floats on water Can divide 72 by 4 without pencil or paper Understands belfrey and espionage Can repeat 6 digits forward and 5 digits in reverse	Voice changes Mature spermatozoa (11–17 yr) Acne may appear in girls Acne may appear in boys Cessation of skeletal growth Involution of lymphoid tissue Muscle constiues 43% total body weight Permanent teeth calcified Eruption of permanent third molars (17–30 yr)	"Revolt" Loosens tie to family Cliques Responsible independence Work habits solidifying Heterosexual interests Recreational activities Preparation for occupational choice Occupational commitment Elaboration of recreational outlets Marriage readiness Parenthood readiness	Legal delinquency Anorexia nervosa Dysmenorrhea Sexual promiscuity Drug overdose Suicidal attempts Acute confusional state Motor vehicle accidents Schizophrenic disorders (adult type) Affective disorders: manic-depressive psychoses Involutional reactions: depression, suicide Senile disorders: chronic brain syndromes, etc.

individual experiences over time. Adult developmental aspects are included because their needs may complement their children's or conflict with them.

Nurses review with families the individual developmental stages that are occurring concurrently among children and adults and are affecting their daily family interactions. They also assist families to accommodate to children's and adults' changing abilities. Table 11 – 2 presents social-emotional, cognitive, and physical dimensions of individual development. There are 12 columns. The first and second columns, *period* and *age,* are orienting time lines: the period column identifies eight stages from infancy through late adulthood, and the age column is divided into chronological years from birth through 18 years, plus the adult years beyond. Column 3, *social-emotional stages,* represents Erikson's theory (1973), which is a life-span view of social-emotional development across the eight stages of human life. Column 4, the *radius of significant relations,* shows how the world of individuals expands as they move beyond their immediate families. Column 5, *stage-sensitive family developmental tasks,* provides the orientation of families as they raise and launch children (Duvall & Miller, 1985). Column 6, *human needs,* is a hierarchy of individual requirements ranging from basic physiological needs to the need for self-actualization (Maslow, 1970). Column 7, *values orientation,* reflects moral development from undifferentiated to complex stages (Kohlberg, 1984; Thomas, 1992a). Individual family members all have their own values, but their values are related to the values of their family and community. Column 8 shows the *cognitive stages of development* (Piaget & Inhelder, 1969; Thomas, 1992b). The *developmental landmarks* shown in column 9 are milestones that families use to measure their children's progress. Column 10, *physical maturation,* unfolds as children grow. Column 11 lists the *developmental steps (lines)* that individuals experience. Column 12 outlines *developmental problems* associated with changes throughout the life span. Nurses can use this table to identify expected developmental progression and potential areas of concern for families.

Patterns of Health, Disease, and Illness

Families experience health, disease, and illness. Healthy behaviors promote optimal physical and social-emotional well-being. Disease is pathology. Illness is the family daily activities associated with treating the disease. Family interactions shape these patterns.

Health

In their daily activities families create **health patterns**, which are interactive family and individual understandings and behaviors associated with optimal physical, mental, and social well-being, not merely with the absence of disease and incapacitation (derived from Dorland, 1974, p. 683; and Meister, 1991). Healthy behaviors in families include both promotional and protective actions. For example, parents may promote children's growth towards self-actualization through after-school programs that encourage school friendships and creativity. Parents prevent disease through childhood immunizations and avoid injuries through poison prevention efforts. Families' normative behaviors are the healthy patterns they follow as they promote and protect the health of their children and the family as a whole.

Disease

Families interpret symptoms as disease and may then seek assistance from the health care system (Doherty & McCubbin, 1985). Kleinman (1988) points out that disease is culturally defined and that families are influenced by the opinions of health professionals. Diseases and conditions are abnormal patterns, or pathology, of physical, social-emotional, or family processes. For example, an abnormal physical pattern is displayed in sickle cell anemia, a genetic disease that is characterized by periodic pain and bleeding into cellular tissues (Shapiro, 1993). Child abuse is a pattern of inappropriate parenting (Sykes, Hodges, Broome, & Threatt, 1987). Families learn to recognize symptoms and signs of disease in order to prevent, treat, and care for their children's health.

Illness

A distinction must be made between disease and illness. Illness **patterns** are the processes families go through to manage a disease and the medical treatments that become a part of their daily lives (Corbin & Strauss, 1988). Family responses vary with the patterns of illness, which are classified as **acute**, **chronic**, and **life-threatening** (Rolland, 1984). Families reorganize themselves and have different illness tasks for each pattern. They temporarily alter daily routines to deal with the crisis of acute diseases and injuries such as communicable diseases, bone fractures, and appendicitis. After disease treatment, however, families usually return to predisease family routines.

In contrast, families permanently reorganize to accommodate repeated, ongoing, incurable diseases such as juvenile arthritis, diabetes, and asthma, as well as abnormal conditions such as cerebral palsy, seizures, mental retardation, or child abuse. Family careers continue to unfold as siblings and affected children grow and develop. For example, siblings may be jealous of the attention that a chronically ill child receives from parents; and chronically ill adolescents often ignore treatments and aggravate their disease as they search for identity and try to avoid appearing different from their peers.

Families again reorganize during life-threatening illness. They frequently experience the unexpectedly shortened life span of children due to causes such as sudden infant death syndrome, fatal ingestion of household poisons or medications by a toddler, cystic fibrosis, or childhood cancer. When death is inevitable, families grieve, mourn, and begin healing after the death of their child. Family rituals such as funerals help families remember and make the transition to ongoing life as they heal and continue through their family careers. All family members are affected and need to be included in the dying, mourning, and healing processes.

In summary, as caretakers, families promote health and cope with acute, chronic, and life-threatening illnesses in their children. Health issues for families with children are influenced by (1) the interacting dynamics of family career, (2) individuals' development, and (3) patterns of health, disease, and illness. The Family Interaction Model allows nurses to analyze the intersecting points of these three processes and develop nursing interventions that will assist families to address children's health issues.

HEALTH PROMOTION

Families' daily routines influence their children's physical, mental, and social health, as well as the health of the family unit. Patterns of physical health are promoted by daily activities of hygiene, nutrition, exercise, and sleep. Patterns of mental and social health are promoted by helping children and adults reach developmentally appropriate landmarks in the family environment. Patterns of **family well-being** are facilitated by balancing the needs of individuals and the family with the resources and options available to meet these needs (Meister, 1991). Nurses help families intergrate physical, social-emotional, and cognitive health promotion into family routines; in doing so, they also affirm positive patterns of health or provide alternative ones. Thus nurses reduce the risk of illness by shaping the family environment to encourage optimal healthy behaviors (Doherty & McCubbin, 1985).

Families sometimes experience conflict between family tasks and the needs of individual family members, and they must try to balance these. For example, working parents of an infant must decide if and when to place their child in day care. Working parents of school-age children and adolescents must decide if the children can be at home without adult supervision during the after-school period before the parents return home from work. In both situations the family task is to provide economic resources for shelter and food, and the children's need is for a trusted caretaker and safe environment. Various families settle these conflicts differently. Nurses can help families resolve the issues through anticipatory guidance, which involves providing information about what to expect in various situations and how to deal with unwanted developmental problems and life changes (Pridham, 1993).

It is important to recognize that families are a major determinant of children's well-being. Nurses and other health professionals should view their work as a collaboration with parents, not as an authoritarian paternalistic relationship in which parents are perceived as secondary to nurses (Carey, 1989; Pesznecker, Zerwekh, & Horn, 1989; Pridham, 1993; Roberts, 1981). Too often in the past, professionals decided what was best for families' children (Darbyshire, 1993). Today, nurses are exploring parents' perceptions and definitions of health situations in order to develop more relevant health care plans (Gedaly-Duff & Ziebarth, 1994).

Health promotion for children occurs during **parenting** activities, and many American families are assisted in parenting by other child caretakers. Health promotion of child-rearing families through the daily activities of parenting, grandparenting, and day-care and after-school facilities is explained in the following discussion.

Parenting

Families with children promote health by practicing behaviors that advance their own physical, mental, and social well-being and that of their children. Everyday parenting activities nurture and socialize children to be healthy, responsible adults. However, parents sometimes are not aware of or do not use developmental principles. Sameroff and Feil (1985) found, for example, that parents whose socioeconomic status (SES) was higher explained their children's behavior with developmental understanding and were flexible in their parenting actions, but parents of lower SES used fewer explanations of development and expected their children to conform. Nurses might conclude that the parents with developmental understanding and flexible parenting are "better" parents; however, these parents are also often overanxious and worry about everything. Parents who expect conformity of their children often have themselves experienced an environment that has few choices. Sameroff and Feil (1985) concluded that such parents are preparing their children to survive in a harsh environment. Because parents' understanding of their roles and child development clearly varies, it is important for nurses to explore how parents understand their role in order to tailor health promotion activities so that they are meaningful to families.

Extreme forms of inappropriate parenting is also termed "child abuse" or "neglect." "Abuse" is a comprehensive term that includes physical, emotional, and sexual harm (Schuster & Ashburn, 1992). For example, a 2-year-old child is physically abused for a temper tantrum because the temper tantrum is perceived as disrespect of the parent rather than the toddler's struggle for autonomy. A parallel example is the teenager who is verbally and physically abused at home because the assertive behavior of the adolescent is perceived by the parent as disrespectful of social values. The parent does not see the adolescent is struggling for a self-identity separate from school and family. The parent hitting the child hard enough to cause bruising is considered physical abuse and an inappropriate way to socialize the toddler to control his or her temper. An apppropriate way to discipline the child is to use a "time-out," or 5 minutes in a quiet place immediately after the tantrum.

Discipline is setting rules and guidelines so children know what is expected of them. Parents may punish their children for disregarding the rules. In American culture, physical harm resulting from punishment is considered abuse. This difference between discipline and abuse may be uncertain because of different cultural traditions but nurses must be alert to helping families learn appropriate discipline measures.

Nurses can assist parents in health promotion. They teach parenting classes for children of various ages and provide programs aimed at preventing the injuries associated with various ages, such as poisonings in infant and toddlers. In addition, nurses screen childrearing families for potentially harmful parenting situations such as child abuse.

Grandparenting

Grandparents also influence health promotion in childrearing families, though grandparenting is not fully acknowledged as a way to promote health in childrearing families (Kivett, 1991). Grandparents indirectly influence the philosophy and values that parents bring to their parenting, because parenting values are derived in part from families of origin. In addition, grandparents provide a continuity of experience, both for the nuclear fostered and for the extended family of aunts, uncles, and cousins. Such continuity can be fostered by family gatherings and contributes to family well-being. During illness, a grandparent can serve as a valued backup, watch dog, safety valve, and stabilizing force for children and their families. Nurses who understand the influence of grandparenting on childrearing families' health include them in their nursing interventions.

Grandparents also have a direct influence on promoting health in families with children. Grandparents may participate as daily and/or weekly child care providers for working single-parent and two-parent families. In such a situation parents and grandparents must develop rules of childrearing that differ from the behaviors of visiting grandparents, who often indulge their grandchildren and are sometimes seen as "spoiling" the child. Grandparents may become major influences if, for instance, they find themselves raising their grandchild while a teenaged parent finishes high school. In some cases grandparents are primary parents to their grandchildren — for example, in the case of drug-addicted babies born to addicted parents (Jendrek, 1993; Kelley, 1993; Minkler & Roe, 1993). In these situations, nurses teach grandparents health promotion strategies for their grandchildren and their families and also discuss strategies for reducing caregiver stress (Kelley, 1993).

Grandparents can also promote health during situational transitions such as divorce, when they can provide emotional and physical support to divorced parents and children. In other cases, grandparents may be completely separated from their grandchildren by divorce. Nurses may then be involved in examining the complex issues of "grandparent visitation rights" (Purnell & Bagby, 1993).

Day-Care and After-School Facilities

Day-care and after-school facilities also influence the health of families with children as more families rely on outside help to nurture and socialize their children while the parents are working. One task of families is to nurture children. Families raise children without expectation of monetary reward, as a "gift" to society. Today many families can no longer "give" all the work of childraising without turning to day-care and after-school facilities for assistance. In 1970, 29% of women with children under age 6 were in the labor force; by 1990, that figure was 52% (Bianchi, 1995). In the year 2000, it is projected that, if current trends continue, 75% of all mothers will return to work before their child's first birthday (Dawson & Cain, 1990). Nurses can help families review the types of day-care and after-school options available, select compatible philosophies for health promotion, and examine the site for health protection features. They can also participate on community boards that regulate these facilities.

Health promotion for school-age children in the home and at after-school facilities is gaining increasing attention. Between 2 and 5 million children, or 20% of all children between the ages of 5 and 13 years, are estimated to be "latchkey" children, who need care before and after school while parents work (Bianchi, 1990, p. 28). The situation of these children raises concerns about loneliness, injuries, and violence. Nurses, parents, and teachers must develop before- and after-school programs at the schools, and homework telephone services with teachers and teachers' aides.

In selecting day-care and after-school options, protection against injuries and infections is a question that must be addressed. Nurses can provide families with a series of questions to help them check safety precautions and see how the facility will handle their children's minor illnesses. For example, are indoor and outdoor activity areas safe for active children? Are there functioning toilets and wash sinks that children can reach? What is the policy for children who arrive ill or develop an illness during their stay?

Minority/ethnic families and families with children with disabilities require special consideration when choosing day-care and after-school options. Children with special health needs are integrated into federally supported day-care facilities such as Head Start (American Academy of Pediatrics, Committee on Children with Handicaps, 1973). For minority/ethnic childrearing families, culture and language development may be issues.

Symbolic interaction theory (Mead, 1934) suggests that children learn meanings, responses to, and values about health through their interactions with their families and communities. Thus parents', grandparents', and childcare workers' responses may shape children's experience. The childrearing activities done by parents, grandparents, and day-care and after-school caretakers are important in health promotion. The case example shows how nurses can facilitate and teach health activities in these contexts (Fig. 11 – 2).

ACUTE ILLNESS

While American families experience health during 85% of their family careers, they will experience illness for 15% of the time (US Department of Health and Human Services, National Center for Health Statistics, 1993). Families with children frequently experience acute illness and injury. In fact, injuries are the leading cause of morbidity (illness) and mortality (death) in children. The patterns of illness and injury in children are revealed by the following statistics. In 1991, 27 children per 100,000 between the ages of 1 and 15 years died from accidents and injuries, while only 7 per 100,000 died from cancer (US Department of Health and Human Services, National Center for Health Statistics, 1993, pp. 18 – 19). Moreover, for every injury resulting in death, 1000 other injuries occur that require treatment (Guyer & Gallagher, 1985). Three million children experience surgery every year (Tyler, 1990). Families with children also experience respiratory infectious diseases, which are a leading cause of mortality in children and account for approximately 50% of visits to health care settings (Pillitteri, 1992).

This case example illustrates a family's efforts to "normalize" their child's kindergarten situation given her juvenile rheumatoid arthritis (JRA) pain. The nurse is approached by the child's parents to help the child's classmates accept their child in the school's daily activities. The nurse develops a teaching plan that considers the family experiences of each child, the class general social-emotional and cognitive abilities, and the nature of pain in healthy situations.

Special care is taken by the nurse to plan with the family and child with JRA how to approach the topic of pain in the classroom. Children frequently do not want to appear different from their classmates. The child with JRA may not want to talk directly about her pain in the group. The nurse makes a plan with the child and her family about how they will discuss pain in the group.

First, the nurse leads a discussion on children's experience of pain in their daily lives, which encourages comparison of different families and children's expression of pain.

Next, the meaning of pain is explored. American families understand cries of pain as a signal that something is wrong. Children learn that pain usually means danger and to be alert to prevent further injury. Using a "faces" pain tool to measure pain, children learn that hurts have different degrees of intensity (Beyer & Aradine, 1988; Wong & Baker, 1988).

Finally, the children learn that they can cope with pain. With cuts or scratches that are considered minor, families manage pain differently. Some children report blowing to soothe the area, and putting Bandaids on the hurt part. By including the child with JRA, the children learn that pain does not always go away. They learn that some pain can be helped by Bandaids, and that JRA pain is helped by special exercises and medicines.

In this case, the nurse recognizes the developmental task of integrating the preschooler with a chronic illness into school life. The nurse discusses pain in developmentally appropriate ways for preschoolers and helps the children learn that pain can be coped with in several ways. Thus, in cooperation with the family, the nurse begins to "normalize" the pain experience for the child with JRA, and helps her classmates learn positive ways to manage pain.

FIGURE 11-2
Case example of health teaching.

Acute illness in children is characterized by the sudden onset of signs and symptoms; treatment can usually restore children and their families to the predisease state. Childhood acute illnesses include communicable infections such as chickenpox, conditions such as appendicitis, and injuries such as bone fractures.

In a health care system that is encouraging day surgery procedures, early discharge, and home care, parents are managing their children's minor diseases and illnesses to a greater extent than are health professionals (Feetham, 1986). Typically, families whose children undergo a short-stay procedure such as an adenoidectomy or tonsillectomy will care for their children at home following the first 4 to 8 hours after surgery. Gedaly-Duff and Ziebarth (1994) studied mothers' experiences in identifying and managing their children's acute pain associated with surgery. They found that mothers learned to manage their children's pain through trial and error. One mother was fearful of both overdosing and undermedicating for the pain. She said:

> I was concerned about giving him too much . . . and I went too long, he was extremely uncomfortable. After that I said, "It's not worth it" . . . it took longer for the medication to get back into his system . . . so then I gave it every three hours, . . . like the label said. . . .

In this study, parents were uncertain about whether their children were adequately treated for pain.

Families in the above study also altered their routines. Parent work schedules were rearranged and most mothers took time off to care for their children. Mothers also described apprehension about the lack of sleep in the household because of their acutely ill child's irritability. Siblings were attentive, anxious, or misbehaving at times because of the extra attention given their ill sister or brother.

To help families experiencing acute illness, nurses must first recognize families' past experiences with and knowledge about acute illness. Second, nurses must alert families to potential disruptions among parents and siblings because of conflicts between family members' needs. Third, nurses can plan with families how to alter their family routines to accommodate the temporary changes required by the acute illness. Fourth, nurses can teach families the developmentally related reactions children have to acute illness — for example, how to assess pain by using age-appropriate methods (Gedaly-Duff, 1991). Finally, nurses can teach families to recognize the patterns and potential complications (bleeding and pain) of acute illness and they can give parents the information they need to manage fever and pain.

CHRONIC ILLNESS

While most childrearing families experience acute illnesses and become familiar with managing these crises, many families are not prepared to care for children with chronic illness and to accommodate to the associated unknowns and uncertainties.

Depending on the definition of "chronic illness," which may include or exclude cancer and mental illness, the number of families with children experiencing chronic illness is estimated to be from 20% to 31% (Newacheck & Taylor, 1992). Chronic illness is characterized by ongoing, repeated relapses of incurable but manageable disease such as juvenile arthritis, diabetes, asthma, and conditions such as cerebral palsy, and mental retardation. Families accommodate to the effects of chronic illness on their children and the family through a process called "reality negotiation" (Ersek, 1992). This process is illustrated by a family that does not comply with prescribed treatments and medications (Jennings, Callahan, & Caplan, 1988) because the family is concretely testing the reality of an incurable diagnosis by experiencing the relapse.

Nurses can support families directly and indirectly during the process of adjusting to a child's chronic illness. For example, families frequently compare their situations to those of other families while waiting to be seen in outpatient clinics (Gedaly-Duff, 1990b), or the nurse can conduct family workshops (Gedaly-Duff, 1990c) that discuss issues such as sibling responses, the burden of taking care of the ill child at home, and family progression through developmental stages.

Families use a variety of strategies to normalize the disease experience and cope with the chronic illness (Knafl & Deatrick, 1986). Gedaly-Duff (1990b), for example, found that initially families were unaware that they had made changes in daily routines to accommodate to their child's chronic disease. Upon reflection, however, families described routines for giving medicine and rituals such as stopping for a special hamburger associated with the family trip for monthly clinic visits.

Parents are flexible in their approach to the health care of their children and are concerned that the children develop to their fullest potential in spite of the disease. For example, the mother of a 5-year-old girl once said:

> Sometimes I'll see her knee seems to be swollen, but I won't say anything. I won't ask her because I figure that if it's really bad, she'll let me know. I mean, she knows she can tell me that, and then we'll figure out what it is we should do. But I'm not going to plant the seed in her mind. . . . She might always have a little bit of pain. She's not going to be very productive as a human being if she props it up on a pillow.

Nurses and families can together create new routines to accommodate disease and continue with the family's life. For example, a 5-year-old's kindergarten class can be scheduled for the afternoon so that he can treat his juvenile rheumatoid arthritis (JRA) with a warm bath before he gets dressed in the morning. Or a motorized tricycle can be taken to a Fourth of July picnic so that the 4-year-old with JRA can ride alongside his playmates. Grandparents can help organize a handicapped softball team to enable their grandson with JRA to play ball (Gedaly-Duff, 1990b). Researchers suggest that chronically ill adolescent children have better self-esteem when their families emphasize independence and participation in recreational activities (Hauser, Jacobson, Wertleib, Brink, & Wentworth, 1985). Nurses can collaborate with families with chronically ill children to carefully monitor achievement of developmental landmarks (Garrison & McQuiston, 1989; Yoos, 1987).

Families are in a difficult situation when their chronically ill children are hospitalized (Robinson, 1985). The families have been the primary caregivers at home but now they are placed in a dependent role, as if they did not understand their child's illness pattern. Nurses who have worked with families of chronically ill children know that they are knowledgeable about how their children respond to disease as well as about their developmental capabilities. Thus it is important for nurses to be "family centered" in working with families of chronically ill children. To help families care for their chronically ill children, the nurse can:

1. Learn how the family's past experiences and expectations of disease and illness are affecting the current illness situation

2. Determine whether the family is responding to diagnosis of a new condition or is experienced in caring for their child's chronic illness

3. Help families to promote health in spite of illness by meeting the continually evolving needs of family members

4. Help families accommodate to the child's developmental limitations related to the disease or condition

In carrying out these specific tasks, the nurse supporting the family of a chronically ill child must consider the nature of the illness and its demands on relationships (Woods, Yates, & Primono, 1989).

LIFE-THREATENING ILLNESS

Families know that chronic illness, like acute injuries and diseases, may be life-threatening; however, the death of a child is a rare and shocking experience for families. Of children in the United States under the age of 14 years, 3 in 10,000 (32 per 100,000) died from all causes in 1990 (US Department of Health and Human Services, National Center for Health Statistics, 1993). Fewer than one child in 10,000 (8.9 per 100,000) under 14 years old died from cancer (US Department of Health and Human services, National Center for Health Statistics, 1993). Even though children's deaths are often reported in television and newspaper media, the death is a distant event. The daily lives of American families do not prepare them for a child's death.

A serious illness is characterized by hospitalization, life-threatening circumstances, and uncertainty. As health professionals, nurses can support and guide families through this traumatic experience. Koch (1985) found that families with children who were recently diagnosed with cancer experienced increased negative affect, role behavior changes, rules prohibiting emotional expression, worsening problems, and a gathering together of family members. Siblings are sometimes overlooked in the crisis of a dying sister or brother, but they need to be included in the family circle. Nurses and other health professionals can encourage family expression of emotions, perhaps teaching them how to express these emotions in a nonthreatening fashion. Indeed, nurses often find themselves helping parents, siblings, and grandparents work through their fears and resolutions of life and death issues (Hagestad & Lang, 1986; Strom & Strom, 1992).

Nurses can use the Family Interaction Model to support families during life-threatening illness situations. First, nurses should assess families' past experiences with a child's death. Generally families have few models for learning how to cope with this situation. Second, nurses can help families learn how children understand and cope with life-threatening illnesses (Waechter, 1971). Thus most families have little experience in caring for a terminally ill child, and they may not know how to manage their child's pain and discomfort in the final days. Nurses can teach them strategies for comfort care (US Department of Health and Human Services, Agency for Health Care Policy and Research, 1994) and anticipate the stages families will experience and plan support for them at the point of death (Benner & Wrubel, 1989). Finally, nurses can facilitate families' grieving and mourning of the child's death.

IMPLICATIONS FOR PRACTICE, EDUCATION, RESEARCH, AND HEALTH CARE POLICY

Family child health nurses interact with families and other health professionals and use a family perspective to guide (1) direct health care delivery, that is, practice; (2) education, both for families and for other health care providers; (3) research, to systematically explore family child health nursing; and (4) health policy proposals and evaluation.

The Family Interaction Model, which incorporates relevant components of family life, family development and transitions, and family health issues, promotes a comprehensive and holistic approach to the nursing of families. Using this model, nurses are able to collaborate with families who are in the processes of health promotion, disease prevention, and illness management.

Implications for Practice

Family child health nursing must be practiced in collaboration with the families themselves and with other health professionals. In family-centered care nurses work with families to promote health, prevent disease, and cope with acute, chronic, and life-threatening illnesses. The Family Interactional Model suggests a number of implications for practice. First, nurses who interact with American families find that many parents work outside the home, and much of their children's time is spent at day-care or after-school care facilities. In addition, families of school-age and adolescent children may focus on school and school-related activities. Igoe (1993), Igoe and Giordano (1992), and others are therefore recommending that more of child health care take place in this arena — as school-based and school-linked health care. For example, families could receive care for their school-enrolled child as well as other members of the family at school-based health clinics.

The Family Interaction Model also has implications for balancing health promotion and the management of health issues. It is well known that anticipating health problems can prevent their occurrence and minimize their effects. With their close and often frequent contacts with families and their children, nurses are in a position to form a partnership with families for wellness promotion. Nurses who practice health promotion can also assist clients to assume self-care responsibilities appropriate to their abilities and developmental levels (Kandzari & Howard, 1981).

A recent report by the National Institute for Nursing Research (1993) indicates that most causes of morbidity and mortality in children and adolescents are due to behavior and lifestyle and are therefore preventable. Nurses who are aware of these risk factors can intervene with children and families to help prevent or at least minimize situational and developmentally related problems.

Nurses can identify health issues or risks for the family and its members by expanding assessment of children (Steele, 1988) to a more comprehensive family assessment. Nurses who explore comprehensively the situations of family members will detect those individual members who are at risk. For example, in a family whose child has been newly diagnosed with a disease, a sibling may begin to fail at school. Here, the nurse can assess the whole family, identify the new behavior, and facilitate a family conference so that each child understands what is happening. This keeps the focus on the family. The family also realizes that other family members need attention.

Implications for Research

Family nurses need to explore ways in which the family interactional approach can be implemented and evaluated. For example, the effectiveness of anticipatory guidance, a commonly used yet underexplored interventional strategy, could be tested (Pridham, 1993). Research could also focus on identifying risk factors for families, to assist nurses and other health care providers to focus their interactions with clients. One question might be: What is the impact of a child's developmental delay on a family with impaired parents? In such a situation, family nurses could identify patterns that are cues for future problems and also explore the efficacy of interventions. Using an interactional approach, they can identify factors in family and child health that are not apparent when the individual is the focus for investigating patterns of health, disease, and illness. This facilitates early screening and interventions, which are efficient and cost-saving strategies.

Implications for Education

Use of the Family Interaction Model must be based on thorough knowledge of the development and patterns of health, disease, and illness, as well as communication between and among all persons involved. Family-focused care that balances health promotion, disease prevention, and illness management needs to be emphasized in formal and informal settings, as well as in academic and community programs (Hanson, Heims, & Julian, 1992). Practicing nurses as well as those receiving their initial nursing education need to explore comprehensive approaches to family child health.

Implications for Policy

Policies govern the health of families at agency, institutional, regional, state, and national levels and influence family health in multiple and diverse ways.

Family nurses influence public policies through their professional organizations as well as through their individual efforts. A professional organization such as the American Nurses' Association can develop standards of practice and provide position papers to public servants developing health policies and laws. Policy analysis is therefore the job of every nurse (Gilliss, 1991).

For example, public policies often place single-parent families in conflicting circumstances (Bowen, Desimone & McKay, 1995). A parent may find a job, but make too much money to qualify for state-assisted health insurance, and not have enough to pay for other types of health insurance. As a result of economic and social policy, family nurses are caring for significant numbers of families with children who are living in poverty or homeless (Malloy, 1992).

Family child health nurses practice in many settings; therefore they need to be aware of policies that apply in and between these settings. For example, a family with a chronically ill child may interact with nurses in an agency, in a hospital, and in the home. At a public policy level, family nurses must advocate for not only "adequate" but "growth-promoting" day-care facilities for the American working family. Safe and health-promoting options are needed for families with children from infancy to adolescence.

SUMMARY Key points to remember are that family nurses focus on the relationship of family life to children's health and illness, and that they assist families to achieve well-being. Through family-centered care, nurses enhance family life and the development of their members to their fullest potential. Using the Family Interaction Model allows nurses to take a comprehensive and collaborative approach to families and incorporates relevant components of family life and interaction, family development and transitions, and family health and illness. It also enables them to screen for potentially harmful situations, instruct families about health issues, and help families to cope with acute illness, chronic illness, and life-threatening conditions.

STUDY QUESTIONS

1. The family child health nurse determines the most *appropriate* health promotion activities with a family with young children through analysis of:
   a. Children's health practices
   b. Patterns of parenting, and family and child developmental tasks
   c. Parents' and grandparent's health beliefs
   d. Patterns of disease and illness reorganization task management

2. Family child health nurses practice family-centered health care, which is most accurately characterized as:
   a. Fostering partnerships between members of different families
   b. Providing consistently high-quality care for all families
   c. Forming partnerships between families and nurses
   d. Viewing the nurse as the constant in family and child health

3. The Family Interaction Model has three major concepts. Which one of the following is *not* one of these major concepts?
   a. Task development cycles
   b. Individual development
   c. Family career
   d. Patterns of health, disease, and illness

4. Which of these principles should family child health nurses incorporate in their care in order to help a family with a child who has diabetes?
   a. Patterns of illness are usually predictable in families.
   b. Protection is paramount in each interaction.
   c. Patterns of illness and patterns of disease are different.
   d. Reorganization of family routines is discouraged.

5. Using the Family Interaction Model, the family child health nurse knows that one of the more important assessments of families experiencing a chronic illness of their child is:
   a. Definition of the disease with which the child has been diagnosed
   b. How the family's past crises have altered their growth
   c. Definition of the limitations that the family is experiencing
   d. How the family's past experience with the illness affects the current situation

REFERENCES

American Academy of Pediatrics, Committee on Children with Handicaps. (1973). Day care for handicapped children. *Pediatrics, 51,* 948.

Andrews, M. P., Bubolz, M. M., & Paolucci, B. (1980). An ecological approach to study of the family. *Marriage and Family Review, 3,* 29–49.

Benner, P., & Wrubel, J. (1989). Remembering Lara. In *The primacy of caring* (pp. 298–307). Menlo Park, CA: Addison-Wesley.

Besser, F. (1977, February 10). Great Ormond Street anniversary. *Nursing Mirror,* pp. 60–63.

Beyer, J., & Aradine, C. (1988). Convergent and discriminant validity of a self-report measure of pain intensity for children. *Children's Health Care, 16,* 274–282.

Bianchi, S. M. (1990). America's children: Mixed prospects. *Population Bulletin, 45,* 1–43. Washington, DC: Population Reference Bureau.

Bianchi, S. M. (1995). The changing demographic and socioeconomic character of single parent families. *Marriage and Family Review, 20,* 71–98.

Bowen, G. C., Desimone, L. M., & McKay, S. K. (1995). Poverty and the single mother family: A macroeconomic perspective. *Marriage and Family Review, 20,* 115–142.

Burlingham, D., & Freud, A. (1942). *Young children in war time.* London: Allen & Unwin.

Burr, W. R., Herrin, D. A., Day, R. L., Beutler, I. F., & Leigh, G. K. (1988). Epistemologies that lead to primary explanations in family science. *Family Science Review, 1,* 185–210.

Cain, V. S., & Hofferth, S. L. (1989). Parental choice of self-care for school-age children. *Journal of Marriage and the Family, 51,* 65–78.

Carey, R. (1989). How values affect the mutual goal setting process with multiproblem families. *Journal of Community Health Nursing, 6,* 7–14.

Corbin, J. M., & Strauss, A. (1988). Illness trajectories. In *Unending work and care: Managing chronic illness at home* (pp. 33–48). San Francisco: Jossey-Bass.

Darbyshire, P. (1993). Parents, nurses and paediatric nursing: A critical review. *Journal of Advanced Nursing, 18,* 1670–1680.

Dawson, D. A., & Cain, V. S. (1990). Child care arrangements: Health of our nation's children, United States, 1988. Advance data from vital and health statistics; no 187. Hyattsville, Maryland: National Center for Health Statistics.

Dickoff, J., James, P., & Wiedenbach, E. (1968). Theory in a practice discipline, I. Practice oriented theory. *Nursing Research, 17,* 415–435.

Doherty, W., & McCubbin, H. (1985). Families and health care: An emerging arena of theory, research, and clinical intervention. *Family Relations, 34,* 5–11.

Dorland's illustrated medical dictionary (25th ed.). (1974). Philadelphia: W.B. Saunders.

Duvall, E. M., & Miller, B. C. (1985). Developmental tasks: Individual and family. In E. M. Duvall & B. C. Miller, *Marriage and family development* (pp. 41–64). New York: Harper & Row.

Erikson, E. H. (1973). *Childhood and society.* New York: W. W. Norton.

Ersek, M. (1992). Examining the process and dilemmas of reality negotiation. *Image: The Journal of Nursing Scholarship, 24,* 19–25.

Faville, K. (1925). The nurse as counselor in troubled homes. *The Red Cross Courier, 4,* 14–15, 22.

Feetham, S. L. (1986). Hospitals and home care: Inseparable in the '80s. *Pediatric Nursing, 12,* 383–386.

Ferraro, A. R., & Longo, D. C. (1985). Nursing care of the family with a chronically ill, hospitalized child: An alternative approach. *Image: The Journal of Nursing Scholarship, 17,* 77–81.

Garrison, W. T., & McQuiston, S. (1989). *Developmental clinical psychology and psychiatry: Vol. 19. Chronic illness during childhood and adolescence.* Newbury Park, CA: Sage Publications.

Gedaly-Duff, V. (1990a, March). Family management of childhood pain. Phase 2: Parent's experiences in care of their children's repeated pain episodes associated with chronic illness such as juvenile rheumatoid arthritis. Paper presented at the meeting of the Robert Wood Johnson Clinical Nurse Scholar program, University of Pennsylvania, Philadelphia.

Gedaly-Duff, V. (1990b). [Family management of childhood pain. Phase 2: Parents' experiences in care of their children's repeated pain episodes associated with chronic illness such as juvenile rheumatoid arthritis.] Unpublished raw data.

Gedaly-Duff, V. (1990c). *A family affair.* Workshop conducted for the American Juvenile Arthritis Organization, Second Regional Conference "Families in Touch," Worcester, PA.

Gedaly-Duff, V. (1991). Developmental issues: Preschool and school-age children. In J. P. Bush & S. W. Harkins (Eds.), *Children in pain: Clinical and research issues from a developmental perspective* (pp. 195–230). New York: Springer-Verlag.

Gedaly-Duff, V., & Ziebarth, D. (1994). Mothers' management of 4- to-8-year-olds' adenoid-tonsillectomy pain: A preliminary study. *Pain, 57,* 293 - 299.

Gilliss, C. L. (1991). Family nursing research, theory and practice. *Image: Journal of Nursing Scholarship, 23,* 19 - 22.

Godfrey, A. (1965). A study of nursing care designed to assist hospitalized children and their parents in their separation. *Nursing Research, 4,* 52 - 69.

Goslin, E. (1978). Hospitalization as a life crisis for the preschool child: A critical review. *Journal of Community Health, 3,* 321 - 346.

Guyer, B., & Gallagher, S. S. (1985). An approach to the epidemiology of childhood injuries. *Pediatric Clinics of North America, 32,* 5 - 15.

Hagestad, G. O., & Lang, M. E. (1986). The transition to grandparenthood. *Journal of Family Issues, 7,* 115 - 130.

Hanson, S. M. H., Heims, M. L., & Julian, D. J. (1992). Education for family health care professionals: Nursing as a paradigm. *Family Relations, 41,* 49 - 53.

Harrison, H. (1993). The principles for family-centered neonatal care. *Pediatrics, 92,* 643 - 650.

Hauser, S., Jacobson, A., Wertlieb, D., Brink, S., & Wentworth, S. (1985). The contribution of family environment to perceived competence and illness adjustments in diabetic and acutely ill adolescents. *Family Relations, 34,* 99 - 108.

Igoe, J. (1993). School-linked family health centers in health care reform. *Pediatric Nursing, 19,* 67 - 68.

Igoe, J. B., & Giordano, B. P. (1992). *Expanding school health services to serve families in the 21st century.* Washington, DC: American Nurses Publishing.

Jendrek, M. P. (1993). Grandparents who parent their grandchildren: Effects on lifestyle. *Journal of Marriage and the Family, 55,* 609 - 621.

Jennings, B., Callahan, D., & Caplan, A. L. (1988). Ethical challenges of chronic illness. *Hastings Center Report,* Special Supplement February/March, 1 - 16.

Kandzari, J. H., & Howard, J. R. (1981). Learning wellness: A challenge for the family. In *A developmental approach to assessment* (pp. 1 - 9). Boston: Little, Brown.

Kelley, S. J. (1993). Caregiver stress in grandparents raising grandchildren. *Image: Journal of Nursing Scholarship, 25,* 331 - 337.

Kivett, V. R. (1991). The grandparent-grandchild connection. In S. P. Pfeifer & M. B. Sussman (Eds.), *Families: Intergenerational and generational connections* (pp. 267 - 290). New York: Haworth Press.

Kleinman, A. (1988). The meaning of symptoms and disorders. In *The illness narratives* (pp. 3 - 30). New York: Basic Books.

Knafl, K. A., & Deatrick, J. A. (1986). How families manage chronic conditions: An analysis of the concept of normalization. *Research in Nursing and Health, 9,* 215 - 222.

Koch, A. (1985). "If only it could be me": The families of pediatric cancer patients. *Family Relations, 34,* 123 - 127.

Kohlberg, L. (1984). *The psychology of moral development.* San Francisco: Harper & Row.

Lash, M., & Wertlieb, D. (1993). A model for family-centered service coordination for children who are disabled by traumatic injuries. *The ACCH Advocate, 1,* 19 - 27, 39 - 41.

Mahaffy, P. (1965). The effects of hospitalization on children admitted for tonsillectomy and adenoidectomy. *Nursing Research, 14,* 12 - 19.

Malloy, C. (1992). Children and poverty: America's future at risk. *Pediatric Nursing, 18,* 553 - 557.

Maslow, A. H. (1970). *Motivation and personality* (2nd ed.). New York: Harper & Row.

Mead, G. H. (1934). *Mind, self, and society.* Chicago: University of Chicago Press.

Meister, S. B. (1991). Family well-being. In A. L. Whall & J. Fawcett (Eds.), *Family theory development in nursing: State of the science and art* (pp. 209 - 231). Philadelphia: F.A. Davis.

Miles, M., Carter, M., Riddle, I., Hennessey, J., & Eberly, T. (1989). The pediatric intensive care unit environment as a source of stress for parents. *Maternal-Child Nursing Journal, 18,* 199 - 206.

Minkler, M., & Roe, K. M. (1993). *Grandmothers as caregivers: Raising children of the crack cocaine epidemic.* Newbury Park, CA: Sage Publications.

National Institute of Nursing Research (NINR). (1993). *Health promotion for older children and adolescents: A report of the NINR priority expert panel on health promotion.* Bethesda, MD: US Department of Health and Human Services, USPHS, NIH.

Newacheck, P. W., & Taylor, W. R. (1992). Childhood chronic illness: Prevalence, severity, and impact. *American Journal of Public Health, 82,* 364 - 371.

Paget, M. (1982). Your son is cured now; you may take him home. *Culture, Medicine and Psychiatry, 6,* 237 - 259.

Pesznecker, B. L., Zerwekh, J. V., & Horn, B. J. (1989). The mutual-participation relationship: Key to facilitating self-care practices in clients and families. *Public Health Nursing, 6,* 197 - 203.

Piaget, J., & Inhelder, B. (1969). *Psychology of the child.* New York: Basic Books.

Pillitteri, A. (1992). *Maternal and child health nursing.* Philadelphia: J. B. Lippincott.

Pridham, D. F. (1993). Anticipatory guidance of parents of new infants: Potential contribution of the internal working model construct. *Image: Journal of Nursing Scholarship, 25,* 49 – 55.

Prugh, D. G. (1983). The development of the child's personality. In *The psychosocial aspects of pediatrics* (pp. 73 – 89). Philadelphia: Lea & Febiger.

Purnell, M., & Bagby, B. H. (1993). Grandparents' rights: Implications for family specialists. *Family Relations, 42,* 173 – 178.

Rankin, S. H. (1989). Family transitions. In C. L. Gilliss, B. L. Highley, B. M. Robers, & I. M. Martinson (Eds.), *Toward a science of family nursing* (pp. 173 – 186). Menlo Park, CA: Addison-Wesley.

Roberts, F. B. (1981). A model for parent education. *Image: The Journal of Nursing Scholarship, 13,* 86 – 89.

Robinson, C. A. (1985). Double bind: A dilemma for parents of chronically ill children. *Pediatric Nursing, 11,* 112 – 115.

Rolland, J. S. (1984). Toward a psychosocial typology of chronic and life-threatening illness. *Family Systems Medicine, 2,* 245 – 262.

Sameroff, A. J., & Feil, L. A. (1985). Parental concepts of development. In I. E. Sigel (Ed.), *Parental belief systems* (pp. 83 – 105). Hillsdale, NJ: Larence Erlbaum.

Schultz, P. R., & Meleis, A. I. (1988). Nursing epistemology: Traditions, insights, questions. *Image: Journal of Nursing Scholarship, 20,* 218 – 220.

Schuster, C. S., & Ashburn, S. S. (1992). Psychosocial development during the toddler and preschool years. In *The process of human development* (3rd ed., pp. 231 – 250). Philadelphia: J. B. Lippincott.

Shapiro, B. (1993). Management of painful episodes in sickle cell disease. In N. Schechter, C. Berde, & M. Yaster (Eds.), *Pain in infants, children, and adolescents* (pp. 385 – 410). Philadelphia: Williams & Wilkins.

Shelton, T., Jeppson, E., & Johnson, B. (1987). *Family-centered care for children with special health care needs.* Washington, DC: Association for the Care of Children's Health.

Spitz, R. (1945). Hospitalism. *Psychoanalytic Study of the Child, 1,* 53 – 74.

Steele, S. M. (1988). Assessing developmental delays in preschool children. *Journal of Pediatric Health Care, 2,* 141 – 145.

Strom, R. D., & Strom, S. K. (1992). Grandparents and intergenerational relationships. *Educational Gerontology, 18,* 607 – 624.

Sykes, M. K., Hodges, M. C., Broome, M., & Threatt, B. J. (1987). Nurses' knowledge of child abuse and nurses' attitudes toward parental participation in the abused child's care. *Journal of Pediatric Nursing, 2,* 412 – 417.

Thomas, R. M. (1992a). The contents of child development theories. In *Comparing theories of child development* (3rd ed., pp. 26 – 52). Belmont, CA: Wadsworth.

Thomas, R. M. (1992b). Gesell's descriptive growth gradients. In *Comparing Theories of Child Development* (3rd ed., pp. 59 – 77). Belmont, CA: Wadsworth.

Thompson, R. (1986). Where we stand: Twenty years of research on pediatric hospitalization and health care. Children's Health Care, *14,* 200 – 210.

Turk, D. C., & Kerns, R. D. (1985). The family in health and illness. In D. C. Turk & R. D. Kerns (Eds.), *Health, illness, and families: A life-span perspective* (pp. 1 – 22). New York: John Wiley & Sons.

Tyler, D. (1990). Pain in infants and children. In J. J. Bonica (Ed.), *The management of pain* (Vol. I, pp. 538 – 551). Philadelphia: Lea & Febiger.

US Department of Health and Human Services. Agency for Health Care Policy and Research (AHCPR). (1994). *U. S. guideline for management of cancer pain* (AHCPR Pub. No. 94-0592). Rockville, MD: Agency for Health Care Policy and Research, Public Health Service, US Department of Health and Human Services.

US Department of Health and Human Services. National Center for Health Statistics. (1993). Highlights. Health, United States, 1992. In *Health, United States, 1992 and healthy people 2000 review* (DHHS Pub. No. PHS 93-1232, pp. 3 – 7, 52 – 60, 68). Hyattsville, MD: Public Health Service.

US Department of Health and Human Services. US Public Health Service. National Institutes of Health. National Institute of Nursing Research. (1993). *Health promotion for older children and adolescents: A report of the NINR priority expert panel on health promotion* (NIH Publication No. 93-2420). Bethesda, MD: US Department of Health and Human Services.

Waechter, E. (1971). Children's awareness of fatal illness. *American Journal of Nursing, 71,* 1168 – 1172.

Wald, L. D. (1904). The treatment of families in which there is sickness. *American Journal of Nursing, 427 – 431,* 515 – 519, 602 – 606.

White, J. (1991). *Dynamics of family development* (pp. 48 – 59). New York: Guilford Press.

Wong, D., & Baker, C. (1988). Convergent and discriminant validity of a self-report measure of pain intensity for children. *Children's Health Care, 16,* 274 – 282.

Wood, C. (1988). The training of nurses for sick children. *The Nursing Record, December 6,* pp. 507 – 510.

Woods, N. F., Yates, B. C., & Primono, J. (1989). Supporting families during chronic illness. *Image: Journal of Nursing Scholarship, 21,* 46 – 50.

Yoos, L. (1987). Chronic childhood illnesses: Developmental issues. *Pediatric Nursing, 13,* 25 – 28.

BIBLIOGRAPHY

Burr, W. R., Day, R. D., & Bahr, K. S. (1993). *Family science.* Pacific Grove, CA: Brooks/Cole.

Carr, P. (1990). Needs to know, wants to know, ought to know. *Home Healthcare Nurse, 8,* 34.

Church, J. L., & Baer, K. J. (1987). Examination of the adolescent: A practical guide. *Journal of Pediatric Health Care, 1,* 65 – 72.

Cone, T. (1976). Highlights of two centuries of American pediatrics, 1776 – 1976. *American Journal of Diseases of Children, 130,* 762 – 775.

Cormany, E. E. (1993). Family-centered service coordination: A four tier model. *Infants and Young Children, 6,* 12 – 19.

Doherty, W. J. (1985). Family interventions in health care. *Family Relations, 34,* 129 – 137.

Dowd, E., & Vlastuin, L. (1990). Home care. In M. Craft & J. Denehny (Eds.), *Nursing interventions for infants and children* (pp. 240 – 256). Philadelphia: W. B. Saunders.

Feetham, S. L., Meister, S. B., Bell, J. M., & Gillis, C. L. (1993). *The nursing of families: Theory/research/education/practice.* Newbury Park, CA: Sage Publications.

Fosanelli, P. (1984). Latch key children. *Journal of Developmental and Behavioral Pediatrics, 5,* 173 – 177.

Fowler, J. W. (1981). *Stages of faith: The psychology of human development and the quest for meaning.* New York: Harper & Row.

Gedaly-Duff, V. (1988). Pain theories and their relevance to nursing practice. *Nurse Practitioner, 13*(10), 66 – 68.

Gedaly-Duff, V. (1988). Preparing young children for painful procedures. *Journal of Pediatric Nursing, 3,* 169 – 179.

Gedaly-Duff, V., & Burns, C. (1992). Reducing children's pain-distress associated with injections using cold: A pilot study. *Journal of the American Academy of Nurse Practitioners, 4,* 95 – 100.

Gesell, A., Ilg, F. L., Ames, L. B., & Rodell, J. L. (1974). *Infant and child in the culture of today.* New York: Harper & Row.

Gilliss, C. L. (1990). Health care and the family. In D. H. Olson & M. K. Hanson (Eds.), *2001: Preparing families for the future.* NCFR Presidential Report. Minneapolis, MN: National Council for Family Relations.

Gortner, S. R. (1990). Nursing values and science: Toward a science philosophy. *Image: Journal of Nursing Scholarship, 22,* 101 – 105.

Igoe, J. (1990). A blueprint for health promotion: Children's rights and community action. *Pediatric Nursing, 16,* 410 – 411.

Ingle, G. (1977). The need for a new medical model: A challenge for biomedicine. *Science, 196,* 129 – 136.

Kail, R., & Bisanz, J. (1982). Information processing and cognitive development. In H. W. Reese & L. P. Lipsett (Eds.), *Advances in child development and behavior* (Vol. 17). New York: Academic Press.

Kivett, V. R. (1993). Racial comparisons of the grandmother role. *Family Relations, 42,* 165 – 172.

Levinson, D. J. (1977). The mid-life transition: A period in adult psychosocial development. *Psychiatry, 40,* 99 – 112.

Mishel, M. H., & Murdaugh, C. L. (1987). Family adjustment to heart transplantation: Redesigning the dream. *Nursing Research, 36,* 332 – 338.

Neugarten, B. L. (1979). Time age, and the life cycle. *American Journal of Psychiatry, 136,* 887 – 894.

Nye, F. I. (1988). Fifty years of family research. *Journal of Marriage and the Family, 50,* 305 – 316.

O'Grady, R. S., & Glass, M. (1989). Children day care for healthy younger families. In C. L. Gilliss, B. L. Highley, B. M. Roberts, & I. M. Martinson (Eds.), *Toward a science of family nursing* (pp. 226 – 247). Menlo Park, CA: Addison-Wesley.

Popenoe, D. (1993). American family decline, 1960 – 1990: A review and appraisal. *Journal of Marriage and the Family, 55,* 527 – 555.

Rollins, J. A. (1993). Nurses as gangbusters: A response to gang violence in America. *Pediatric Nursing, 19,* 559 – 567.

Rosenstock, I. M. (1988). Enhancing patient compliance with health recommendations. *Journal of Pediatric Health Care, 2,* 67 – 72.

Sears, R. (1975). Your ancients revisited: A history of child development. In E. M. Hetherington (Ed.), *Review of child development research* (Vol. 5, pp. 1 – 73). Chicago: University of Chicago Press.

Thorne, S. E., & Robinson, C. A. (1989). Guarded alliance: Health care relationships in chronic illness. *Image: Journal of Nursing Scholarship, 21,* 153 – 157.

Tubman, J. G. (1993). Family risk factors, parental alcohol use, and problem behaviors among school-age children. *Family Relations, 42,* 81 – 86.

US Bureau of the Census. (1991). *Statistical abstract of the United States* (111th ed.). Washington, DC: US Government Printing Office.

US Department of Labor, Women's Bureau. (1982, August). *Employers and child care: Establishing services through the workplace* (Pamphlet 23-Bab-441). Washington, DC: US Government Printing Office.

Van Ingen, P. (1927). Child health in the past. *American Journal of Diseases of Children, 34,* 95 – 105.

Warner, K. E., & Warner, P. A. (1993). Is an ounce of prevention worth a pound of cure? Disease prevention in health care reform. *Journal of Ambulatory Care Management, 16*(4), 38 – 49.

Wegner, G. D., & Alexander, R. J. (1993). *Readings in family nursing.* Philadelphia: J. B. Lippincott.

Werner, E. E. (1979). Cross-cultural tests of Piaget's theory of cognitive development. *Cross-cultural child development: A view from the planet earth* (pp. 211 – 234). Belmont, CA: Brooks/Cole.

Wright, L. M., & Leahey, M. (1990). Trends in nursing of families. *Journal of Advanced Nursing, 15,* 148 – 154.

Zigler, E., & Hall, N. (1988). Daycare and its effect on children: An overview for pediatric health professionals. *Developmental and Behavioral Pediatrics, 9,* 38 – 45.

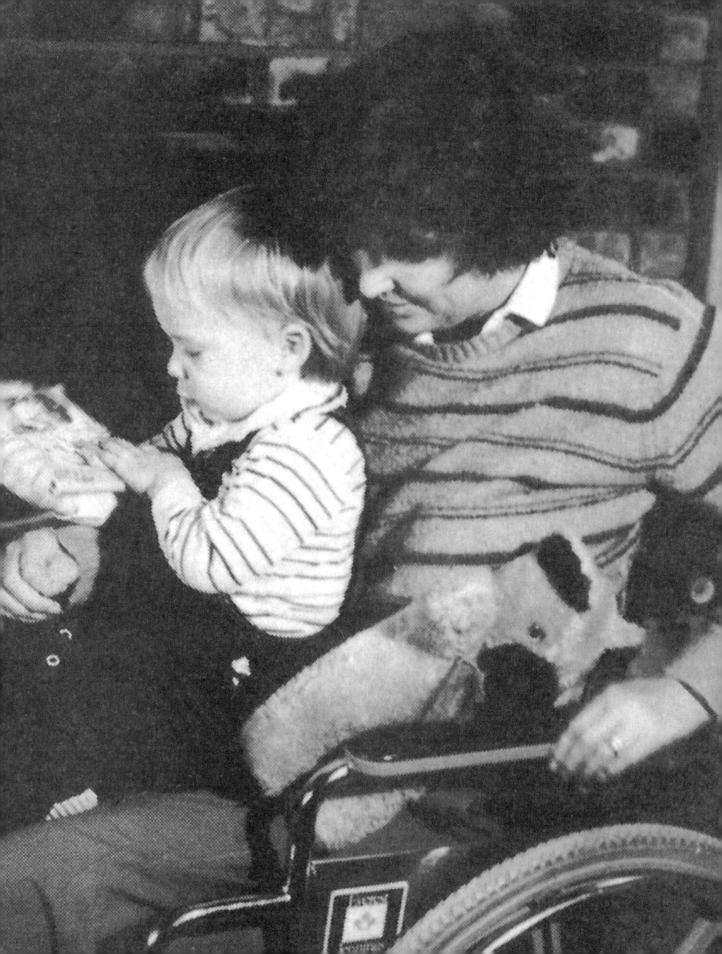

Family Nursing in Medical-Surgical Settings

When adults are ill and need hospitalization, they are generally admitted to a medical or surgical unit in a hospital. Regardless of the reason for the patient's hospital admission, the experience is a stressful one for patients and their families: both need nursing care.

This chapter describes issues for nurses to consider as they plan care for families in medical-surgical settings. There is a summary of the stressors that families face during hospitalization and a discussion of the use of the therapeutic quadrangle to analyze family needs during an illness episode.

Students will be particularly interested in the section that deals with caring for families before illness, during acute and chronic illness, and during the terminal illness experience.

The discussion of the application of theoretical models to family medical-surgical nursing addresses typical student concerns about the connection between theory and practice. In addition, broad categories of family nursing interventions for use during any phase of illness are described, including family support, promotion of family integrity, and family mobilization. The case study that is presented realistically portrays the agony and growth often experienced by families dealing with AIDS. The chapter closes with a discussion of the implications of developments in family nursing on medical-surgical education, research, and health care policy.

CHAPTER 12

Family Nursing in Medical-Surgical Settings

Nancy Trygar Artinian, PhD, RN

OUTLINE

OBJECTIVES

Upon completion of this chapter, the reader will be able to:

1. Discuss various approaches to assessing the impact of illness or injury on families.
2. Use the Structural-Functional Model, Family Systems Model, and Family Stress Model to design and implement care for families in medical-surgical settings.
3. Identify family needs and related interventions during the preillness, acute, chronic, and terminal phases of care.
4. Analyze factors to consider when determining hospital visitation policies.
5. Discuss family participation in do-not-resuscitate decisions.
6. Describe how nurses can help families prepare advance directives.
7. List advantages and disadvantages to having families present to watch nurses and physicians carry out resuscitative efforts.
8. Identify Thorne and Robinson's stages in relationships between the family and health care team.
9. Identify factors that may influence family readiness for hospital discharge.
10. Determine the potential impact of family nursing knowledge on medical-surgical nursing practice, education, research, and health care policy.

In the past, most nurses considered family nursing to be the domain of community health, mental health, or maternal-child nurses. "This trend is changing as more nurses are discovering that holistic care to clients, regardless of the setting, involves providing care to the entire family unit as well as caring for clients in the context of their families" (Ross & Cobb, 1990b, p. 13). Although other specialties are still more likely to incorporate families in nursing care, nurses in medical-surgical settings are beginning to recognize the importance of family nursing.

Several factors contribute to the increasing concern for families in medical-surgical settings. First, there is a growing body of evidence that families influence patient recovery (Frederickson, 1989; King, Reiss, Porter, & Norsen, 1993; Kulik & Mahler, 1989; O'Connor, 1983; Yates, 1989). Second, there is a growing consumer demand for unfragmented, holistic, humane, and sensitively delivered health care. Finally, the prospective payment system for health care results in early hospital discharge of patients to the care of their families. In such cases family-focused care throughout the patient's hospitalization helps prepare the family to give care after discharge.

FAMILY STRESSORS DURING HOSPITALIZATION

Families experience many stressors during hospitalization. Not only are hospital environments foreign, but nurses and doctors are strangers speaking another language. To add to the stress, families are separated from their ill member soon after entering the hospital doors and asked to go to a small, sometimes crowded, waiting room. There, they wait endlessly for someone to give them information as they deal with emotions such as fear, anger, guilt, or all three.

Illness or injury requiring hospitalization of a loved one has been termed a non-normative stressor event for families, that is, it is unexpected and unpredictable. Experiencing such an event may help some families to grow but cause conflicts in others. In the case of illness or injury, home routines are disrupted and some family members may need to assume responsibilities they have never had before. In addition, parents may struggle with how much to tell their children, or children may fear they are going to lose a parent.

Figley and McCubbin (1983) have described the characteristics of non-normative events that can be used to assess the impact of illness or injury on families. The degree to which these characteristics exist determines the degree of family stress. These characteristics are: (1) the amount of time the family has had to prepare for the event, in this case illness or injury; (2) the family's previous experience with the illness or injury; (3) the availability of resources to assist the family to manage the illness and injury; (4) the prevalence of the illness or injury event; (5) the extent of loss associated with the illness or injury (e.g., loss of life, loss of body part, loss of roles, loss of income, etc.); and (6) the amount of family disruption or number of family changes caused by the event.

THE THERAPEUTIC QUADRANGLE

Medical-surgical nurses need to assess the impact of hospitalization on families and deliver care accordingly. The therapeutic quadrangle is one aid they can use to analyze family care needs (Fig. 12-1). The therapeutic quadrangle has four interrelated parts: the illness, the family, the health care team, and the patient (Rolland, 1988). Caring for families in medical-surgical settings requires analyzing all these elements of the therapeutic quadrangle; and

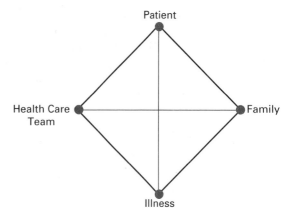

FIGURE 12-1

The therapeutic quadrangle. (From Rolland, JS: A conceptual model of chronic and life-threatening illness and its impact on families. In Chilman, CS, Nunnally, EW, and Cox, FM (Eds): Chronic Illness and Disability: Families in Trouble Series, vol. 2. Sage, Newbury Park, CA, p. 39, with permission.)

understanding illness, family, health care team, and patient-related factors will help nurses design and implement tailor-made plans for family care.

Illness

There is a great deal of variability associated with illness, and this variability is characterized by differences in the onset, course, outcome, and degree of incapacitation of the illness (Rolland, 1988). The onset of illness may be sudden or gradual. Strokes and myocardial infarctions have sudden onsets; arthritis and emphysema have gradual onsets. The type of onset may explain the amount of family readjustment needed. The course of the disease may be progressive, constant, or relapsing. Cancers, rheumatoid arthritis, and emphysema are progressive; a spinal cord injury is constant; and multiple sclerosis and asthma are relapsing. Relapsing illnesses require a different kind of family adaptability from that needed in an illness with a progressive or constant course (Rolland, 1988); in addition, the extent to which an illness is likely to cause death also affects the family. Metastatic cancer and AIDS are progressive and usually fatal, whereas hypertension and arthritis are not likely to end in death if treated properly. Illness outcome influences the degree to which the family experiences anticipatory grief (Rolland, 1988). Thus, the expectation of future loss can alter family perceptions and problem-solving abilities. "The tendency to see the family member as practically 'in the coffin' can set in motion maladaptive responses that divest the ill member of important responsibilities" (Rolland, 1988, p. 25). The degree of illness incapacitation also determines the specific adjustments required of a family. Incapacitation can result from impairment of cognition (e.g., Alzheimer's disease), sensation (e.g., blindness), movement (e.g., stroke with paralysis), or energy production (e.g., cardiovascular and pulmonary diseases). Illness incapacitation can also result from social stigma (e.g., AIDS).

The complexity, frequency, and efficiency of treatment, the amount of home- and hospital-based care required by the disease, and the frequency and intensity of symptoms vary widely across illnesses and have important implications for family adaptation (Rolland, 1988). The phases of an illness, which are designated as crisis, chronic, and terminal, also affect family adjustment to the illness.

Family

The family is the second element in the therapeutic quadrangle. Family flexibility, cohesion, structure, cultural background, past experience with illness, resources, problem-solving ability, coping skills, and perceptions are just a few of the qualities that influence the family's relationships with the other elements in the therapeutic quadrangle.

There are a number of family tasks to consider in relation to illness. Moos (1984) described these illness-related tasks as (1) learning to deal with pain, incapacitation, or other illness-related symptoms of their ill member; (2) learning caregiving procedures; and (3) establishing workable relationships with the health care team.

Health Care Team

The third element in the therapeutic quadrangle is the health care team. Health team members vary in the priority they assign to family care, in their sensitivity to family needs, and in their knowledge and ability to assess and intervene with families.

Patient

The final element in the therapeutic quadrangle is the patient. The identity of the sick person (e.g., mother, father, grandmother, spouse, sister, and so on) and the way the patient handles illness affect family adjustment. The point in the individual's life span at which the illness occurs also influences the family's adjustment. Often illness in the prime of life is unexpected, whereas illness in old age may be anticipated. In general, the more emotionally significant the sick family member, the more disruptive the illness will be. For example, if the ill person is the one everyone in the family depended on or turned to when they needed advice or other type of help, the more likely the loss of their contributions to the family will be acutely missed.

APPLICATION OF THEORETICAL MODELS

Family theoretical models can help nurses in medical-surgical settings plan systematic care for families. Theoretical models are systematic ways of looking at the world to describe, explain, predict, or prescribe nursing care (Meleis, 1991). The usefulness of a theoretical model comes from the organization it provides for thinking, observation, and interpretation of what is seen. A model may also provide a structure and rationale for activities, point out solutions to practical problems, and provide general criteria for deciding when a problem has been solved (Huckabay, 1991). Family theoretical models can help medical-surgical nurses develop systematic insights into families and thus provide a basis for family assessment. They may be used to diagnose processes in the patient-family situation and provide direction for family nursing interventions (Fawcett, 1984).

Some family theoretical models are more helpful to medical-surgical nurses than others. In this setting, the short hospital stays involved, the sometimes overwhelming needs of patients, and the many other demands on their time influence nurses' abilities to plan and deliver care to families. For the family, the first priority is to help them cope with the immediacy of the hospitalization. Therefore, models that are concise and easy to use and do not depend on long-term relationships with families probably are most useful to acute-care nurses. The goal is to help nurses assess and provide care for families within a short period of time. Three models are particularly useful in this.

Structural-Functional Model

The Structural-Functional Model focuses on the relationship between a family as a whole and its individual members. This perspective looks at the arrangement of members within the family, the relationships between the members, and the relationships of the members to the whole (Friedman, 1992) (Table 12 – 1). The model is concerned with family behavioral outcomes that result from the organization of the family. The focus is the family structure and its effectiveness in performing its functions.

The structure of the family refers to how the family is organized, the manner in which members are arranged, or how members relate to each other (Friedman, 1992). Some nurses view family structure as family form. Various family forms exist in today's society, including traditional nuclear families, single-parent families, stepfamilies, cohabitating couples, and homosexual unions. Other structural dimensions of the family may include role structure, value systems, communication patterns, power structure, and support networks (Friedman, 1992).

The family's structure facilitates the achievement of family functions, or what the family does. Friedman (1992) identified seven family functions:

1. Affective function (meeting the emotional needs of family members)
2. Socialization and social placement function (socializing children and making them productive members of society)
3. Reproduction function (producing new members for society)
4. Family coping function (maintaining order and stability)

TABLE 12–1

SUMMARY OF THE STRUCTURAL-FUNCTIONAL MODEL

Overview

Focuses on family structure and family function and how well the family structure performs its functions.

Concepts

Structure: Family form, roles, values, communication patterns, power structure, support network (Friedman, 1992).
Function: Affective, socialization, reproductive, coping, economic, physical care, and health care functions (Friedman, 1992).

Assumptions

The family is a system and a small group that exists to perform certain functions (Friedman, 1992).

Clinical Application

Assess, diagnose, and intervene with the family according to major concepts.

Assessment

What impact did the illness event have on family structure and function? How did the illness alter family structure? What family roles were changed? What family functions have been affected? What are family members' physical responses to the illness event?

Interventions

Assist the family to modify its organization so that role responsibilities can be distributed. Respect and encourage adaptive coping skills used by the family. Counsel family members on additional effective coping skills. Identify typical family coping mechanisms. Tell the family it is safe and acceptable to use typical expressions of affection. Provide family visitation. Encourage family members to recognize their own health needs. Help family members find ways to meet their health needs while helping them feel that their concern for the patient has not diminished. Assist the family to use existing support structures.

SOURCE: From "Selecting a Model to Guide Family Assessment," by N. T. Artinian, 1994, *Dimensions of Critical Care Nursing*, *13*, 4 – 12. Copyright 1994, with permission.

5. Economic function (providing sufficient economic resources and allocating resources effectively)
6. Providing physical necessities (food, clothing, shelter)
7. Health care function (maintaining health)

The structural-functional perspective provides a useful framework for assessing families in a medical-surgical setting. The illness of a family member alters the family structure
and may have an impact on family role relations. For example, illness may prevent one
family member from carrying out his or her usual roles, so that it becomes necessary for
another member to take on more responsibilities to compensate. If a single mother is ill,
she cannot carry out her various roles, and a grandparent or sibling may have to assume
her child care responsibilities. Illness may incapacitate the family if the power structure is
patriarchal and it is the husband-father who is ill. Communication may cease if the wife-
mother is the person in the family through whom all communication passes and she is ill.

Using the structural-functional framework, assessment focuses on the impact of the
illness on family structure and on the family's ability to carry out its functions. This model
highlights functions that are important to assess during crisis, such as family coping, affective functioning, economic functioning, and health care functioning. Interventions become necessary when a change in the family structure alters the family's ability to function. Interventions include reinforcing, modifying, or changing the family organization or
structure to strengthen, modify, or change its functioning (Berkey & Hanson, 1991). For example, a nurse may use the Structural-Functional Model to plan care for a family whose 18-
year-old daughter has been left a paraplegic by a motor vehicle accident. Assessment revealed the family is unable to carry out the coping function, that is, they were unable to
manage the stress associated with their perception that their daughter's life was over. An
intervention may include assisting the family to explore an alternate value structure related to family/individual productivity and achievement.

Family Systems Model

Another model that can be easily applied in medical-surgical settings is the Family Systems
Model, which focuses on the interaction of the various members of the system rather than
simply describing the functions of the members (Friedman, 1992). Both family process
and family outcomes are important in the Family Systems Model (Table 12–2). Assumptions of the family systems perspective include the following (Mercer, 1989):

- The family system is greater than and different from the sum of its parts.
- There are logical relationships between the subsystems. The subsystems interact
  with one another, and the whole family system interacts with other systems.
- Family systems increase in complexity over time, evolving to allow greater adapt-
  ability, tolerance to change, and growth by differentiation.
- Family systems change constantly in response to stresses and strains from within as
  well as from the outside environment.
- There are structural similarities in different family systems.
- Patterns in a family system are circular rather than linear.
- A family system is an organized whole; individuals within the family are parts of the
  system and are interdependent.
- Family systems have homeostatic features to maintain stable patterns.

A system is a set of interacting elements (von Bertalanffy, 1968). As a small group of
interrelated and interdependent individuals, the family may be considered a system; within
it there may be many subsystems. A subsystem can be formed by two or more interrelating

TABLE 12–2

SUMMARY OF THE FAMILY SYSTEMS MODEL

Overview

Focuses on the interactions of members of the family system and the interaction of the family system with other systems. A change in one member of the family system influences the entire system.

Concepts

Subsystems, boundaries, openness, energy, negentropy, entropy, feedback, adaptation, homeostasis, input, output, internal system processes (Ross & Cobb, 1990a).

Assumptions

The family system is greater than the sum of its parts. Subsystems are related and interact with one another and the whole family system interacts with other systems. Family systems have homeostatic features and strive to maintain a dynamic balance (Mercer, 1989).

Clinical Application

Assess, diagnose, and intervene with family according to major concepts.

Assessment

How did the change caused by the illness event affect all the members of the family? How are members of the family system relating to one another? How is the family system relating to the health care team and hospital environment? What are the "inputs" into the family system? Is the family system internally processing inputs? What are the family system outputs? How open is the family system? Does the family system have homeostasis? Determine how family behavior affects the patient. Determine how patient behavior affects the family.

Interventions

Encourage nurse-family interactions through establishing trust and using communication skills to check for discrepancies between nurse and family expectations. Establish a mechanism for providing the family with information about the patient on a regular basis. Foster the family's ability to get information. Listen to the family's feelings, concerns, and questions. Orient the family to the hospital environment. Answer family questions or assist them to get answers. Discuss strategies for normalizing family life with family members. Provide mechanisms for the patient and family members to interact with one another (e.g., pictures, videos, audiotapes, open visiting). Monitor family relationships. Facilitate open communication among family members. Collaborate with the family in problem solving. Provide knowledge that will help the family make decisions.

SOURCE: From "Selecting a Model to Guide Family Assessment," by N. T. Artinian, 1994, *Dimensions of Critical Care Nursing*, *13*, 4–12. Copyright 1994, with permission.

family members, and family members may be part of various subsystems (Ross & Cobb, 1990). Mother-father, parent-child, or brother-sister are examples of family subsystems. Family systems are also part of larger suprasystems. Communities, health care systems, political systems, and educational systems are examples of suprasystems.

Families are open systems. The degree of openness varies, that is, the amount of interaction the family has with its environment may differ from family to family, and from time to time. Family openness is regulated by boundaries that filter the exchange of energy to and from the environment. These boundaries are not physical boundaries but are the attitudes, values, or rules that influence a family's exchange with its environment. Boundaries inhibit or facilitate human transactional processes between systems. For example, a family may have a rule such as "we do not air our dirty linen in public." If their family member is hospitalized due to injury resulting from alcoholism or domestic violence, they may be reluctant to respond to the nurse's or doctor's assessment questions.

Survival of the family system depends on an exchange of energy with its environment. Energy may infuse into the family in the form of goods, services, information, or other resources; or it may be released from the family in the form of motivations, skills, goods, or services. Families process energy through activities such as interacting, valuing, goal setting, decision making, and problem solving. Energy that promotes order within the family is called negentropy; energy that results in disorganization or chaos is called entropy (Ross & Cobb, 1990).

An important feature of this model is the concept of feedback, which "refers to the process by which a system monitors the internal and environmental responses to its behavior (output) and accommodates or adjusts itself" (Friedman, 1992, p. 117). Using feedback, the family can identify its needs and determine whether it is achieving its goals (Friedman, 1992). Family systems receive and respond to feedback in order to maintain a dynamic balance, or homeostasis, and reduce strain. Adaptation is considered a component of feedback because it is the family system's way of adjusting to the input (Friedman, 1992). For example, a family may realize they are anxious because they do not have enough information about their ill member's condition. As a result they adjust their behavior of waiting passively for information and begin to actively pursue the information they need in order to relieve their stress.

The family system perspective encourages medical-surgical nurses to expand their view of the patient to include family members. Using a family systems perspective they can explore the effects of the illness or injury on the entire family system; that is, they can place emphasis on wholeness rather than reduction into parts. Assessment includes family system members, family subsystems, family boundaries, openness, family inputs and outputs, family interactions within the system, and family processing, adaptation, or change capabilities. It also includes answering questions such as: Who makes the decisions about care for family members? What is the educational level of family members? What information does the family need, or want? What significant family members need to be involved in decision making? Interventions may be designed to assist individual system functioning, family subsystem functioning, or the functioning of the whole family. Interventions may also facilitate family processing capabilities (e.g., family problem solving or family decision making) or enhance the interchanges among members or among systems, with the goal of restoring family stability. For instance, infusing energy into the family by giving information about possible treatment options may facilitate family process by helping them solve a problem that previously caused many disagreements.

Family Stress Model

The Family Stress Model fits medical-surgical situations because of the stress on the family that is due to the medical or surgical problem and to the hospitalization. Reuben Hill (1949), the father of family stress theory, conducted research on war-induced separation and reunion within families, and from that research two important perspectives emerged. First, for families facing a crisis event the process of adjustment is like a roller-coaster. This process begins with the crisis event, which is followed by a downward turn in family functioning, that is, family disorganization. After the family has figured out how to adjust to the crisis, there is an upward recovery curve, which ends with a new level of family organization.

The ABCX Model, which is the second theoretical perspective developed by Hill (1949), identifies how factors A, B, and C can result in crisis X (Table 12–3). "A" is the provoking event or stressor with its associated hardships (Boss, 1988). The stressor event is important enough to cause change in the family system. "B" refers to the family's strengths or the resources available to help the family deal with the stressor event. Family resources may include finances, religious beliefs or other coping mechanisms, social support, physi-

TABLE 12–3

SUMMARY OF THE FAMILY STRESS MODEL

Overview

Focuses on stressors, resources, and perceptions to explain the amount of family disruption due to a stressful event.

Concepts

"A"—stressful event with associated hardships; "B"—physical, psychological, material, social, spiritual, informational resources of family; "C"—family's subjective definition of the stressful event; "X"—crisis, the amount of disruptiveness or incapacitation within the family due to the stressful event (Boss, 1988).

Assumptions

The family is a system (Boss, 1988). Unexpected and ambiguous illness events are more stressful (Boss, 1988; Eshleman, 1991). Stressful events within the family are more disruptive than stressor events that occur outside the family. Lack of experience with a stressor event leads to increased perceptions of stressfulness (Eshleman, 1991).

Clinical Application

Assess, diagnose, and intervene with the family according to the major concepts.

Assessment

Identify the family's understanding and beliefs about the situation. What family hardships are associated with the illness event? What are other situational stressors for the family? Did the family have time to prepare for the event? Has the family had experience with the event? What resources are available to the family? Are the resources sufficient to meet the demands of the event? What are the family's perceptions of the event? Do they perceive the event to be a threat or challenge? Do the family members blame themselves for the event? How incapacitated is family functioning?

Interventions

Help the family to cope with imposed hardships. If appropriate, provide spiritual or informational resources for the family. Introduce the family to other families undergoing similar experiences. Discuss existing social support resources for the family. Assist the family to capitalize on its strengths. Assist the family to resolve feelings of guilt. Help the family visualize successfully handling all the hardships associated with the situation. If possible, encourage the family to focus on the positive aspects of the situation or cognitively reappraise the situation as positive.

SOURCE: From "Selecting a Model to Guide Family Assessment," by N. T. Artinian, 1994, *Dimensions of Critical Care Nursing,* *13,* 4–12. Copyright 1994, with permission.

cal health and stamina, or family flexibility. The third variable, "C," is very important; it refers to the family's view of the seriousness of the stressor event, or the subjective meaning the family attaches to the event. In fact, the family's definition of an event determines how they will deal with it and how stressful it will be for them.

Factors A, B, and C all influence the family's ability to prevent the changes associated with the stressor event. Changes created by illness may lead to a crisis, "X," which refers to the disruptiveness or incapacity within the family system caused by the stressful event (Burr, 1982). Crisis proneness reflects both a deficiency in family resources and a tendency to define hardships as crisis producing. Assumptions of the Family Stress Model include the following (Boss, 1988; Burr, 1982; Danielson, Hamel-Bissell, & Winstead-Fry, 1993; Eshleman, 1991):

- The family is a system.
- Unexpected events, or events that are not planned, are usually perceived as more stressful than expected events.

- Events *within* the family that are defined as stressful (e.g., a family member's illness) are more disruptive than stressor events that occur *outside* the family (e.g., war, flood, or depression).
- Lack of previous experience with a stressor event leads to greater perceived stressfulness.
- Ambiguous stressor events (i.e., events about which clear facts are not available) are more stressful than nonambiguous stressor events.

A medical-surgical nurse assessing the impact of illness or injury on the family first examines the stressor event. A number of questions should be considered: Did the family have time to prepare for the event, or was it unexpected? What family hardships and demands are associated with the event? Has the family previously experienced similar stressful events?

Assessment also includes a review of the physical, psychological, spiritual, and social resources available to the family. Identification of the meaning that the illness or injury has for the family is also important — for example, whether the family views the situation as a threat or a challenge, whether they blame themselves or place blame outside themselves. Assessment also includes evaluation of the level of crisis the family is experiencing, and how much the crisis has disrupted or incapacitated the family.

In the Family Stress Model, interventions target A, B, or C variables. For example, the nurse enhances family resources or helps the family to modify their subjective perceptions of the event.

It is important to note that the ABCX Model is not the only Family Stress Model. The Double ABCX Model is a derivation of the ABCX Model (McCubbin & Patterson, 1982), and it may be more useful to nurses when their focus is on helping families adapt and recover from illness over time. The Double ABCX Model adds postcrisis variables to Hill's original model to describe life stressors that accumulate over time as the family adapts to chronic illness. The model also adds social and psychological factors that families use to successfully adapt to the illness event.

A more recent Family Stress Model is the Resiliency Model (McCubbin & McCubbin, 1993), which builds on the ABCX Model and Double ABCX Model. This model guides health care professionals in determining what family types, capabilities, and strengths are needed to manage a stressful illness event, with emphasis on family adaptation (McCubbin & McCubbin, 1993). The time constraints imposed by short hospital stays may prevent medical-surgical nurses from making full use of the last two Family Stress Models. However, they are worth exploring further when patients and families face chronic illness.

In sum, personal philosophy, hospital unit philosophy, the nature of the nurse's clinical practice, and patient and family needs will influence the nurse's use of models to guide practice.

CARING FOR FAMILIES DURING VARIOUS PHASES OF AN ILLNESS

Pre-Illness: Health Promotion

Medical-surgical nurses may care for families during periods of pre-illness, acute illness, chronic illness, and terminal illness. Caring for families during the pre-illness period has two aims. The first is to help all family members develop healthy lifestyles. Studies have shown that families play a key role in determining the health-promoting behaviors of their members (Crooks, Iammarino, & Weinberg, 1987), and that family support is important in changing both health attitudes and behaviors (Kirks, Hendricks, & Wyse, 1982). During the pre-illness period, nurses caring for patients at high risk for familial diseases such as heart disease, stroke, or cancer can suggest to the whole family ways to lower the risk of developing these diseases. Not only can this be done in the same amount of time that it takes to teach the patient alone, but the family benefits as a whole and, at the same time, can help the patient make needed changes in lifestyle.

A second aim during the pre-illness period is to prevent a stress-filled hospitalization from negatively affecting the family's health (Artinian, 1989; Turk & Kerns, 1984). Hathaway and colleagues (Hathaway, Boswell, Stanford, Schneider, & Moncrief, 1987) conducted a study to determine how the health-related activities and health of significant others are altered by patients' hospitalizations. The sample ($n = 50$) included wives, daughters, mothers, fathers, husbands, in-laws, cousins, and a nephew. The investigators found that significant others altered their health practices and experienced a worsening of health because of the patient's hospitalization. The health practices most severely affected were exercise, sleep, nutrition, and relaxation. Of the respondents, 40% believed they were less healthy than before the patient's hospitalization, 40% currently experienced a health problem, and 20% believed the problem had either started or gotten worse since the hospitalization of the patient. Blood pressure problems were reported most frequently, followed by severe headaches, severe weight problems, arthritis, stomach problems, and other miscellaneous conditions. When asked what could be done to help patients' families cope with hospitalization, significant others suggested caring attitudes by the staff, counseling, religious activities, overnight sleeping arrangements, long-term parking, waiting room amenities, a nursery, and resources for diversional activities.

During hospitalization of a family member nurses can facilitate family health promotion by including families in admission assessments, involving families in plans of care, determining the effects of patient hospitalization on the family, developing caring, open relationships with families, and intervening to address family needs.

Acute Illness

The acute phase refers to the immediate aftermath of illness — for example, the period immediately following a heart attack (Steinglass, 1992). Families with members who are acutely or critically ill are often seen in intensive or cardiac care units or emergency rooms under conditions where they are greatly stressed because a member of their family is experiencing a life-threatening illness or injury.

Rolland (1988) described five tasks that families must accomplish during the crisis phase of illness: (1) creating a meaning for the illness event that preserves a sense of mastery over their lives, (2) grieving for the loss of the pre-illness family identity, (3) moving toward a position of accepting permanent change while maintaining a sense of continuity between the past and the future, (4) pulling together to undergo short-term crisis reorganization, and (5) developing family flexibility about future goals.

Admission to a critical care unit signals to the family that the patient is seriously ill and that death or major disability is a possibility. Communication among family members may become distorted because the fear, anger, and guilt that members experience may be too intense for them to handle. "In some families, conflicts may be blocked or submerged during the initial period of a critical illness, but as time goes on and the family resources become depleted, conflict between members may become more obvious" (McClowry, 1992, p. 561).

Many nurses have investigated the needs of families in critical care units (Molter, 1979; Daley, 1984; Boumann, 1984; Leske, 1986; Mathis, 1984; Norris & Grove, 1986). The following needs were frequently important: to have questions answered honestly; to know the facts about what is wrong with the patient; to be informed about the patient's progress, outcome, and chance for recovery; to be called at home about changes in the patient's condition; to receive understandable explanations; to receive information once a day; to have hope; to believe hospital personnel care about the patient; to have reassurance that the patient is receiving the best possible care; and to see the patient frequently. Leske (1992) summarized these as needs for assurance, proximity, information, comfort, and support. In general, families' needs in a critical care unit or during the acute illness period are similar, regardless of their age, gender, relationship to the patient, and patient diagnosis (Leske, 1991).

Leske's five family need categories can be used to direct nursing interventions, which should begin on initial contact with family members. Providing assurance entails establishing a calm and relaxed atmosphere that will support a trusting and empathetic relationship (Leske, 1992). Enhancement of proximity means allowing family members to be near the patient, by exercising flexible family visitation policies. There are several ways to provide family information: educational orientation programs, classes that provide social support and information about illness management and recovery, informational packets, or unit tours. Comfort measures may include waiting rooms conducive to rest and relaxation, the availability of private rooms for conferences between the health team and family, placement of telephone and bathroom facilities near the waiting room, and helping families to take care of their needs, such as adequate rest, nutrition, and personal hygiene. A nurse supports the family by showing compassion, concern, and sensitivity to all family needs (Leske, 1992).

Family Concerns During Hospitalization for Acute Illness

Three specific concerns for families during hospitalization for acute illness are: family visitation policies, do-not-resuscitate decisions, and policies surrounding cardiopulmonary resuscitation.

Family Visitation Policies During the period of acute illness, families usually encounter restrictive hospital visiting policies. They may not be able to visit their loved one in the hospital when it is convenient for them or when their work schedule permits, and frequently they must rearrange their plans and routines to fit the policies set by the hospital. Numerous studies have found that visiting policies in intensive care units (ICUs) restricted the number and length of visits, and the number and ages of visitors, as well as limiting visitors to members of the immediate family (Kirchhoff, 1982; Younger, Coulton, Welton, Juknialis, & Jackson, 1984).

Originally hospital visiting periods were limited so that the patient could rest and recover. Recent studies challenge the premise that visiting in the ICU should be restricted because of adverse effects on patients. Research findings suggest that family-patient interactions do not alter hemodynamic stability any differently than nurse-patient interactions (Fuller & Foster, 1982). Moreover, one recent study found that "Restricting visits to short time periods and terminating visits prematurely contribute to adverse hemodynamic responses in critically ill patients" (Titler & Walsh, 1992, p. 625). In fact, patient-family interactions have been shown to be therapeutic (Bruya, 1981).

Research has uncovered several factors that should be considered when planning visiting periods with families. Zetterlund (1971) reported that visits longer than the period desired by the patient had untoward effects, and Simpson (1991) found that age, patients' personality characteristics, and patients' perceptions of the illness influenced patients' visiting preferences. For instance, older patients preferred longer visits, and extroverted patients preferred more frequent visits. Surprisingly, the more severely ill patients perceived themselves to be, the more visitors they preferred.

The diversity of patients' responses to visiting policies suggests that policies should be tailored to patient and family preferences. Hamner (1990) suggested that visiting preferences should be included in patient-family assessments. One way to do this is to ascertain the answers to questions such as "How would you like visiting times to be handled while you are here?" "Who would you like to be allowed/disallowed to visit?" "When do you want to see visitors?" "How often?" "How long?" in order to tailor visiting policies to meet patient-family needs.

Family Participation in Do-Not-Resuscitate Decisions   Families may have to face decisions regarding the use of life-saving or life-extending measures during the acute illness period. Frequently illness occurs without preparation, and sometimes families must deal with illnesses or injuries in which there is no hope for recovery. In the acute illness period, patients and families are in a crisis situation with little time to discuss the options regarding life-saving measures. Often there is little, if any, discussion about resuscitation preferences while the patient is competent to make a decision, so that frequently health care professionals and families must make end-of-life decisions without the guidance of the patient. Bedell, Pelle, Maher, and Cleary (1986) found that 86% of decisions regarding resuscitation measures involved the family, while only 22% of the patients were included in the decision making.

Several issues should be kept in mind with regard to do-not-resuscitate (DNR) orders. First, physicians may discuss many variations of DNR orders with families. Sometimes it is appropriate, for example, to withhold chest compressions and intubation but still administer antiarrhythmic and vasopressor drugs. At other times no life-saving measures may be administered. Nurses can help families by clarifying the various options presented to them and offering opportunities for discussion. Needless to say, decisions about DNR status are difficult to make.

The appropriate timing of discussion of DNR orders is also difficult to determine. It is hard for the physician to know when it is best to discuss the DNR status of the patient with the family. Because nurses develop special insights due to the time they spend at the bedside getting to know the patient and family, they can help physicians schedule these important discussions.

Bedell et al. (1986) found that four factors assisted families to make decisions about DNR status. First, an explanation of brain death criteria by the physician eased the family's ability to make a decision, as did the second factor, physician and nurse support for the family. Third, families wanted assurance that comfort measures would continue. Fourth, families found any prior discussion they had had with the patient about life decisions was helpful in the decision-making process.

Nurses can help families prepare for the possibility of a DNR decision through community education about **living wills** and **durable power of attorney for health care**. Such education will enable family members to discuss end-of-life decisions before a crisis event occurs and in less stressful circumstances. Ideally decisions about end-of-life care are made by the patient with the family prior to admission to the hospital.

In December 1991, the Patient Self-Determination Act (PSDA) went into effect. The PSDA requires all health care facilities receiving Medicare or Medicaid funds to provide written information to adult patients abut their rights to make treatment decisions and execute advance directives (Marsden, 1992). Advance directive may be in the form of a living will or in the form of durable power of attorney. A living will is a written statement that tells a person's family, friends, and doctor(s) what medical treatment he or she would want in the future should the person become unable to express his or her wishes. An advance directive is a written statement that allows individuals to select, in advance, someone to speak for them when they can no longer state their wishes. An advance directive applies only to those who are unable to make their own decisions because they are incapacitated, or who, in the opinion of two physicians, are otherwise unable to make decisions for themselves (American Nurses Association, 1992). Different states have different laws about advance directives. For detailed information about state law and for samples of advance directive forms for every state, nurses can contact the organization entitled Choice in Dying (see Appendix A). Patients and families need to be informed about advance directives, to know that the directive is intended to help others make decisions for the patient, and to know that it can be as simple or as complex as they feel necessary. Nurses can help patients and families prepare advance directives by showing sample forms and provide the support and reassurance the family needs as these important decisions are being made. The American Nurses Association (ANA) recommends that nurses ask specific questions as part of the patient/family assessment. These questions are displayed in Table 12–4.

Should Families Witness Cardiopulmonary Resuscitation Efforts? During the acute illness period, the patient may suffer a sudden arrest of heartbeat and/or respirations requiring cardiopulmonary resuscitation (CPR). When a patient has an arrest, the CPR team is called to the bedside. Physicians, nurses, and other health team members crowd around the patient to administer chest compressions, manually ventilate the patient, perform defibrillation, give drugs, or carry out other life-restoring activities. Until the patient's heart rhythm and respirations are restored, this is a tension-filled period.

Martin (1991) suggests that there are advantages to having families present to watch nurses and physicians carry out resuscitative efforts. The advantages for families include recognizing that the patient is dying, knowing that everything possible is being done, being able to touch the patient while he or she is still warm and to say whatever they need to say while there is still a chance the patient can hear, recognizing the futility of further resuscitation efforts, and accepting the reality of death.

On the other hand, there may be disadvantages to having families observe CPR (Osuagwu, 1991; Redheffer, 1989). The experience is traumatic and frightening to watch; families may interfere with protocols and procedures; there is not enough space at the patient's bedside for the CPR team as well as the family; and staff are not available to provide family information and support during the resuscitation. Thus there is no general answer to the question of whether families should witness resuscitation efforts.

TABLE 12–4

PATIENT/FAMILY ASSESSMENT QUESTIONS ABOUT END-OF-LIFE DECISIONS

Have you discussed your end-of-life choices with your family and/or designated surrogate and health care team workers?

Do you have basic information about advance directives including living wills and durable power of attorney for health care?

Do you wish to initiate an advance directive?

If you have already prepared an advance directive, can you provide it now?

SOURCE: From "Nurses to Educate for End of Life Decisions," by American Nurses Association, 1992, *American Nurse, 24.* Copyright 1992, with permission.

Providing hospital and unit policies permit families to witness resuscitation efforts, decisions about family visitation should be made on a case-by-case basis. Martin (1991) provides guidelines for nurses deciding when families are to be permitted in the patient's room during CPR. Martin's guidelines include the following directions:

- Discuss the option with the family and give them a description of what will be going on in the room.
- Check the code status with the doctor and the nurse in charge.
- Assess the room from the point of view of the family.
- Accompany the family member into the room to ensure that the family member gets an accurate explanation and has an appropriate perception of what is being done.
- Do not permit family members to enter the code area while intravenous lines are being placed or while the patient is being intubated.
- Let family members in once the code is under way.
- If a family member cannot handle the visit, escort him or her from the room.

Hopefully nurses will be sensitive to family needs during this stress-filled time and will consider the benefits and risks for families of witnessing CPR.

Chronic Illness

Chronic illness imposes another set of concerns for families. Chronic illness is "the irreversible presence, accumulation, or latency of disease states or impairments that involve the total human environment for supportive care and self-care, maintenance of function, and prevention of further disability" (Lubkin, 1986, p. 6.). Many factors influence the impact of chronic illness on families: the type of illness, the stage of illness, the structure of the family, the role of the patient, the life cycle stage of the patient, and the life cycle stage of the family (Biegel, Sales, & Schulz, 1991).

The entire family system is affected when chronic illness strikes. "Normal patterns of interaction are disrupted, and there are often reassignments in tasks and roles assumed by particular family members" (Biegel et al., 1991, p. 20). The family must reorganize itself around the chronic illness or disability (Steinglass, 1992). Families may make changes related to work schedules, household tasks, provision of family income, or in interpersonal areas such as solidarity and belonging, sexuality and love (Leventhal, Leventhal, & Nguyen, 1985).

Families and patients face both social and psychological challenges during the course of chronic illness (Biegel et al., 1991, pp. 20–21). These include:

- Preventing medical crises and their management once they occur
- Controlling symptoms
- Carrying out prescribed regimens
- Preventing or living with the sense of isolation caused by lessened contact with others
- Adjusting to changes in the course of the disease
- Normalizing interactions with others and finding the necessary money to pay for treatments or to survive, despite partial or complete loss of employment
- Confronting attendant psychosocial, marital, and familial problems

Families in the chronic phase may have to deal with a member's illness for a long period of time — an illness that may be constant, progressive, or episodic in nature. A key family task is to maintain normal life in the "abnormal" presence of this chronic illness and the resulting heightened uncertainty (Rolland, 1988).

As they manage their family member's illness on a day-to-day basis, families become expert caregivers. Exacerbation of a chronic illness, when it leads to hospitalization, brings expert family caregivers in contact with the health care team. Thorne and Robinson (1988), who analyzed relationships between the family and the health care team from the perspective of the family members, found that these relationships moved through three stages. These stages reflected shifts in family trust of health care professionals.

The first stage, naive trusting, was described by family members who had not had much experience with chronic illness yet. These family members trust that health care professionals have the same perspective about caring for their ill member that they did. Families believed that their involvement on a day-to-day basis as the primary health care providers would be acknowledged and respected, and that professionals would be cooperative and collaborative. Family members naively trusted that health care professionals would act in their ill member's best interests. Over time, however, family members learned that their long experience was often disregarded, as was their involvement and expertise in illness management.

The second stage, the disenchantment phase, was characterized by dissatisfaction with care, frustration, and fear. Families found that it was difficult to be effectively involved in care because they had difficulty obtaining information. As trust diminished, family relationships with health care professionals became adversarial, and families saw their ill member as vulnerable and needing protection.

During the last stage, the guarded alliance phase, families renegotiated trust with health care professionals. They actively sought information and understood the differences in their perspective and that of health care professionals. Families were able to state clearly their own expectations and perceptions, an ability which led to more satisfying care. Families and health care professionals developed a partnership in care. Nevertheless, families still experienced the frustration of waiting, fear that they would not know the right questions to ask, and anger at the recognition that their own expertise was devalued.

Leahey and Wright (1987) have described interventions for families experiencing chronic illness that focus on the family's cognitive, affective, and/or behavioral levels of functioning. Cognitive interventions include giving information about the chronic illness and its treatment, giving advice about potential family responses to the illness (e.g., need for respite, possible strain on family relationships), giving information about community resources, and helping with family decision making. Affective interventions are designed to modify intense emotions, such as guilt or anger, that may block a family's problem-solving efforts (Leahey & Wright, 1987). They include validating family members' emotional responses and helping them understand that those responses are normal; discussing with families ways to reduce their isolation; referring families to an appropriate support group; helping families open channels of communication; and helping families identify and mobilize their strengths and resources. Interventions targeted at behavioral functioning are designed to help family members interact more effectively (Leahey & Wright, 1987). "This goal can be accomplished by assigning specific behavioral tasks to some or all family members" (Leahey & Wright, 1987). For example, families may need help to coordinate care and negotiate responsibilities for particular caregiving activities (Gilliss, Rose, Hallburg, & Martinson, 1989). They may also need caregiving training in order to feel comfortable with the tasks at hand.

Other nursing interventions may be directed toward helping health care personnel work with families who are coping with chronic illness. Findings from Thorne and Robinson's (1988) research suggests strategies to improve relationships between the family and the health care team. Nurses need first to recognize the stage of their relationship (naive trust, disenchantment, or guarded alliance) with these families. Activities to promote cooperative caring must be negotiated between the nurse and the family, and being sensitive to what caregivers have experienced prior to hospitalization and recognizing their experience is essential to this process. Helping families access the information they need is also important; in fact it is a prerequisite to developing a shared understanding that will help in the development of goals upon which there is mutual agreement.

Caring for families with chronic illness presents many challenges for medical-surgical nurses. The problems and concerns that families experience differ from those in the acute illness stage. Nurses need to keep these differences in mind as they plan care.

Terminal Illness

Sometimes nurses in medical-surgical settings encounter families who are coping with the terminal phase of an illness. Knowledge about the process of dying can help nurses work effectively with families during this very difficult time. The more the nurse knows about the family the better, since how families deal with death is affected by the family's cultural background, stage in the life cycle, values and beliefs, the nature of the illness, whether the loss is sudden or expected, the role played by the dying person in the family, and the emotional functioning of the family before the illness (Rosen, 1990).

Families move through phases of adaptation in response to the news that a family member has a fatal illness (Rosen, 1990), and various emotional responses may emerge during these phases, including disorganization, anxiety, emotional lability, or turning inward. The first phase is the preparatory phase. This phase begins when symptoms first appear and it continues through the initial diagnosis. During the preparatory phase, families experience fear and denial and may refuse to accept the prospect of death. Some family members decide to withhold all information from those whom they consider vulnerable, such as children or elderly parents (Rosen, 1990). During this period of initial symptoms, diagnosis, and treatment plan, the family may be highly disorganized and display emotional lability.

Once the family accepts the prospect of loss and begins to live with the reality of the fatal illness and the caretaking tasks of the illness, they move into the middle phase. Families live the day-to-day challenge of dealing with physical symptoms, treatment, and care (Rosen, 1990). The family becomes less disorganized; indeed it reorganizes to assume new roles. On the other hand, the tedium of daily care may tax the physical and financial resources of the family. Further, if hospitalizations are lengthy or frequent, the logistics of visitation may create discord among family members (Rosen, 1990) — some members of the family may feel others are visiting too little or too much — and unresolved family issues from the past may emerge.

The final stage, acceptance, comes when the family accepts the imminent death and concludes the process of saying farewell. Family emotions that surface during the first phase but subsided during the middle phase may resurface. Family members may draw together in anticipation of their loved one's death (Rosen, 1990).

Nurses can help families with a dying relative by informing them that it is natural to pass through phases of adaptation and they can expect to address complex issues in each phase of a fatal illness. Helping families accept their feeling and directing them to appropriate resources such as hospice, family support groups, social workers, and family conferences may be useful.

Caring for families when a member is dying is not easy. Rarely do nurses feel comfortable and confident discussing death with patients or families. Two issues are especially difficult for nurses: conveying news of sudden death and offering families the option of organ donation.

Conveying News of Sudden Death to Families

Family grief reactions may be manifested as guilt, self-reproach, anxiety, loneliness, fatigue, shock, numbness, sleep and appetite disturbances, crying, overactivity, or confusion (Swanson, 1993). Informing the family of the death of a loved one is a challenging task. A health care professional's initial contact with the family about a death or about dying has a significant impact on the family's grief reaction. "Bad news, conveyed in an inappropriate, incomplete, or uncaring manner may have long-lasting psychological effects on the family" (Swanson, 1993, p. 352). Table 12–5 presents guidelines for nurses to keep in mind at the time when families are told of the sudden death of a family member.

Offering Families the Option of Organ Donation

Discussing organ donation with a family whose loved one has suddenly died is difficult. "Often the deceased is a young, previously healthy person who died suddenly in a tragic accident" (Hoffman & Malecki, 1990, p. 24). In a study of 124 nurses, Malecki and Hoffman (1987) found that those who felt uncomfortable about requesting donation got more negative responses from potential donor families than nurses who were sad but comfortable and confident.

If organ donation is viewed as a consoling act, rather than an imposition on a grieving family, offering the option of organ donation becomes easier. Organ donation benefits the family of the donor as well as the organ recipient. Hoffman and Malecki (1990) have noted that donation of organs can help families cope with their loss. Perceiving that organ donation can help someone else live, that functioning organs are not wasted, that something

TABLE 12–5

CONVEYING NEWS OF SUDDEN DEATH TO FAMILY MEMBERS: RECOMMENDATIONS FOR NURSES

Obtain as much information as possible regarding the patient and the circumstances surrounding the death. Be knowledgeable before talking with the family.

Ask the family members to come to a private area.

Go to where family members are gathered; walk in; introduce yourself and sit down. Address the closest relative.

Briefly describe the events at the time of death. Use open and factual terminology. Avoid euphemisms such as, "he has passed on" or "he is no longer with us." Use the words death, dying, or dead.

Allow a period for the shock to be absorbed. Use direct eye contact, physical comforting, and emotional sharing. Convey sensitivity and caring.

Respect the family's cultural background and use of rituals, customs, or styles to deal with death.

Allow as much time as necessary for questions and sharing. Avoid rushing.

Inform the family of the process of caring for their family member after death (e.g., signing the death certificate, the request for organ donation, and transfer to the morgue).

Allow the family the opportunity to view the body. Prepare the family if technological equipment is still attached.

Accompany the family to the patient's room. Stay with the family to assess their reactions. Allow some private time if feasible.

Offer the opportunity to discuss additional questions.

SOURCE: From "Psychological issues in CPR," by R. W. Swanson, 1993, *Annals of Emergency Medicine, 22*(2, part 2), 350–353. Copyright 1993, with permission.

TABLE 12–6

HOW TO OFFER FAMILIES THE OPTION FOR ORGAN AND TISSUE DONATION

Take the family to a quiet, private area without distraction. Asking for donation at the bedside of the deceased is poor nonverbal communication. It shows disrespect for the donor as a person, emphasizing instead the organs and tissues in question.

Once in a private location, appear physically comfortable. Openness and empathy can be conveyed with relaxed body language, such as uncrossed legs and open hands placed in the lap. A nurse's personal discomfort with the issue may convey disapproval. The information then loses its objectivity. Obviously uncomfortable nurses put themselves in unnecessarily stressful roles as "persuaders" or "nonpersuaders." The role of the nurse is to present information, not to persuade. A nurse who is opposed to donation should not be requesting it.

Begin the discussion by offering sympathy to the family member(s) about the death in your own words. For example, "I'm sorry that your husband died," or "I'm sorry that John has been pronounced dead."

Focus on the deceased's wishes. Had the deceased ever signed a donor card? Had he or she ever discussed organ donation? This can lessen the stress on the survivor if such a decision has already been made.

Answer questions simply and honestly. In order to do this, nurses do not need to be experts on procurement. A nurse who needs assistance should contact the organ procurement organization (**OPO**). Donor families have common concerns about donation. Nurses should be generally familiar with these areas of concern.

Consent for any type of donation must be obtained from the next of kin or guardian. Consent forms can be obtained from OPO, and signatures must be witnessed by two persons. When the next of kin is not present a consent may be obtained over the telephone with two witnesses to the conversation. If the next of kin cannot be located, the OPO and the hospital will make a decision in conjunction with the medical examiner or coroner.

The medical examiner or coroner must give final consent in cases of death under their jurisdiction (e.g., homicides, suicides, or any questionable death). It may be prudent to first obtain the medical examiner's or coroner's consent before approaching the family, in case the postmortem investigation precludes donation. In "John Doe" cases, in which the identity of the potential donor is unknown, donation will usually not occur because of the lack of available medical history.

To avoid nonverbal pressure on the family, keep the consent form out of sight until the decision to donate has been made.

SOURCE: From "Organ Procurement and Preservation," by M. Hoffman and M. Malecki. In K. M. Sigardson-Poor and L. M. Haggerty (Eds.), 1990, *Nursing Care of the Transplant Recipient*, pp. 13–34. Philadelphia: W. B. Saunders. Copyright 1990 by W. B. Saunders. Reprinted with permission.

positive can come out of death, or that a family member can live on in someone else through donation can help families cope with their loss. Table 12-6 provides guidelines for offering the option of organ and tissue donation to a bereaved family and Table 12-7 lists common concerns that families have about donation.

INTERVENTIONS FOR FAMILIES IN A MEDICAL-SURGICAL SETTING

Medical-surgical nurses must intervene with families during all phases of an illness. "Nursing interventions for families are nursing treatments that assist families and their members to promote, attain, or maintain optimal health and functioning or to experience a peaceful death" (Craft & Willadsen, 1992, p. 520) Craft and Willadsen have identified nine categories of family nursing interventions: family support, family process maintenance, promotion of

TABLE 12–7

COMMON CONCERNS FAMILIES HAVE ABOUT ORGAN DONATION

Many families require repeat explanations of brain death. The nurse should be prepared to discuss the definition of brain death in simple terms. For example: "Brain death means total, irreversible loss of brain function. Your loved one appears to be breathing but is being mechanically maintained. If we were to turn off the ventilator, he would not even be able to take a breath. We have performed a number of tests to come to this conclusion. Do you have any questions or concerns about brain death that I can help clarify?"

Donor families fear that their loved ones will be disfigured by surgical recovery of the organs and tissues. All organs and tissues are removed under sterile conditions in an operating room, just as they would be on a living person, with the utmost respect for the donor's body. Funeral arrangements, including an open casket, are not affected by donation. Because some families may not broach this issue, it is helpful to say, "In case you were wondering, there will be no disfigurement. You will be able to have an open-casket viewing if you so choose."

All of the major religions support donation and transplantation. Enlist the counseling support of hospital clergy when necessary.

Cultural differences play a part in the decision-making process of donor families, particularly among minority groups. It is important to keep their orientation in mind, including their views of the American health system. Enlist the support of a social worker and interpreter when necessary.

Once a donor is accepted by the OPO and the family consents, all costs incurred related to the donation are the responsibility of the OPO. The family incurs no costs in making the donation. They are, however, still responsible for funeral costs.

Families may ask if the donation will delay their funeral plans. The best person to answer such a question is the procurement coordinator. The answer will depend on which teams are retrieving organs and tissues and what their travel time will be to the donor hospital. It is best to be as honest as possible with the family about this issue, reassuring them that the OPO will do everything possible to be efficient.

It is often difficult for family members to decide when to "say good-bye" to their loved one. It may be helpful for the nurse to determine when the family can do no more (possibly after consent has been obtained) and to gently suggest that the family go home. Under no circumstances should family members be forced to leave before they are ready. Every consideration should be given to their comfort.

The family may ask to view the body after the organs have been removed. The procurement coordinator should be advised of their request to ensure that the body is properly prepared for viewing.

SOURCE: From "Organ procurement and preservation," by M. Hoffman and L. M. Malecki. In K. M. Sigardson-Poor and L. M. Haggerty (Eds.), *Nursing Care of the Transplant Recipient*, pp. 27–28. 1990, Philadelphia: W. B. Saunders. Copyright 1990 by W. B. Saunders. Reprinted with permission.

family integrity, family involvement, family mobilization, caregiver support, family therapy, sibling support, and parent education. The first five categories are particularly relevant for medical-surgical family nursing; they are defined in Table 12–8.

Family Support

Families in medical-surgical settings are experiencing life changes and stressors, and are frequently in need of support. Nurses can support the family in several ways. Effective, open, and honest communication is important, that is, listening to family concerns, feelings, and questions, and answering all questions or assisting the family to get answers. Helping the family acquire information is another supportive activity. Respecting and supporting family coping mechanisms, fostering realistic hope, assisting families to make decisions through providing information about options, and providing opportunities to visit are other supportive activities. Family conferences to allow ventilation of family feelings, permitting the family to make some decisions about patient care, and clarifying information are also supportive. Henneman, McKenzie, and Dewa (1992) note that flexible visiting

TABLE 12–8

CATEGORIES AND DEFINITIONS OF FAMILY NURSING INTERVENTIONS IN MEDICAL-SURGICAL SETTINGS

Category of Family Nursing Intervention	Definition
Family support	Promotion of family interests and goals
Maintenance of family process	Minimizing effects of family disruption
Promotion of family integrity	Promotion of family cohesion and unity
Family involvement	Family involvement in the emotional and physical care of the patient
Family mobilization	Utilization of family strengths to influence patient's health in a positive direction

SOURCE: From "Interventions Related to Family," by M. J. Croft and J. A. Willadsen, 1992, *Nursing Clinics of North America*, *27*, 517–540. Copyright 1992, with permission.

hours and information booklets are two practical and specific methods to support families.

Family Process Maintenance

The illness and hospitalization of a family member upsets family routines and activities. Identifying how the acute illness episode has altered family roles and consequently disrupted typical family processes is a necessary part of maintaining family process. Offering flexible opportunities for visiting will help to meet the needs of family members as well as the patient and can also promote maintenance of typical family processes. Family members may want to discuss with the nurse other strategies for normalizing family life.

Promotion of Family Integrity

Stressful hospitalizations may adversely affect the emotional bonding that family members have with one another. Nurses can promote family cohesion and unity through allowing for family visitation and facilitating open communication among family members. Scheduling a family conference to encourage all family members to voice their concerns about care management with one another and with the health care team is a way to facilitate open communication. Telling family members that it is safe and acceptable to use typical expressions of affection may also be appreciated. For example, a wife may appreciate knowing she won't disrupt the technological equipment at her husband's bedside or disrupt equipment attached to his body if she kisses his cheek or holds his hand. Providing opportunities for private family visits can make the visits more satisfying.

Family Involvement

Family members may be comforted by giving physical care to their loved one during hospitalization, especially if the family member has routinely provided physical care for the patient at home. Before encouraging family members to become involved in patient care, however, it is important to identify their preferences, the patient's preferences, and family members' capabilities. Family members can be involved with care in a number of ways, such as helping during meal times, assisting with brushing teeth or other comfort measures, and assisting with patient positioning or range of motion.

Family Mobilization

Family caregivers may be experts in caring for the patient because of their many years of experience with a chronic illness. Nurses can acknowledge this family expertise and use the family's strengths through family mobilization techniques. For example, discussing how family strengths and resources can be used to enhance the health of the patient and establishing realistic goals with the patient and family are both ways to mobilize families. Collaborating with family members in planning and implementing patient therapies and lifestyle changes is another. Families may want to share information about the patient's favorite position when lying in bed, preferences in music, bedtime habits, or preferred comfort measures. Determining family cultural practices and incorporating these into plans for care is yet another way to mobilize the strengths of the family.

PREPARING FAMILIES FOR PATIENT DISCHARGE

While hospitalization is stressful for families, leaving the hospital is also stressful. As a result of the **prospective payment system** and other efforts to control health care costs, patients nowadays are discharged quickly from the hospital (Brooten et al., 1988). As a result, patients and families must manage most of the patient's recovery at home. Early discharge requires careful attention to discharge planning to help patients and families anticipate problems after discharge.

Numerous investigators have described the preparation of patients for discharge (Duryée, 1992; Garding, Kerr, & Bay, 1988; Steele & Ruzicki, 1987), but few researchers have looked at preparing families for discharge. In a study involving patients who experienced a coronary artery bypass graft, Artinian (1993) found that spouses identified four factors as helpful in readying them for their partner's hospital discharge: (1) availability of social support, (2) use of coping strategies, (3) personal resources, and (4) knowledge of what to expect.

Consideration of these four factors suggests ways to prepare other types of families for discharge. For instance, available social support can include persons who are available to give necessary information about recovery at home. Such predischarge recovery information should include the trajectory of an uncomplicated recovery, how to distinguish between normal and unusual symptoms during recovery, signs and symptoms of complications, and activities family members can do to make the patient comfortable. Giving a phone number of someone the family can call if they have concerns is also helpful. Supplying bandages, canes, medicines, or other materials to families before they go home may be of assistance in the immediate postdischarge recovery period, because families do not want to have to run to the store and leave the patient alone as soon as they return home. Postdischarge contact also may support family management of recovery at home. Various strategies for doing this have been described, including follow-up contact by telephone (Beckie, 1989; Garding, Kerr, & Bay, 1988; Gortner et al., 1988; Nicklin, 1986).

Families need coping skills to manage recovery at home. These skills include problem-solving ability, ability to seek help if needed, ability to manage worry and anxiety, and ability to acquire needed information. Nurses need to assess these family coping strategies in order to devise interventions that will fit the individual family's needs.

Four categories of personal resources can help family members feel ready to take a patient home from the hospital. These categories, health and energy, time, self-confidence, and positive beliefs (Artinian, 1993), need to be assessed by the nurse. For example, if the family member taking the patient home has numerous chronic health problems leaving them with feelings of fatigue, discharge activities and recovery at home may seem overwhelming to them. Assessing family members' perceptions of their own health may indicate whether the family needs additional help to manage care at home. Families who lack time to prepare for discharge because of multiple responsibilities may need encouragement to arrange for help or to plan ahead. Assessing family confidence about recovery and managing caregiving activities at home may be beneficial. Or, if a family member does not have positive beliefs about the patient's recovery, and does not believe the patient is physically ready to go home, they also will not feel ready. Because optimistic beliefs can help families feel ready for discharge, it is useful to point out to families the positive signs of recovery. The goal of preparing families for discharge is to help them know what to expect and how to assist in the patient's recovery. Focusing on the four categories previously outlined help the nurse prepare the patient's family for this task.

Case Study: A Family Facing AIDS

AIDS The following study illustrates one family's experience with the various illness phases of the chronic illness AIDS. Increasing numbers of families are coping with AIDS today. The number of adult and adolescent AIDS cases reported in the United States as of December 1992 was approximately 250,000 (Davis, 1993), and AIDS continues to spread. Persons and families with AIDS are double victims: first of debilitating disease and second of social stigmatization (Davis, 1993).

The clinical symptoms of AIDS are the end result of infection by the human immunodeficiency virus (HIV), which infects the body's cells and then disrupts the immune system. HIV can lie dormant in the body for a long time, and clinical manifestations of AIDS may not appear for 5 years or longer after infection (Rice, 1992). According to the Centers for Disease Control and Prevention (CDC), the diagnosis of AIDS is made when individuals meet the following criteria: (1) laboratory evidence of HIV; (2) laboratory evidence of unexplained immunodeficiencies; and (3) documentation of an indicator or opportunistic disease such as Kaposi's sarcoma, mycobacterium tuberculosis, *Pneumocystis carinii* pneumonia, or others (Rice, 1992).

"Medical treatment of AIDS is aimed at the early detection and treatment of opportunistic infections and malignancies, the management of symptoms, and prevention of complications" (Jones, 1993, p. 381). Nursing diagnoses for AIDS may include Infection, risk for; Gas Exchange, impaired; Tissue Integrity, impaired; Nutrition, altered, less than body requirements; Diarrhea; Pain; Anxiety; Thought Processes, altered; Knowledge Deficit (patient and family); Self-Esteem disturbance; Fluid Volume deficit, risk for; Social Isolation (patient and family); Fluid Volume deficit; Powerlessness; Coping, Individual, ineffective; Family Coping, ineffective; and Family Processes, altered.

The Depps The following case study illustrates the Depp family's experience with AIDS.

Alex Depp, a 26-year-old single white teacher, was diagnosed with AIDS a year ago. He has been HIV positive for 4 years. His only admitted risk factor for AIDS is promiscuous homosexual activity when he was younger. Alex's immediate family consists of his mother and his sister Jane. Both Alex's mother and Jane were deeply saddened when they learned Alex had AIDS. They believed he would die before he could accomplish what he wanted to do with his life. Soon after Alex's AIDS diagnosis, Jane noticed frequent mood swings in her mother and they began to have constant arguments over small things.

Alex regularly experiences night sweats, fatigue, and weakness, and he has ongoing weight loss, diarrhea, and malaise. Yesterday he was admitted to the hospital for a diagnostic bronchoscopy to determine the cause of his persistent nonproductive cough, dyspnea, tachypnea, fever, chills, and chest pain. He had one episode of *Pneumocystis carinii* pneumonia (PCP) in the past, and was at that time diagnosed with AIDS. For the last year Alex has feared that the next opportunistic infection would bring about his death.

Before his diagnosis of AIDS, Alex was a healthy, active man. He became debilitated and has been unable to work because of extreme fatigue. He is dependent on his mother and sister for help with the activities of daily living. Alex's mother left her job as a cashier in a grocery store, in part to care for Alex and in part because she found it difficult to deal with her coworkers' concerns that she was handling food. Alex's sister is a student. She is angered by the fact that her friends distanced themselves from her after she told them about her brother's illness. Her anger is compounded by guilt and fear—guilt because she once rejected her homosexual brother, and fear because she is concerned that she may get AIDS from spending so much time caring for Alex.

Alex underwent bronchoscopy without complications. The bronchial biopsy confirmed PCP. To treat the causative organism, Alex was placed on intravenous Pentam, an antiprotozoal drug used to fight PCP infections. After a brief stay in the ICU, Alex was transferred to one of the hospital's medical units. Because his arterial oxygen levels continued to be low, he was given oxygen. Other care included liquid nutritional supplements, positioning in semi- to high Fowler's position, frequent nose and mouth care to prevent candidiasis, and clustering activities so there are periods of time to designate as rest periods.

Throughout his hospital stay Alex's mother and sister felt that no one listened to them. They wanted to talk to the doctor and nurse every day about Alex's condition, but this never seemed possible. At times the family felt the staff was afraid of Alex because they rarely came into the room and they stood at the door of the room to talk to them. Sometimes they waited 20 minutes for Alex's light to be answered. Alex's mother was bothered by the fact that bedclothes and linens were moist from Alex's fever and sweats. She wondered why the staff didn't change his gown and sheets more often.

Alex was discharged from the hospital 3 weeks after his admission. Six months later he contracted PCP again. He was readmitted to the hospital, where he died 3 days later of respiratory failure. Alex's mother, Jane, and their minister were at his bedside when he died. Nurses noted that the family appeared to accept the reality of Alex's death and mobilized themselves to participate in Alex's funeral and other tasks that would assure their ultimate adjustment.

Discussion   The Depp family illustrates many features common to families coping with the phases of illness and in particular with AIDS. Alex's mother, Jane, and Alex—that is, the Depp family system—were all affected by AIDS. The frequent arguments that occurred between Jane and her mother after they learned of the AIDS diagnosis may have served as a distraction from the harsh reality of

Alex's eventual death. It may have been the family's way to avoid addressing their imminent loss. This behavior is common during the preparatory phase of a family's adaptation to a fatal illness.

After the family initially adapted to the prospect of loss, they began to live with the reality of the chronic nature of AIDS. During this "settling-in" or middle phase, Jane and her mother adjusted to illness-related stressors and their caregiving roles. They focused on preventing opportunistic infections and spent time managing Alex's symptoms of fever, night sweats, malaise, and weight loss. Jane and Alex's mother also took over some of the other family functions that had once been assumed by Alex.

Families adjusting to the chronicity of illness endure many stressors. In families facing AIDS, decisions about who to tell about the diagnosis can create great stress (Serovich, Greene, & Parrott, 1992) and families may disagree about the level of disclosure that feels safe to them. Alex's mother, for example, learned that it was not safe to disclose the news of her son's illness to her coworkers. As a consequence, the boundaries of the Depp family system changed. Many families of patients with AIDS desire privacy because of the possibility of stigma and discrimination.

Like Jane Depp, almost everyone who has a family member with AIDS or HIV infection will experience the fear of becoming infected, even when they know rationally that there is no basis for the fear (Macklin, 1988). Partners may hesitate to share a bed, relatives may hesitate to share a meal, grandmothers may hesitate to babysit, and family members in general may not want to become involved (Macklin, 1988). In other words, a diagnosis of AIDS affects internal family system processes.

Like Alex, persons with AIDS may have fears that affect the whole family and stress family relationships. They may be hesitant to be tested for fear of learning the results and reluctant to express physical affection such as hugs or kisses for fear of infecting loved ones; they may fear abandonment, picking up an infection that the immune system cannot handle, or that treatment for infection will not be effective; they may fear painful treatments, death, or the process of dying (Macklin, 1988).

Jane Depp experienced guilt, which is another stressor that families of persons with AIDS may experience. Jane's guilt was due to her having once rejected her now very ill brother because he was gay. Guilt may also result from abandoning a partner because of fear of infection. Frequently, well partners experience guilt because they have been spared (Macklin, 1988).

It is not uncommon for families of patients with AIDS to experience anger. The anger may be at fate for the illness, at the disease itself, at the partner for behaviors that led to the infection, or, as in Jane Depp's case, at friends for being judgmental and unsupportive (Macklin, 1988). In addition, families may grieve about the loss of a healthy and active family member, the loss of dreams for the future, the loss of family normalcy, the loss of the pre-AIDS relationship, the loss of personal freedom as the person with AIDS becomes more homebound, and the impending actual loss of the person with AIDS (Macklin, 1988; Brown & Powell-Cope, 1991).

Uncertainty pervades the lives of families of persons with AIDS. As in Alex's case, the uncertainty may be related to not knowing which opportunistic infection will herald death. Due to Alex's immune system defects, infectious agents that rarely cause disease in persons with normal intact systems could unexpectedly cause death in Alex. There may also be uncertainty about when death will occur, or even uncertainty about staying in a relationship (Brown & Powell-Cope, 1991). Persons with AIDS may be uncertain that they want to put their families through the difficulties associated with their illness and they may consider dissolving relationships. Family members may not be able to cope with the stigma and other illnesses associated with hardships and they may consider withdrawing from relationships.

According to the Family Stress Model, a stressful event is accompanied by many hardships. For instance, families frequently suffer economic hardship as a result of an AIDS diagnosis. In the Depp family, Alex and his mother gave up full-time jobs. Families may find themselves poverty-stricken because of the loss of earning power, the loss of health insurance, the high cost of treatment, lack of financial assistance, and missed financial opportunities (Brown & Powell-Cope, 1991; Macklin, 1988). Some family members must take sick leave, vacation days, or personal days due to caring for the person with AIDS. Other family hardships may be associated with taking on additional family responsibilities, such as caregiving responsibilities.

During Alex's hospitalization, Jane and her mother experienced the acute illness phase of AIDS. They displayed behaviors characteristic of Thorne and Robinson's (1988) disenchantment stage in the relationship between the family and the health care team. They were dissatisfied with care and frustrated by the difficulty of obtaining information. Nursing interventions classified as family support (e.g., effective communication, answering questions), family involvement (e.g., changing some of the bed linens), and family mobilization (e.g., permitting the Depps to describe how they cared for Alex at home) might have helped.

The Depps' guess that hospital staff were afraid of Alex because they talked to them from the door of the room was probably correct. During a hospital stay families and persons with AIDS may meet health care personnel who are fearful of catching AIDS from patients. Some staff believe they have the right to refuse to care for persons with AIDS. Others believe that caring for persons with AIDS would be upsetting to their own significant others (Scherer, Haughey, Wu, & Kuhn, 1992).

Nurses caring for Alex and other similar patients need help to cope with their fears about caring for persons with AIDS. Discussion groups can afford nurses the opportunity to voice their feelings and foster the development of positive attitudes, and staff members who are more comfortable in caring for AIDS patients and their families can serve as role models or preceptors for nurses who object to caring for patients like Alex (Scherer, Haughey, Wu, & Kuhn, 1992).

The Depps appeared to cope effectively with the terminal phase of illness. Jane and her mother coped by clinging together in anticipation of Alex's death, and nurses helped by permitting their minister to stay with them at the bedside.

This case study illustrates one family's experiences with the various phases of illness, each of which presents different challenges to families. Medical-surgical nurses must be prepared to help families face the challenges and concerns of all these stages.

IMPLICATIONS FOR EDUCATION, RESEARCH, AND HEALTH CARE CARE POLICY

The body of knowledge about medical-surgical family nursing is growing, and there are many opportunities for nurses to apply this knowledge to practice. It is no longer appropriate to study medical-surgical nursing only from the perspective of individual patient care. Faculty need to clearly define family health care practice in medical-surgical settings (Hanson & Heims, 1992) and incorporate family care into medical-surgical nursing courses and appropriate practice settings. Family assessment frameworks that lead to specific strategies for intervention also need attention in medical-surgical nursing curriculums (Hanson, Heims, & Julian, 1992). Relegating the bulk of family content to specialty courses such as community health nursing or childbearing family nursing misleads students about the practice of family nursing. Nursing staff on medical-surgical units also need to be educated about family nursing, especially as many staff members were educated at a period when family nursing was not considered important in medical-surgical settings.

Identification of family practice problems (e.g., difficulties associated with delivering care to families) and investigating the validity, relevance, cost, and benefits of potential solutions to those problems will help to promote research-based practice (Lindquist, Brauer, Lekander, & Foster, 1990). Designing, implementing, and testing family nursing interventions will foster the growth of medical-surgical family nursing knowledge. However, research findings about families only become valuable to families after they pass through the research utilization process. The goal of research utilization is to improve nursing care, which results in optimal family outcomes. Through research utilization, knowledge about families that is obtained from research is transferred into clinical practice. Nurses who seek to improve family care through research utilization engage in critically analyzing research literature about families, select from the literature interventions that are appropriate for their practice setting, implement the interventions, then evaluate the family outcomes.

Health care policies clearly influence nursing practice. Family nursing practice in medical-surgical settings can be enhanced through hospital and unit-based philosophy statements that include the family. Policies about family visitation, family participation in care, family presence during CPR, families staying overnight in patient rooms, and families bringing in favorite foods should be evaluated in light of a family care philosophy.

SUMMARY   There is a growing demand for family-focused care within medical-surgical settings. Hospital environments are foreign to family members, a situation which adds to the stress of illness and injury for patients and families. When planning interventions, nurses caring for families need to consider the nature of the illness, family characteristics, the health care team's philosophy about family care, and the characteristics of the patient. Family theoretical models, including the Structural-Functional Model, Family Systems Model, and Family Stress Model, can provide a basis for family assessment and intervention.

Medical-surgical nurses may care for families during periods of pre-illness, acute illness, chronic illness, or terminal illness. During pre-illness, nurses need to acknowledge the stress of hospitalization and direct interventions at health promotion. During the acute illness phase, nursing interventions should focus on providing assurance, enhancing the proximity of patient and family, managing information, facilitating comfort, and reinforcing support. Families in the chronic phase have been dealing with illness for a long time; thus acknowledging these families' experiences with illness management is important. Common family concerns in chronic illness, such as guilt, fear, uncertainty, anger, and lack of knowledge about the illness, care requirements, or resources, may require interventions. During the terminal phase, interventions are directed toward helping families move through the phases of adaptation in response to the fatal illness of a family member. In any illness stage, family support, family process maintenance, promotion of family integrity, family involvement, or family mobilization may be helpful.

Efforts to control health care costs have resulted in a pattern of early patient discharge from the hospital. Research suggests that the availability of social support, use of coping strategies, availability of personal resources, and knowing what to expect once at home positively influence a family's perception of readiness for discharge. Nurses should assess these family characteristics in order to determine family needs at discharge.

Nurses in medical-surgical settings need to use the growing body of knowledge about medical-surgical family nursing in practice. They also need to advocate for changes in hospital policies and procedures to reflect this knowledge, and update this knowledge through future research. Only when medical-surgical nurses include families in plans for care can they hope to provide unfragmented, holistic, humane, and sensitively delivered health care.

STUDY QUESTIONS

1. Which of the following factors have led to the growth of family nursing in medical-surgical settings:
   a. Consumer demand for unfragmented and holistic care
   b. Early hospital discharge
   c. Empirical evidence that families influene patient recovery
   d. All of the above

2. All of the following characteristics are likely to increase the degree of family stress associated with hospitalization *except*:
   a. Sudden illness onset with no time to prepare
   b. Repeated family experience with the illness
   c. Few sources of guidance for the family
   d. Significant disruption of family functioning as a result of the hospitalization

3. Nurses caring for families in medical-surgical settings need to consider the following factors of the "therapeutic quadrangle":
   a. Illness, family, doctor, patient
   b. Illness, doctor, nurse, patient
   c. Illness, family, health care team, patient
   d. Family, health care team, social work services, chaplain services

4. The focus of the Structural-Functional Model is on:
   a. Guiding analysis of stressors, resources, and family perceptions to explain family crisis outcomes
   b. Examining the amount of interaction a family has with its environment
   c. Examining family process and resultant family outcomes

   d. Examining family behavioral outcomes that result from the organization of the family

5. Helping families maintain healthy lifestyles is a major aim for nurses during the:
   a. Pre-illness phase
   b. Acute illness phase
   c. Chronic illness phase
   d. Terminal illness phase

6. Establishing a calm and relaxed atmosphere that will support a trusting and empathetic relationship describes which of the following family nursing interventions:
   a. Proximity enhancement
   b. Information management
   c. Assurance provision
   d. Comfort facilitation

7. Minimization of family disruption effects describes which category of family nursing interventions?
   a. Family support
   b. Family process management
   c. Promotion of family integrity
   d. Family involvement

8. Which of the following family behaviors is rarely displayed during the chronic phase of illness?
   a. Accepting the imminence of death
   b. Carrying out prescribed treatment regimens
   c. Finding the necessary money and resources to facilitate care
   d. Preventing the social isolation caused by lessened contact with others

9. Relationships between the family and the health care team move through stages. The stage characterized by family renegotiation of trust with health care professionals is called the stage of:
   a. Naive trust
   b. Disenchantment
   c. Guarded alliance
   d. None of the above

10. What factors should be considered when determining hospital visiting policies?
    a. Patient preferences
    b. Family preferences
    c. Nursing care needs
    d. All of the above

11. Which of the following is *not* an advantage to having families present when nurses and physicians carry out resuscitative efforts?
    a. Assurance that the patient is dying
    b. Less nursing staff time is needed for giving explanations, since the family has witnessed activities firsthand.
    c. It helps the family accept the reality of death.
    d. It provides the family with an opportunity to say what they need to say while there is still a chance the patient can hear.

12. Families of patients with AIDS may experience:
    a. Social stigmatization
    b. Guilt
    c. Economic hardship
    d. All of the above

REFERENCES

American Nurses Association. (1992). Nurses to educate for end-of-life decisions. *American Nurse, 24,* 9.

Artinian, N. T. (1989). Family member perceptions of a cardiac surgery event. *Focus on Critical Care, 16,* 301–308.

Artinian, N. T. (1993). Spouses' perceptions of readiness for discharge after cardiac surgery. *Applied Nursing Research, 6,* 80–88.

Artinian, N. T. (1994). Selecting a model to guide family assessment. *Dimensions of Critical Care Nursing. 13,* 4–12.

Beckie, T. (1989). A supportive-educative telephone program: Impact of knowledge and anxiety after coronary artery bypass graft surgery. *Heart & Lung, 18,* 46–55.

Bedell, S., Pelle, D., Maher, P., & Cleary, P. (1986). Do-not-resuscitate orders for critically ill patients in the hospital. *Journal of the American Medical Association, 256,* 233–237.

Berkey, K. M., & Hanson, S. M. H. (1991). *Pocket guide to family assessment and intervention.* St. Louis, Mosby Year Book.

Biegel, D. E., Sales, E., & Schulz, R. (1991). *Family caregiving in chronic illness.* Newbury Park, CA: Sage Publications.

Boss, P. (1988). *Family stress management.* Beverly Hills, CA: Sage Publications.

Boumann, C. C. (1984). Identifying priority concerns of families of ICU patients. *Dimensions of Critical Care Nursing, 3,* 313–319.

Brooten, C., Brown, L. P., Munro, B. H., York, R., Cohen, S. M., Roncoli, M., & Hollingsworth, A. (1988). Early discharge and specialist transitional care. *Image: Journal of Nursing Scholarship, 20,* 64–68.

Brown, M., A., & Powell-Cope, G. M. (1991). AIDS family caregiving: Transitions through uncertainty. *Nursing Research, 40,* 338–345.

Bruya, M.A. (1981). Planned periods of rest in the intensive care unit: Nursing activities and intracranial pressure. *Journal of Neurosurgical Nursing, 13,* 184–194.

Burr, W. R. (1982). Families under stress. In H. I. McCubbin, A. E. Cauble, & J. M. Patterson (Eds.), *Family stress, coping and social support.* Springfield, IL: Charles C. Thomas.

Burr, W. R., Hill, R., Nye, F. I., & Reiss, I. L. (1979). *Contemporary theories about the family, Vol. 1.* New York: The Free Press.

Craft, M. J., & Willadsen, J. A. (1992). Interventions related to family. *Nursing Clinics of North America, 27,* 517–540.

Crooks, C. E., Iammarino, N. K., & Weinberg, A. D. (1987). The family's role in health promotion. *Health Values, 11,* 7–12.

Daley, L. (1984). The perceived immediate needs of families with relatives in the intensive care setting. *Heart & Lung, 13,* 231–237.

Danielson, C. B., Hamel-Bissell, B., & Winstead-Fry, P. (1993). *Families, health & illness.* St. Louis, MO: C. V. Mosby.

Davis, M. C. (1993). Understanding AIDS. *Caring Magazine, 12,* 5–13.

Donley, R. (1988). The health care system. In J. M. Flynn & P. B. Heffron, *Nursing: From concept to practice* (2nd ed., pp. 115–134). Norwalk, CT: Appleton & Lange.

Duryée, R. (1992). The efficacy of inpatient education after myocardial infarction. *Heart & Lung, 21*, 217–226.

Eshleman, J. R. (1991). *The family: An introduction* (6th ed.). Boston: Allyn & Bacon.

Fawcett, J. (1984). *Analysis and evaluation of conceptual models of nursing*. Philadelphia: F. A. Davis.

Figley, C. R., & McCubbin, H. I. (Eds.). (1983). *Stress and the family: Vol. 2. Coping with catastrophe*. New York: Brunner/Mazel.

Frederickson, K. (1989). Anxiety transmission in the patient with myocardial infarction. *Heart & Lung, 18*, 617–622.

Friedman, M. M. (1992). *Family nursing: Theory and practice* (3rd ed.). Norwalk, CT: Appleton & Lange.

Garding, B. S., Kerr, J. C., & Bay, K. (1988). Effectiveness of a program of information and support for myocardial infarction patients recovering at home. *Heart and Lung, 17*, 355–362.

Gilliss, C. L., Rose, D. B., Hallburg, J. C., & Martinson, I. M. (1989). The family and chronic illness. In C. L. Gilliss, B. L. Highley, B. M. Roberts, & I. M. Martinson (Eds.), *Toward a science of family nursing* (pp. 287–299). Menlo Park, CA: Addison-Wesley.

Gortner, S. R., Gilliss, C. L., Shinn, J. A., Sparacino, P. A., Rankin, S., Leavitt, M., Price, M., & Hudes, M. (1988). Improving recovery following cardiac surgery: A randomized clinical trial. *Journal of Advanced Nursing, 13*, 649–661.

Hamner, J. B. (1990). Visiting policies in the ICU: A time for change. *Critical Care Nurse, 10*, 48–53.

Hanson, S. M. H., & Heims, M. L. (1992). Family nursing curricula in U.S. schools of nursing. *Journal of Nursing Education, 31*, 303–308.

Hanson, S., Heims, M., & Julian, D. (1992). Education for family health care professionals: Nursing as a paradigm. *Family Relations, 41*, 49–53.

Hathaway, D., Boswell, B., Stanford, D., Schneider, S., & Moncrief, A. (1987). Health promotion and disease prevention for the hospitalized patient's family. *Nursing Administration Quarterly, 11*(3), 1–7.

Henneman, E. A., McKenzie, J. B., & Dewa, C. S. (1992). An evaluation of interventions for meeting the information needs of families of critically ill patients. *American Journal of Critical Care, 1*(3), 85–93.

Hill, R. (1949). *Families under stress*. New York: Harper & Brothers.

Hoffman, M., & Malecki, M. (1990). Organ procurement and preservation. In K. M. Sigardson-Poor & L. M. Haggerty, *Nursing care of the transplant recipient* (pp. 13–34). Philadelphia: W. B. Saunders.

Huckabay, L. M. D. (1991). The role of conceptual frameworks in nursing practice, administration, education and research. *Nursing Administration Quarterly, 15*(3), 17–28.

Jones, A. (1993) Hematology/immunology. In J. Hartshorn, M. Lamborn, & M. L. Noll, *Introduction to critical care nursing* (pp. 348–385). Philadelphia: W. B. Saunders.

King, K. B., Reiss, H. T., Porter, L. A., & Norsen, L. H. (1993). Social support and long term recovery from coronary artery surgery: Effects on patients and spouses. *Health Psychology, 12*, 56–63.

Kirchhoff, K. (1982). Visiting policies for patients with myocardial infarctions—a national survey. *Heart & Lung, 11*, 571–576.

Kirks, B. A., Hendricks, D. G., & Wyse, B. W. (1982). Parent involvement in nutrition education for primary grade students. *Journal of Nutrition Education, 14*, 137–139.

Kulik, J. A., & Mahler, H. I. (1989). Social support and recovery from surgery. *Health Psychology, 8*, 221–238.

Leahey, M., & Wright, L. M. (1987). Families and chronic illness: Assumptions, assessment, and intervention. In L. M. Wright & M. Leahey, *Families and chronic illness* (pp. 55–76). Springhouse, PA: Springhouse.

Leske, J. S. (1986). Needs of relatives of critically ill patients: A follow up. *Heart and Lung, 15*, 189–193.

Leske, J. S. (1991). Internal psychometric properties of the Critical Care Family Needs Inventory. *Heart & Lung, 20*, 236–344.

Leske, J. S. (1992). Needs of adult family members after critical illness. *Critical Care Nursing Clinics of North America, 4*, 587–596.

Leventhal, H., Leventhal, E. A., & Nguyen, T. V. (1985). Reactions of families to illness: Theoretical models and perspectives. In D. C. Turk & R. D. Kerns (Eds.), *Health, illness and families: A life-span perspective* (pp. 108–145). New York: John Wiley & Sons.

Lindquist, R., Brauer, D. J., Lekander, B. J., & Foster, K. (1990). Research utilization: Practice considerations for applying research to nursing to practice. *Focus on Critical Care, 17*, 342–347.

Lubkin, I. M. (1986). *Chronic illness: Impact and intervention*. Boston: Jones & Bartlett.

Macklin, E. D. (1988). AIDS: Implications for families. *Family Relations, 37*, 141–149.

Malecki, M., & Hoffman, M. (1987). Getting to yes: How nurses' attitudes affect their success in obtaining consent for organ and tissue donations. *Dialysis and Transplantation, 16*, 276–278.

Marsden, C. (1992). Making patient self determination a reality in critical care. *American Journal of Critical Care, 1*, 122–124.

Martin, J. (1991). Rethinking traditional thoughts. *Journal of Emergency Nursing, 17*(2), 67–68.

Mathis, M. (1984). Personal needs of family members of critically ill patients with and without brain injury. *Journal of Neurosurgical Nursing, 16*, 36–44.

McClowry, S. G. (1992). Family functioning during a critical illness: A systems theory perspective. *Critical Care Nursing Clinics of North America, 4*, 559–564.

McCubbin, M. A., & McCubbin, H. I. (1993). Families coping with illness: The Resiliency Model of family stress adjustment and adaptation. In C. B. Danielson, B. Hamel-Bissell, & P. Winstead-Fry, *Families, health, and illness* (pp. 21 – 63). St. Louis, MO: C. V. Mosby.

McCubbin, H. I., & Patterson, J. M. (1982). Family adaptation to crisis. In H. I. McCubbin, A. E. Cauble, & J. M. Patterson (Eds.), *Family stress, coping and social support* (pp. 26 – 47). Springfield, IL: Charles C. Thomas.

Meleis, A. I. (1991). *Theoretical nursing: Development and progress* (2nd ed.). Philadelphia: J. B. Lippincott.

Mercer, R. T. (1989). Theoretical perspectives on family. In C. L. Giliss, B. C. Highley, B. Roberts, & I. M. Martinson (Eds.), *Toward a science of family nursing.* Menlo-Park, CA: Addison-Wesley.

Mishel, M. H., & Murdaugh, C. L. (1987). Family adjustment to heart transplantation: Redesigning the dream. *Nursing Research, 36,* 332 – 338.

Molter, N. C. (1979). Needs of relatives of critically ill patients. *Heart and Lung, 8,* 332 – 339.

Moos, R. H. (Ed.). (1984). *Coping with physical illness. 2: New perspectives.* New York: Plenum Press.

Nicklin, W. M. (1986). Post discharge concerns of cardiac patients as presented via a telephone callback system. *Heart & Lung, 15,* 268 – 272.

Norris, L. O., & Grove, S. K. (1986). Investigation of selected psychosocial needs of family members of critically ill adults. *Heart & Lung, 15,* 194 – 199.

O'Connor, A. M. (1983). Factors related to the early phase of rehabilitation following aortocoronary bypass surgery. *Research in Nursing and Health, 6,* 107 – 116.

Osuagwu, C. C. (1991). ED codes: Keep the family out. *Journal of Emergency Nursing, 17,* 363 – 364.

Potter, P. A., & Perry, A. G., (1989). *Fundamentals of Nursing.* St. Louis, MO: C. V. Mosby.

Redheffer, G. M. (1989). A trauma nurse's opinion. *Nursing, 19*(3), 45.

Rice, R. (1992). The patient with AIDS. In R. Rice (Ed.), *Home health nursing practice* (pp. 203 – 217). St. Louis, MO: Mosby-Year Book.

Rolland, J. S. (1988). A conceptual model of chronic and life-threatening illness and its impact on families. In C. S. Chilman, E. W. Nunnally, & F. M. Cox (Eds.), *Chronic illness and disability: Families in trouble series, Vol. 2* (pp. 17 – 68). Newbury Park, CA: Sage Publication.

Ross, B., & Cobb, K. L. (1990a). *Family nursing: A nursing process approach.* Redwood City, CA: Addison-Wesley Nursing.

Ross, B., & Cobb, K. L. (1990b). Introductions to the family as a client. In B. Ross & K. L. Cobb, *Family nursing: A nursing process approach* (pp. 1 – 24). Redwood City, CA: Addison-Wesley Nursing.

Rosen, E. J. (1990). *Families facing death.* New York: Lexington Books.

Scherer, Y. K., Haughey, B. P., Wu, Y. B., & Kuhn, M. M. (1992). AIDS: What are critical care nurses' concerns? *Critical Care Nurse, 12*(7), 23 – 29.

Serovich, J. M., Greene, K., & Parrott, R. (1992). Boundaries and AIDS testing: Privacy and the family system. *Family Relations, 41,* 104 – 109.

Simpson, T. (1991). Critical care patients' perceptions of visits. *Heart & Lung, 20,* 681 – 688.

Steele, J. M., & Rizicki, D. (1987). An evaluation of the effectiveness of cardiac teaching during hospitalization. *Heart & Lung, 16,* 306 – 311.

Steinglass, P. (1992). Family systems theory and medical illness. In R. J. Sawa (Ed.), *Family health care* (pp. 18 – 29). Newbury Park, CA: Sage Publications.

Swanson, R. W. (1993). Psychological issues in CPR. *Annals of Emergency Medicine, 22,* (2; part 2), 350 – 353.

Thorne, S. E., & Robinson, C. A. (1988). Health care relationships: The chronic illness perspective. *Research in Nursing and Health, 11,* 293 – 300.

Titler, M., Cohen, M. Z., & Craft, M. J. (1991). Impact of adult critical care hospitalization: Perceptions of patients, spouses, children, and nurses. *Heart & Lung, 20,* 174 – 182.

Titler, M. G., & Walsh, S. M. (1992). Visiting critically ill adults: Strategies for practice. *Critical Care Nursing Clinics of North America, 4,* 623 – 632.

Turk, D. C., & Kerns, R. D. (Eds.). (1985). *Health, illness, and families: A life-span perspective.* New York: John Wiley & Sons.

von Bertalanffy, L. (1968). *General system theory.* New York: George Braziller.

Whall, A. L., & Fawcett, J. (1991). The family as a focal phenomenon in nursing. In A. L. Whall & J. Fawcett, *Family theory development in nursing: State of the science and art.* Philadelphia: F. A. Davis.

Yates, B. C. (1989). Stress and social support during recovery from a cardiac illness event. *Oklahoma Nurse, 34*(5), 7.

Younger, S. J., Coulton, C., Welton, R., Juknialis, B., & Jackson, D. L. (1984). ICU visiting policies. *Critical Care Medicine, 12* 606 – 608.

Zetterlund, J. E. (1971). An evaluation of visiting policies for intensive and coronary care units. In M. Duffey, E. H. Anderson, B. S. Bergersen, M. Lohr, & M. H. Rose (Eds.), *Current concepts in clinical nursing,* vol. 3 (pp. 316 – 325). St. Louis, MO: C. V. Mosby.

BIBLIOGRAPHY

Doherty, W. J., & Baird, M. A. (Eds.). (1987). *Family-centered medical care: A clinical case book.* New York: Guilford Press.

Doherty, W. J., & Campbell, T. L. (1988). *Families and health.* Newbury Park, CA: Sage Publications.

Feetham, S. L., Meister, S. B., Bell, J. M., & Gilliss, C. L. (Eds.). (1993). *The nursing of families: Theory/research/education/practice.* Newbory Park, CA: Sage Publications.

Hickey, M. L. (Ed.). (1992). Family issues in critical care. *Critical Care Nursing Clinics of North America, 4,* 549–649.

Leahey, M., & Wright, L. M. (1987). *Families & life-threatening illness.* Springhouse, PA: Springhouse Corporation.

Leske, J. S. (Ed.). (1991). Family interventions. *AACN Clinical Issues in Critical Care Nursing, 2,* 181–354.

Sawa, R. J. (Ed.). (1992). *Family health care.* Newbury Park, CA: Sage Publications.

Wright, L. M., & Leahey, M. (1987). *Families & chronic illness.* Springhouse, PA: Springhouse Corporation.

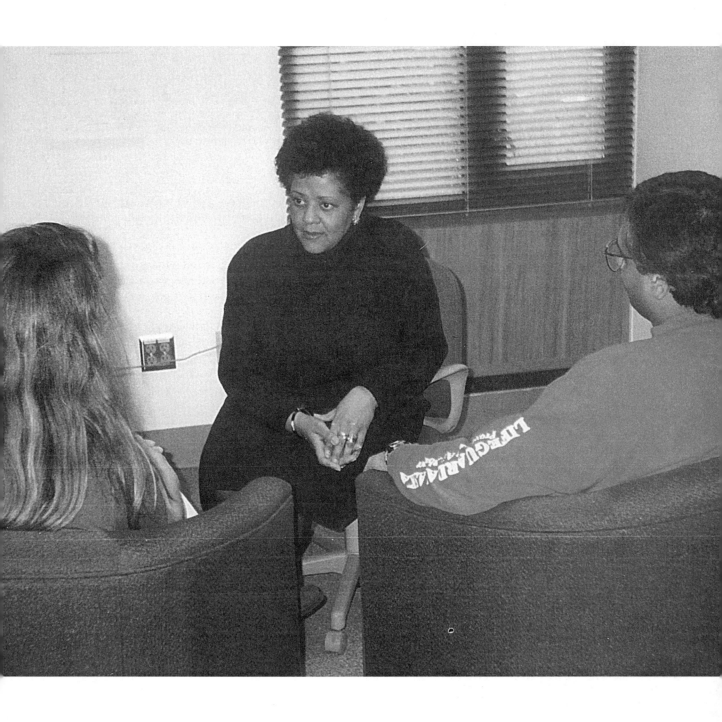

Family Mental Health Nursing

The experience of most nursing students in psychiatric mental health settings involves *individuals* with either acute or chronic conditions. In contrast, this chapter examines the intricacies of *family* mental health nursing.

A historical overview of trends in family mental health nursing is followed by an outline of common theoretical perspectives. The topics covered include Bowen's theory, structural, contextual, and communication theory, the multiple systems view, and nursing conceptual models, so that students are provided with an excellent background on the theoretical bases of family mental health nursing practice.

The chapter continues with a discussion of the importance of health promotion and identifies strategies that, regardless of the practice setting, will assist the nurse in creating a healthy environment for families. The case examples are realistic and address family mental health treatment on both inpatient and outpatient units.

The discussion of chronic mental illness is timely and demonstrates a sensitivity to the cultural issues that pervade our care of families and individuals with mental health problems. The use of case studies helps the student to understand chronic mental health problems and the multiple roles of the family mental health nurse. The chapter concludes with a consideration of the implications of the family approach to mental health nursing for practice, education, research, and health policy.

CHAPTER 13

Family Mental Health Nursing

Margaret P. Shepard, PhD, RN ▪ *Helene J. Moriarty, PhD, RN, CS*

OBJECTIVES *Upon completion of this chapter, the reader will be able to:*
1. Describe family mental health nursing.
2. Explain how conceptualizations of the family and family interventions have evolved over the past 200 years in psychiatric and mental health nursing.
3. Identify and describe five common theoretical perspectives used in family mental health nursing.
4. Identify the goals for family mental health nursing interventions in health promotion, acute illness, and chronic illness.

Psychiatric and mental health nursing is a specialized area of nursing practice that is based on the science of theories of human behavior and on the art of the therapeutic use of self (American Nurses Association [ANA], 1994). The practice is directed to both preventive and corrective efforts against mental disorders and their sequelae. It is concerned with promotion of optimum mental health for society, communities, families, and individuals. Family nursing is an integral component of psychiatric and mental health nursing, though not all nurses in this field practice family nursing. Family mental health nursing recognizes the interaction between families and the mental health of family members. It addresses the psychiatric and mental health care needs of the individual client in the context of the family, while also addressing the needs of the family as a whole.

Health care reform, shortened hospital stays, and more manageable medication protocols have all influenced clients' treatment needs and the system of care delivery in psychiatric and mental health treatment (Baker, 1993). Increasingly, short-term psychiatric hospital admissions are designed for intensive management of acute symptoms, and early discharge places the client with continuing symptoms back in the care of the family and the community. While there are many benefits in caring for mentally ill clients outside the hospital, this increases the burdens on the families of the mentally ill (Maurin & Boyd, 1990). Extended care for an ill family member strains family resources and often leaves the family ill-equipped to manage the stigma, guilt, and loss that may be experienced (Baker, 1989). Family caregiving brings an extraordinary number of stressors, placing relatives in what may be a situation of risk. Stressors experienced by the family include difficulties in coping with disturbed behavior, the uncertainty and unpredictability of symptoms, and loneliness and isolation due to the stigma of having a mentally ill family member (Chafez & Barns, 1989). Family caregivers require support to manage these stressors, as well as information about symptom management and community resources, to effectively manage the mentally ill family member at home. Mental health nurses practicing family-centered care are in a position to meet the needs of the client within the context of the family and to meet the needs of the family as a whole.

Contemporary psychiatric mental health nursing practice includes the domains of prevention, intervention, and rehabilitation (ANA, 1976). Thus, nurses practicing mental health and psychiatric care may be found in many settings, providing many levels of care. Two practice levels of psychiatric and mental health nursing have been delineated by the ANA (1994). These are the psychiatric–mental health registered nurse and the psychiatric–mental health advanced practice registered nurse. Both are prepared to use the nursing process and theoretical frameworks to address a broad range of physical and psychosocial problems presented by clients and their families. And both collaborate with a variety of other professions working with and on behalf of the client. The clinical examples in this chapter illustrate the different roles of the nurse in psychiatric and mental health nursing.

HISTORICAL OVERVIEW OF FAMILY NURSING IN PSYCHIATRIC AND MENTAL HEALTH SETTINGS

Psychiatric and mental health nurses have a long history of working with the family. However, conceptualizations of families and family interventions have changed over the last 200 years with advances in knowledge and changes in health care delivery.

During the Colonial period in American history, there was no organized system of care for people suffering with mental illness. Responsibility for the care of the mentally ill lay primarily with the family. In the absence of a family, the mentally disturbed were supported and maintained through the charity of neighbors and the community (Ramshorn, 1978). It was not until the advent of the "asylum," or the public mental hospital, in the nineteenth century that any systematic care was provided for the mentally ill. In this period, the insane were taken away from the stimulation of the home environment and placed in institutions that had orderly and structured routines in order to recuperate. However, because there were few professional tools available to understand and treat mental illness and the debilitating effects of institutionalization had not yet been recognized, patients often stayed in the hospital indefinitely.

Twentieth-century psychiatric treatment was greatly influenced by the Freudian psychoanalytic movement (Bowen, 1976). Before Freud, psychiatric illness was believed to be due to some unidentified brain pathology. Freud's research led to a theory that proposed that psychiatric symptoms were a function of the mind rather than a brain disease. In addition, Freud introduced the concept of transference, which led to one of the cornerstones of psychiatric treatment, the therapeutic relationship. During this period, however, psychiatric treatment was still provided primarily in institutions, within the framework of the medical model. The role of the nurse was to provide custodial care and companionship for patients. Family participation in treatment was discouraged (Peplau, 1993). This mode of treatment persisted until the National Mental Health Act of 1946, which represented the first national commitment to solving the problem of mental illness through funding for research, services, and training. As part of this commitment, the relationship between psychiatric patients and nurses began to be studied, in an effort to identify how the nurse-patient relationship could be therapeutic for patients. The result was the emergence of the clinical specialty of psychiatric nursing (Peplau, 1993).

In the middle of the twentieth century biomedical research led to the development of the phenothiazines, the medications that help to control the major symptoms associated with psychosis. Effective use of these antipsychotic medications made it possible for clients who had formerly been "out of touch with reality" to enter into significant therapeutic relationships with psychiatric staff. Thus, this was an exciting time for mental health nurses, who began to implement therapeutic relationships with their patients. This period also marked the beginning of a trend toward less restrictive treatment and discharge of chronically ill patients to the community and the family. Simultaneously, researchers started to examine the reciprocal relationship between the mentally ill client and the family (Maurin & Boyd, 1990). There was increased recognition that caring for the mentally ill placed a burden on families and that families may play a major role in maintaining the symptoms of mental illness in an individual member.

Efforts to provide community-based services for the mentally ill resulted in the Community Mental Health Centers Act of 1963, which marked a significant shift away from institutional services to community-based services for the mentally ill (Ramshorn, 1978). The act authorized funding for continuous and comprehensive services in community mental health centers and led to what has been called the "deinstitutionalization movement." Large numbers of chronically ill individuals were released from hospitals, and the focus of care shifted toward the community, a change that led to expanded roles for psychiatric nurses as individual, group, and family therapists (Peplau, 1993).

Initially, family therapists tended to blame families for the client's illness, based on the view that the client's symptoms were a manifestation of family pathology. In particular, the mother was often blamed for improperly nurturing her young children, and a disturbed mother-child relationship was thought to be the cause of the psychiatric disturbance in the child. Too often, families felt blamed by nurses and other mental health professionals, through overt or covert implications that they had been responsible for causing or maintaining the individual's symptoms (Walsh, 1987). Other factors related to symptoms received little attention. Experiences such as these only exacerbated family burdens of guilt and shame. Further, there is little empirical evidence supporting the efficacy of treatment strategies that regard the patient as the victim and other family members as villains (Walsh, 1987).

The deinstitutionalization movement was expected to bring sweeping solutions to the problems of the seriously mentally ill. Yet many communities were not able to provide the comprehensive services required to treat this population. As a result, many patients experienced the "revolving door phenomenon": early discharge to the community without adequate treatment strategies and supportive services resulted in frequent readmissions to the hospital (Ramshorn, 1978). In the absence of adequate services, many families had to assume even more responsibility for caring for their mentally ill family member. Frustrated with inadequate services and the tendency of mental health professionals to blame families for individuals' illnesses, families formed consumer advocacy groups such as the National Alliance for the Mentally Ill (NAMI). Groups such as these became very active in lobbying Congress and the public for increased research on mental illness and its treatment. And indeed, research in the last decade has produced major breakthroughs in genetics, immunology, and knowledge of brain function, and has increased scientists' and mental health practitioners' understanding of biological factors related to mental illness. For example, specific structural and functional changes in the brain have been associated with schizophrenia, and DNA markers for the genetic predisposition to certain affective disorders have been identified (McBride, 1990).

Growing recognition of the biopsychosocial correlates of mental illness, shorter hospital stays, and the necessity for families to take primary responsibility for their member's care have led nurses and other mental health professionals to enter into a relationship with families as "partners in care." These professionals now acknowledge the benefits of basing family interventions on respect for the needs of family members and the family's collaborative role in improving patient functioning (Walsh & Anderson, 1987). Mental health professionals are thus combining information about brain function with a consideration of the psychological, social, cultural, and familial factors that also influence human behavior (McBride, 1990). This integrated approach (McKeon, 1990) has propelled nurses and other mental health professionals to identify and study the most effective strategies for mental health promotion in the family (Duffy, 1988), the most effective ways to share information about a member's schizophrenia with the family (Main, Gerace, & Camilleri, 1993), and the most effective ways to support families in caring for a schizophrenic family member in the community (Brooker & Butterworth, 1991; Zastowny, Lehman, Cole, & Kane, 1992).

COMMON THEORETICAL PERSPECTIVES IN FAMILY AND MENTAL HEALTH NURSING

Psychiatric–mental health nurses typically use therapeutic principles from a number of family systems theories to guide their assessments and interventions with families. Psychiatric–mental health advanced practice nurses, many of whom are family therapists, are more apt to base their practice on one *specific* theoretical framework; however, some advanced practice nurses use multiple frameworks. Five major theoretical frameworks are commonly employed in family mental health nursing: Bowen's Family Systems Theory, Structural Family Theory, Contextual Family Theory, Communication Theory, and the multiple systems view. It is important to note that there is some conceptual overlap among theories.

Bowen's Family Systems Theory

One theory commonly used in family mental health nursing is Bowen's Family Systems Theory (Bowen, 1976; Brown, 1991; Gillis, 1973; Kerr & Bowen, 1988). This theory views the nuclear family as part of the multigenerational extended family and theorizes that patterns of relating tend to repeat themselves over generations. The theory does not "pathologize" families but, rather, encourages individuals to see their families in positive ways. Family members are guided to acknowledge that parents and relatives "did the best with what they had" (Brown, 1991).

The theory consists of eight interlocking concepts that describe emotional patterns and interactions: (1) differentiation of self, (2) triangles, (3) the family projection process, (4) the nuclear family emotional system, (5) the multigenerational transmission process, (6) sibling position, (7) emotional cutoff, and (8) societal regression. Understanding families requires understanding these concepts and the relationships among the concepts.

The central concept is *differentiation of self;* it has two aspects. First, it refers to the capacity to be a separate yet related human being, and second it refers to the ability to separate thought from reactive feeling. Differentiation exists on a continuum; the level of differentiation influences the ability to manage anxiety. Those at the higher end of the continuum are able to have intimate relationships while still maintaining a sense of self. They also exhibit more thinking than reactive feeling. Because they are less reactive, they are better able to manage anxiety and to cope with stress. Those at the lower end of the continuum have more fused relationships — they are extremely close to others but are unable to maintain a basic sense of self. They also show less thinking and more reactive feeling. Because they are more reactive, they are more anxious in times of stress and less able to cope with stress.

A *triangle* describes a relational pattern among persons, objects, or issues. It is an emotional configuration of three members; the members may be three persons; or two persons and a group, an issue, or an object. When tension mounts between two persons, one or the other moves toward the third member of the triangle to relieve the anxiety between the twosome. Triangles operate in all families but become problematic over time when they are rigid and entrenched.

The *family projection process* is the process by which parental anxiety is transmitted to children via triangles. The *nuclear family emotional system* describes how anxiety is managed: (1) through marital conflict or distance; (2) through dysfunction of a spouse; or (3) through projection onto a child or children. The *multigenerational transmission process* is the family projection process in action over several generations. *Sibling position* refers to the place and role a child assumes in the family. There is a tendency for siblings in certain positions to take on certain roles and behaviors. For example, the oldest child tends to be a responsible caretaker in the family. *Emotional cutoff* is the process of physically or emotionally separating from the family of origin as a way to handle the anxiety of fusion. *Societal regression* refers to the idea that a high level of anxiety in a society (e.g., from war or economic problems) can lead to reacting emotionally rather than in a thinking way (e.g., through riots).

Using Bowen's Family Systems approach, the therapist may meet with only one family member, with some members, or with all members. No matter who is present, however, the work is seen as family therapy because the therapist takes a multigenerational view of the family. The therapist and family develop a three- to four-generation genogram to examine family processes. The therapist uses this genogram to assess patterns of relationships, patterns of behavior, significant nodal events (life events), level of differentiation, level of anxiety, and triangles.

The goal of therapy is to increase the level of differentiation in the family. Therapy starts by helping family members learn about the family system — to see patterns of relationships and triangles over generations. It also helps individuals take responsibility for changing their position in generational patterns of relating. Family members are encouraged to develop one-to-one relationships with different family members in order to get to know the family system, to know the triangles, and to "detriangulate self." For example, a husband and wife may be encouraged to talk directly to one another about their marital problems rather than using their typical triangle (e.g., the wife complains about the husband to her mother and the husband uses work to escape from the marital tension.) Family members are also assisted to take an "I position"; that is, each member is encouraged to speak for himself or herself rather than speaking for the entire family with statements such as "We feel" or "We think." In addition, therapy helps members to think instead of reacting in an impulsive, reflexive way.

Structural Family Theory

A second family systems theory is Structural Family Theory, developed by Minuchin (1974) and his colleagues (Minuchin & Fishman, 1981; Minuchin, Rosman, & Baker, 1978). This theory emphasizes the relationship between the presenting problem and the structure of the family. Nurses and other health professionals have applied this theory to families facing problems as diverse as diabetes, asthma, eating disorders, juvenile delinquency, family violence, drug abuse, and divorce.

The family structure consists of the "invisible set of functional demands that organize the ways in which family members interact" (Minuchin, 1974, p. 51). Structure encompasses three major areas: (1) power, (2) subsystems, and (3) boundaries. The family's structure may be dysfunctional in any of these areas.

Power refers to the influence that each family member has on family processes. The theory views a hierarchy of power as necessary for effective family functioning. *Subsystems* are sets of family relationships, each with specific functions. For example, in the spousal subsystem, one function of spouses is to support each other in a relationship that fosters individual growth. The parental subsystem performs the tasks of nurturing and socializing children. In the sibling subsystem, siblings learn about peer relationships, power, and alliances. The last area, *boundaries*, includes the rules that differentiate the tasks of different subsystems. For families to function effectively, there must be clear boundaries between subsystems with some connectedness between them. Families with boundary problems may be disengaged or enmeshed. In disengaged families with rigid boundaries, there is little communication and support among family members; only a high level of stress will evoke support from other members. In enmeshed families with diffuse boundaries, the intense togetherness hinders individuation of members; in these families, stress of one member elicits strong reactions from other members.

The goal of structural family therapy is to solve problems by altering the underlying structure of the family. The initial assessment includes these overlapping phases: (1) joining with the family to temporarily become part of the family system; (2) obtaining a description of the problem; (3) exploring the family structure by observing transactions around the problem; and (4) assessing boundary flexibility, sensitivity to members' actions, family developmental stage, family life context (sources of support and stress), and the way in which the identified patient's symptoms are related to dysfunctional family structure.

The structural therapist focuses primarily on the individual and family in the present. This approach, however, does not negate history but acknowledges transactional patterns from the past. Nevertheless, its primary focus is on present interactions. As Minuchin (1974) noted, "Structural family therapy is a therapy of action. The tool is to modify the present, not to explore and interpret the past" (p. 14).

The therapist takes an active role in the therapy, and tries to create change by transforming those aspects of the family structure that are related to the problem. Restructuring techniques result in a shift of power, subsystems, and boundaries. These techniques include: (1) actualizing transactional patterns; (2) marking boundaries; (3) assigning tasks; (4) relabelling communication; (5) modifying mood and affect; (6) escalating stress; and (7) supporting, educating, and guiding (Minuchin, 1974).

Contextual Family Theory

Another major family theory is Contextual Family Theory, which was developed by Boszormenyi-Nagy and his colleagues (Boszormenyi-Nagy & Spark, 1973; Boszormenyi-Nagy & Krasner, 1986; Cotroneo, 1982, 1986; Cotroneo & Moriarty, 1992). This is a multigenerational family theory that links concern for individuation with concern for rootedness and for significant others in one's relationship network. The relationship network includes: (1) one's legacy — the facts, events, and circumstances of the family and culture into which one is born; (2) the quality of current relationships with nuclear and extended family, peers, friends, colleagues, and the world; and (3) relational connections to the next generation (Cotroneo, Hibbs, & Moriarty, 1992). The theory has been applied to families with a wide variety of problems such as disturbed parent-child relationships, divorce, family violence, incest, and chronic mental illness.

In Contextual Family Theory, trust and loyalty are key multigenerational dynamics that shape a person's relationships, commitments, and expectations through the interactive process of giving and receiving care. A fundamental assumption of this theory is that living in a family requires a balance of giving and receiving care (Cotroneo, Moriarty, & Smith, 1992).

In relationships based on trust, family members are able to live as separate persons while at the same time they are connected and available to others as resources. The contextual therapist focuses on behaviors that enhance trust and those that diminish it. The therapist assists family members to identify sources of trust and mistrust in their past and present relationships, and to rebalance mistrust with resources that can be used constructively. This process of building trust requires family members to consider the merit of positions taken by other family members even when these positions oppose each other (this is termed multidirected partiality). The contextual therapist guides families in this process (Cotroneo, Moriarty, & Smith, 1992).

Loyalty, the other key dynamic in this theory, signifies commitments, obligations, and attachments that bind family members to each other over time. Loyalty forms the basis for family members' obligations to care for one another. In addition, whether or not one received the care one deserved and how one received care, shape one's relationships with others outside the family. For example, expectations for care that were not met in the family of origin may be assigned to partners and children, tending to overburden these relationships and often distorting their reality. An assessment of at least three generations is needed to understand how loyalty expresses itself among members of a family (Cotroneo, Moriarty, & Smith, 1992).

The contextual family therapist guides family members in:

1. Examining the balance of give and take, and individuals' sense of fairness or unfairness in past and present relationships

2. Inquiring into the "other side" of family members — for example, exploring one's parents' side

3. Guiding family members to rebalance unfairness and helping adults make a claim on their family of origin for consideration (Cotroneo, Moriarty, & Smith, 1992)

Communication Theory

Communication theorists such as Bateson (Bateson, Jackson, Haley, & Weakland, 1956), Haley (1963, 1976), Jackson (1965a, 1965b), Watzlawick (Watzlawick, Beavin, & Jackson, 1967; Watzlawick, Weakland, & Fisch, 1974) and Weakland (1976) propose that verbal and nonverbal communication among family members influences behaviors within the family. Watzlawick and colleagues (1967) presented four axioms of communication that can serve as guides for assessing communication within families:

1. All behavior, whether nonverbal or verbal, is communication and conveys a message.
2. All communication defines a relationship.
3. Persons communicate' both verbally and nonverbally; the former presents more content whereas the latter informs more about the relationship.
4. All communications are either symmetrical (equality exists and either person is free to take the lead) or complementary (one leads and the other follows).

According to this theory, dysfunctional communications such as disconfirmation, disqualification, and incongruent messages (double-bind) are related to problematic family behaviors. Disconfirmation refers to the invalidation of a family member's perception of himself or herself, or invalidation of his or her experience. Disqualification includes unclear communications such as contraindications, changes of subject, and incomplete sentences. Incongruent messages consist of verbal and nonverbal messages given at the same time, which conflict. Strategic family therapy tries to change dysfunctional communications to clear, direct communications in order to change family behaviors (Haber, Hoskins, Leach, & Sideleau, 1987).

Strategic family therapists, often working with a consultation team of mental health professionals, begin by observing sequences of problematic behaviors and then identifying behaviors that maintain the problems. For example, the therapist asks the family to define a goal for treatment, stated in measurable behavioral terms. The therapist then assigns tasks to families, tries to break dysfunctional communication loops, and uses paradox. Paradoxical instruction "prescribes the symptom" or encourages the family to do more of what it has been doing (i.e., continue the status quo) rather than change. The instruction is based on the assumption that the family will instinctively resist what is suggested by the therapist and, therefore, will do the opposite and begin to change (Haber, Hoskins, Leach, & Sideleau, 1987; Hare-Mustin, 1976; Stanton, 1981).

Multiple Systems View

A multiple systems view incorporates the consideration of many levels in work with families—familial, biological, psychological, cultural, environmental, and spiritual—and explores the interactions of these different levels. Treatment modalities may be offered at these different levels of systems. Use of a specific treatment modality does not necessarily imply an intervention directed toward the etiology of the problem. Rather, treatment modalities may address issues and concerns that are present in individuals and families regardless of the possible etiologies of the problem.

The choice of which systems to work with and the relative importance of each system depends on the problem. Current research indicates that severe mental illnesses, such as schizophrenia and affective disorders, have a biological basis that interacts with other factors to influence the course of the illness (Molz, 1993; Walsh & Anderson, 1987). This suggests the use of pharmacological interventions complemented by psychosocial and environmental supports for patients with these illnesses. There are other individual and family problems, however, where the biological component is less obvious or may not be present — for example, in adjustment disorders, intrafamilial abuse, incest, juvenile delinquency, problems after divorce, problems after bereavement, parent-child relationship problems, and marital problems. In these cases, working with the family and possibly other psychosocial and biological systems is warranted.

Nursing Conceptual Models

In addition to the five theories previously discussed, some family mental health nurses have used nursing conceptual models to guide their assessment, conceptualization, and goal setting with families (Berkey & Hanson, 1991; Clements & Roberts, 1983; Fawcett & Whall, 1991; Herrick & Goodykoontz, 1989). Neuman, King, Orem, Roy, Rogers, Black, and Roberts (Clements & Roberts, 1983) have all discussed how their models address the family and can be applied to nursing practice with families. Some family nurse theorists have noted that there is a lack of congruence between the conceptualizations of family in the nursing models and in the family systems theories. In response to this problem, Whall (1991) reformulated some family systems theories to make them more congruent with the nursing conceptual models.

Herrick and Goodkoontz's report (1989) exemplifies how a nursing model is helpful for family nursing in mental health settings. They described how Neuman's Systems Model guided their assessment of individual, family, and environmental stressors in a family referred to an outpatient clinic for assistance with an emotionally disturbed teenager. The assessment identified multiple stressors present in different family members, in family dynamics, and in the family's environment. Based on this assessment, family therapy was chosen as the appropriate intervention.

HEALTH PROMOTION

"Prevention seeks to lower or eliminate the rate of onset of mental disability by promoting positive coping abilities and by counteracting harmful conditions which may produce disability" (ANA, 1976, p. 14). In family mental health nursing, health promotion falls in the domain of prevention. To help prevent mental illness, psychiatric nurses consult with health agencies and schools, provide mental health education, develop and evaluate community programs, and offer family therapy. The family may be considered the unit of care, or the family may be seen as influencing lifestyle choices that may prevent illness for individual members of the family (Danielson, Hamel-Bissell, & Winstead-Fry, 1993).

Many stressors in life leave families at high risk for problems, within individuals and within the family as a whole. One such stressor is poverty, which has been identified as a major risk factor for mental disorders in children and adolescents (Institute of Medicine, 1989).

Olds, Henderson, Chamberlin, and Tatelbaum (1986) describe a prevention program designed to reduce the risk factors associated with poverty in unmarried pregnant teenagers. Olds and his colleagues randomly assigned 400 first-time parents to one of four treatment groups. The first three groups received no intervention or only limited support during the prenatal and early postnatal periods. The fourth group received nursing visits throughout the pregnancy and up until the child's second birthday. The nurses' visits were designed to enhance family coping by supplementing the family's resources to deal with the stresses of poverty and a new baby. The nurses promoted linkages with formal service agencies, enhanced social support for mothers, taught them about parenting and health, and emphasized the need for personal planning. Finally, the nurses assisted the mothers to clarify their values related to social and family issues. Families in the treatment group had better mental and physical health outcomes than the families in any of the control groups.

In this study, health promotion was directed at the family as a unit and some of the benefits were identified in the children. These children experienced fewer health risk factors as a result of the lifestyle choices made by the family; that is, children in the treatment group were abused and neglected less and they had better development and fewer emergency room visits than children in the other groups.

A second stressor that may place families at risk is divorce and the custody disputes that sometimes arise. Child custody disputes signal parental conflicts that have negative implications for all parties, especially children (Hetherington, 1981; Wallerstein & Kelley, 1980). In situations of intense parental conflict, children are at high risk for emotional and behavioral disturbances such as depression, low self-esteem, school problems, and antisocial behavior (Emery, 1982; Hetherington, Cox, & Cox, 1978; Hetherington, 1981). The contextual approach to custody decisions, which is derived from contextual family systems theory, can be used to minimize or prevent mental health problems in families by helping families negotiate a custody/visitation agreement (Cotroneo, Hibbs, & Moriarty, 1992; Cotroneo, Moriarty, & Smith, 1992). This approach is based on the view that the best interests of children cannot be separated from the welfare of their parents. Examining the interests of children in an intergenerational context reflects the full reality of their relationship network and family loyalties.

In this approach, family meetings are held that include both parents and all siblings; they may also include grandparents, aunts, uncles, and other significant persons. Each family member is asked to identify his or her own needs and commitments regarding parenting. The therapist helps the family examine the full relational context of the parents as well as the children, and particularly the kind of parenting that the parents themselves received. The therapist also helps family members explore family loyalty issues and unfinished family business that may undermine trust. Cotroneo and colleagues speculate that parents who struggled with loyalty conflicts in their families of origin may use marriage and parenting of their children to re-enact that struggle. Thus parents' perception of what is at stake in a custody dispute may be distorted, their capacity for giving and sharing may be impaired (Cotroneo, Hibbs, & Moriarty, 1992).

Topical guidelines for structuring these meetings are outlined in Table 13–1. These meetings redirect the focus from blame to trust building, so that parents can see themselves less as adversaries and more as collaborators in the care of their children. Parents learn to differentiate between issues that belong to the marriage and issues of parenting, and they also address issues from their families of origin. In this context of trust, parents are encouraged to negotiate an arrangement that they can live with and that protects the child's access to both parents (Cotroneo, Hibbs, & Moriarty, 1992).

Cotroneo et al. (1992) have illustrated the use of the approach with a small sample of families and through a case study. The findings suggest that the approach can help families create alternatives to continued disputation. The authors suggest using the approach as soon as a parent files for custody or visitation in order to minimize damage to the child.

Families who are not experiencing severe stressors such as poverty or divorce may choose to work on issues such as stress reduction and strengthening relationships among family members. There is no such thing as a perfect family. All families have issues and con-

TABLE 13–1

TOPICAL GUIDELINES FOR FAMILY MEETINGS AROUND CHILD CUSTODY DISPUTES

1. Current family situation
   a. Response of family members to separation/divorce
   b. Effects on family members
      1. What has been done to help the children deal with the situation?
      2. Contact made with significant legal, religious, psychological, social, and health care resources
2. Family genogram information
   a. Ways in which parents define and validate themselves in relation to significant others, particularly their own families of origin
      1. Patterns of expectations and commitments across three generations
      2. Gender-related issues
      3. Intergenerational history of losses, relational injuries, and injustices
3. An exploration of parenting of children (past, present, and future) and the developmental burdens and demands that are placed on children
   a. Acknowledgment of children for their contributions to the family that may have been taken for granted
   b. Exploration of the worries that children may be experiencing and how they get help when it is needed
   c. Acknowledgment of the parents for the losses, relational injuries, and injustices experienced in their families of origin
   d. Exploration of ways in which family members can work to correct injustices and exploitation in past and present relationships, and repair injuries that have already been sustained
   e. Consideration of the consequences of any imbalances in giving and receiving care and fairness that exist in the family
4. Family task (conjoint session)
   a. Describe the family situation as you see it. What are the conflicts for you?
   b. In thinking about what to do, what are you considering and why?
   c. If you could have things you way (according to your preferences), what would you do now?
   d. If you were to put your plan into action, what would happen? Do you think your plan would be successful? Why? Why not?
   e. What would be the consequences of your plan for you, your spouse/partner, and each individual child?

SOURCE: From "Uses and Implications of the Contextual Approach to Child Custody Decisions," by M. Cotroneo, B. J. Hibbs, and H. Moriarty, 1992, *Journal of Child and Adolescent Psychiatric and Mental Health Nursing, 5* (3), p.17. Copyright 1992 by Nursecom, Inc. Reprinted with permission.

cerns even if they are not experiencing severe distress. A basic goal for mental health promotion is to assist healthy, functioning families to maintain and enhance the health of both the family and family members. Health promotion for these families may take place in community educational programs or through counseling. A nurse working with the family can use a variety of approaches to enhance the family's communication and relationships.

FAMILY MENTAL HEALTH NURSING IN ACUTE ILLNESS

Some clients and families experience acute symptoms, such as suicidal ideation in a major depression. It is estimated that 300,000 people attempt suicide each year (Kneisl & Riley, 1992). Clients and families may also present with an acute exacerbation of a chronic illness; for example, a client with chronic schizophrenia may experience a resurgence of psychotic symptoms. In most epidemiological studies, schizophrenia has been found in one quarter to one half of all patients presenting with psychosis (Helzer & Guze, 1986). Acute symptoms require early diagnosis and treatment, and prompt referral for additional consultation as necessary.

When the nurse is caring for the family as client, acute distress is often associated with a familial crisis (Minuchin & Fishman, 1981). For example, 15-year-old Angela attempted suicide by swallowing "a handfull" of her grandmother's medication for hypertension. During the assessment, the advanced practice nurse learned that Angela thought she was pregnant. She was afraid to tell her parents because she thought it would hurt and disappoint them. Acute distress may also be associated with a severe stressor that triggers psychiatric symptoms such as a panic attack (American Psychiatric Association [APA], 1994). When the nurse cares for the client within the context of the family, the relationship between the individual's symptoms and the family response to the symptoms is considered. In either case, the meaning the family attaches to the symptom can influence the family's decision to seek care (Danielson et al., 1993).

Acute psychiatric and mental health disturbances often compel families to seek immediate care. They may seek care from the general family practitioner or go directly to an emergency room or community mental health center. In many cases the initial screening is done by a nurse who has not been prepared as a psychiatric and mental health nurse. The nurse assesses the presenting problem and then makes appropriate referrals. In the case of Angela, the nurse would first determine if Angela had ingested a potentially lethal dose of medication, which would require immediate medical intervention. If Angela needed to be stabilized in an intensive care unit, she and her family might be seen by the psychiatric consultation liaison nurse. The role of this nurse in a medical treatment setting is to help the client and the family begin to understand the implications of the crisis that has occurred and the options for family treatment.

Once Angela's physiological safety had been established, she might be referred to a psychiatric–mental health advanced practice nurse for a comprehensive assessment. Using a multiple systems perspective, the nurse would assess: (1) Angela's physiological condition; (2) her mental status, including any persistent suicidal ideation; (3) the availability of family resources and support to keep the client safe; (4) the meaning the crisis had for the family; and (5) the need for psychiatric hospitalization.

In acute situations the nurse collaborates with the family and other mental health professionals in planning for the client's care. Initial treatment may focus on assisting the client and family to open lines of communication. After resolution of the crisis, the family may be referred for family therapy to help them develop more effective coping strategies.

Care of the client experiencing acute distress often involves admission to an inpatient psychiatric unit. Traditionally, hospitalization reinforces an individualistic view of care, in which one member is seen in the sick role and the other members of the family are seen as peripheral to the illness. Merely adding family therapy to the treatment program does not make the inpatient experience a family experience. Family-focused care can be more fully integrated into inpatient treatment programs through use of the following five strategies identified by Bowers and McNally (1983):

1. Plan intake conferences at the time of admission. An intake conference with the family makes it possible to assess the family as a unit and the needs of each of its members. It also serves to inform the family that care will be family centered and indicates how they may be involved in treatment.

2. Structure intensive family therapy into the treatment program. Family therapy may help the family view the presenting problem as a family problem rather than as solely the problem of the hospitalized client.

3. Make family conferences a regularly scheduled activity. In inpatient settings, inter-

disciplinary treatment teams typically meet frequently to evaluate the client's progress toward the goals of treatment, but families are not usually included in these meetings. Family conferences involve the family in setting treatment goals and evaluating progress for the individual and family.

4. Plan therapeutic leaves of absence for the individual so that family members may work together outside the hospital setting on family treatment goals.

5. Use psychiatric–mental health advanced practice nurses to supervise family treatment. These specialists, who have education and experience in working with families, can both conduct family sessions and supervise others involved in family meetings and conferences.

A family-centered approach alters the traditional concept of milieu therapy (Bowers & McNally, 1983). Traditionally, the family was seen as "intruders" or visitors to the inpatient milieu and not as a part of the treatment process. Integrating the family into the milieu may involve restructuring traditional components of the milieu; for example, families need to be included in community meetings, medication groups, and discharge groups. New components may also need to be added to milieu treatment — for example, family intake conferences, multifamily therapeutic groups, and joint meetings of client, family, and staff.

CASE STUDY: Family Treatment on an Inpatient Unit

The following case example depicts family-focused inpatient treatment. The therapeutic goals and treatment strategies reflect a multiple systems view in addressing many levels of systems. Interventions at the family level are derived from Bowen's (1978) multigenerational Family Systems Theory.

Jeremy G., an 18-year-old high school senior, was experiencing severe mood swings along with escalating angry, defiant behavior, school failure, and suicidal ideation. At times, Jeremy felt "on top of the world." During these periods, he felt he could accomplish almost anything. At other times, Jeremy reported "sub-zero" self-esteem. An intensive outpatient evaluation indicated that Jeremy was a gifted student and an artistic young man. His longstanding pattern of mood swings supported a diagnosis of a bipolar mood disorder called cyclothymia (APA, 1994).

The family evaluation revealed that his parents had a long history of marital problems. The parents maintained emotional distance from one another, and Jeremy was distant from his father. Jeremy felt that he had tried, for many years, to get along with his father but that his father was "cold and impossible to please." Mr. G. reported having a very distant relationship with his own father. Jeremy and his mother had an unusually close or fused relationship. Jeremy's two sisters, aged 13 and 15 years, were relatively free of the triangular emotional system that occurred between Jeremy and his parents.

Jeremy and his family agreed to a 3-week hospitalization for Jeremy. He was referred for a neurological evaluation and magnetic resonance imaging (MRI) to rule out any biological causes for his mood swings, and he began a trial of tricyclic antidepressant medication for management of cyclothymia. The family agreed to participate in family therapy sessions. The therapeutic goal was to decrease emotional reactivity among family members and increase the family's level of differentiation.

In therapy, family members were encouraged to take an "I position" and to become more thoughtful in their responses to one another, rather than emotionally reactive. In addition, Jeremy was encouraged to participate in age-appropriate peer relation-ships. This helped Jeremy remove himself from the three-person triangular emotional system and begin to improve his self-esteem. Treatment staff helped Jeremy identify his strengths and encouraged him to pursue his dream of going to art school. In addition to attending family sessions and treatment conferences, Jeremy's parents attended a medication group to learn about the medication prescribed for Jeremy. They also attended a parents' group that focused on learning from and sharing with other parents about childrearing issues. In separate sessions, the parents began to focus on their own marital issues. The Gs had managed their problems by submerging them and projecting their marital anxiety onto Jeremy. When the couple began to address their problems in therapy, less anxiety was projected onto Jeremy.

Mr. G.'s parents also attended several family therapy sessions. Mr. G. was encouraged to be less reactive with his own father and to work on developing a one-to-one relationship with him. As he did so, Mr. G. became more open to developing a relationship with his son. As Jeremy began to assume an "I position" in his family, he was able to express his desire for a rewarding relationship with his father. This goal was incorporated into the plans for therapeutic leaves of absence. Jeremy and his father went on several outings together to work on their relationship. Following the 3-week hospitalization, Jeremy was discharged and the family began monthly family therapy sessions to build on the successes in the hospital.

Special Family Considerations: When Hospitalization Involves a Child

When a child with acute psychiatric symptoms requires hospitalization, the staff need to keep in mind how radical and strange hospitalization may seem to the family, who is used to having responsibility for the child. Many hospitals have rules that shut out families from the process of goal setting and treatment for the child (Goren, 1992). Goren (1992) stresses the need for inpatient staff to work in partnership with families because family participation is essential for effective problem solving. She presents the following guidelines for engaging families in inpatient treatment of a child:

1. Recognize the family's competencies. Given that "all families have competencies" (p. 45), staff should point out parents' strengths and emphasize the importance of using these strengths in the child's treatment.

2. Replace therapeutic relationships with therapeutic systems. That is, rather than relying heavily on the traditional one-to-one therapeutic relationship, rely on the therapeutic *system* of child, family, and staff.

3. Involve the child, family, and staff as partners in treatment planning conferences and in developing the treatment contract.

4. Work *through* the family rather than in its place. Given that the family is the natural caregiver for the child, staff should assist the family to intervene with the child.

5. Consider family-support alternatives to out-of-family placement. Rather than removing the child from the family, try to build up the family's strengths and bring in supports from the extended family and community.

6. Decrease the barriers between the hospital and the community and minimize the hospital's interference with parenting. Encourage parents to take part in activities such as meals, classes, and bedtime preparation.

When these guidelines are followed, treatment becomes a process between the staff system and the family system, with the involvement of community services as well. As Goren says, "The child belongs, in the sense of what is ordinary and usual, to the family and community. The responsibility of the staff is to intervene in ways that support the child's 'belongingness' and that increase the likelihood of rapid return to normal life" (1992, p. 46).

Outpatient Care of the Client and Family Experiencing Acute Mental Illness

For some acute problems, outpatient treatment may be appropriate if there is no danger to family members or others. The following case study illustrates outpatient family treatment when a mother reported feeling overwhelmed by raising her children and questioned her ability to raise them. Treatment was based on Structural Family Theory.

Case Study: Family Treatment in an Outpatient Setting

Caroline M., the mother, was a 30-year-old, single African-American who was referred to the community mental health center by a female friend. Caroline lived in a three-bedroom row home with her five children: Paul, aged 12 years; Tametrice, aged 10 years; Sam, aged 8 years; Nina, aged 6 years; and Vera, aged 4 years. Caroline had held various jobs over the last 10 years as kitchen help, a typist, and a factory worker. She had been unemployed for several months, since she quit her job because of her boss's verbal abusiveness. Presently, the family was subsisting on welfare. Caroline came to the clinic because she was very "edgy and nervous." She reported difficulty in expressing her anger toward family and friends and felt physically explosive. She was raising five children with little outside support and felt overwhelmed by this. She cared deeply about her children but questioned her ability to raise them. She had had two previous contacts at the clinic for the same reasons but reported withdrawing from therapy because she "did not like" the therapists. During the present contact, she began work with two nurse cotherapists. Nine sessions were conducted: six sessions with the entire family, two sessions with Caroline, and one session with the children.

During the sessions, the therapists joined with the family to attempt to better understand the family system and assess the family structure. The mother and Paul made up the parental subsystem. As the oldest son, Paul was a "parentified child," who was assuming many parental functions in the family; when Caroline felt overwhelmed by her parental functions, she delegated these to Paul. He attempted to meet his mother's expectations of him in order to receive her love and approval, but she did not acknowledge his contributions. Figure 13–1 depicts some aspects of the family's structure and the therapeutic goals for transforming these aspects. Table 13–2 outlines therapeutic goals for strengthening the parental subsystem, strengthening the sibling subsystem, and supporting the mother's personal needs.

FAMILY MENTAL HEALTH NURSING IN CHRONIC ILLNESS

Chronic mental illness is characterized by diagnosis, duration, and disability (Bachrach, 1991). Health care providers are now also using the term "severe and persistent illness" to denote

Present Map

M and PC (executive subsystem)
....
Children (sibling subsystem)

Therapeutic Goal

M

PC: Other siblings

KEY

M = Mother
PC = Parentified child
... = Diffuse boundary
--- = Clear boundary

FIGURE 13–1
The map under Therapeutic Goal represents a clear boundary between mother and children, with Paul, the parentified child, returning to the sibling subsystem, but maintaining a position of leadship among his siblings.

chronic mental illness. For example, schizophrenia, chemical dependence, and eating disorders are considered chronic illnesses. A mental illness that persists for 2 years or more is considered chronic. A lingering disability such as one that precludes the ability to return to work full-time also characterizes a disorder as chronic. Prevalence rates for chronic mental illness in the United States range from 1.7 million to 2.4 million. Further, it has been estimated that about one third of the homeless population is chronically mentally ill (Price-Hoskins, 1992).

TABLE 13–2

THERAPEUTIC GOALS FOR THE M. FAMILY BASED ON STRUCTURAL FAMILY THEORY

1. Strengthening the parental subsystem:
   a. Acknowledge Caroline's stressors as a single parent.
   b. Teach Caroline about age-appropriate expectations for the children.
   c. Teach her new ways to enforce limits (e.g., through rewards or through withholding privileges).
   d. Assign tasks both inside and outside the therapy session that reinforce the parental subsystem (e.g., designation of assigned days for dishwashing).
   e. Help Caroline to identify her double-bind messages and her inconsistent expectations for the children.
   f. Facilitate mobilization of supports (e.g., family, friends, church, community groups).

2. Strengthening the sibling subsystem:
   a. Emphasize individual differences to mark boundaries between the children, and between mother and children.
   b. Role play or assign tasks to teach siblings ways to resolve conflicts without calling for mother.
   c. Decrease the children's competition for mother's attention by encouraging mother to designate one "special time" for each child to spend with her alone.
   d. Modify Paul's position as parentified child:
      i. Support Paul in his efforts to increase his autonomy outside the family.
      ii. Acknowledge Paul's contributions to the family.
   e. Encourage activities involving only the sibling subsystem by assigning tasks requiring cooperation among siblings (e.g., Paul could teach his siblings about black history or all siblings could make a present for their mother).

3. Supporting Caroline's personal needs:
   a. Explore Caroline's needs for intimacy and social contact (e.g., through her relationships and social activities). Have some individual sessions with Caroline to discuss sexual issues or other issues she wishes to address without the children present.
   b. Explore the impact of Caroline's present conflict with her partner on her ability to cope with her children.
   c. Discuss possible job opportunities and completion of her general equivalency diploma.

Given the prevalence of chronic mental illness, nurses and other health care professionals in many settings are likely to encounter mental illness and its related problems. For example, medical management of a client with diabetes may be complicated by chronic schizophrenia. A woman's pregnancy may be complicated by a 10-year history of bulimia. Treatment of a client's alcohol abuse may need to include consideration for the client's depression.

Because of the encompassing nature of the label chronic mental illness, it is difficult to generalize about treatment needs for this population. One client may lack family support and require supportive services for housing, management of medications, and a daily routine. Another client may receive family and community support, but the family may require assistance in managing the burdens associated with caring for a chronically ill family member.

Cultural Perspectives on Chronicity

The family's cultural beliefs influence their perceptions and management of the client's chronic mental illness. Indeed, cultural psychiatrists (Lefley, 1990) have suggested that the concept of chronicity in mental illness is an artifact of cultural belief systems and expectations regarding the nature of illness. In Westernized cultures, such as the mainstream culture in the United States, chronicity may be a byproduct of the treatment community's belief that serious mental illness is inherently chronic. Also the bureaucratized treatment system tends to reinforce dependence and the "sick role" behavior associated with chronicity. Further, it has been suggested that the incidence of mental illness is higher in cultures that produce high stress and offer low social support. The incidence of chronicity may also be higher in cultures that provide few opportunities for work for chronic patients and few supports to caregivers of the chronically mentally ill.

In some non-Western cultures, mental illness is perceived as external to the patient, and is thought to be caused by supernatural forces or possession (Skultans, 1991). In such cultures patients and families may experience less blame and stigmatization for the illness. Also, the family and community are likely to be more supportive, and family support is perceived as an integral component of treatment.

It is also interesting that in non-Western cultures, where mental illness is believed to be brief and temporary, the incidence of chronicity is lower (Lin & Kleinman, 1988). The differing rates of chronic mental illnesses in Western and non-Western cultures tend to support the view of cultural psychiatrists that chronicity in mental illness is a cultural artifact.

Chronic mental illnesses that demonstrate great cultural variations include the eating disorders — anorexia and bulimia. Both disorders are found almost exclusively among women in Westernized cultures. In the United States, these eating disorders usually appear among girls and women from higher socioeconomic status groups (Minuchin et al., 1978). Family systems theories suggest that certain types of family organization are closely related to the development and maintenance of symptoms of eating disorders. The following case example demonstrates a family mental health nursing approach to assessing eating disorders on an inpatient unit.

Case Study: Family Assessment of Eating Disorders on an Inpatient Unit

Carmella was a 19-year-old woman admitted to an inpatient psychiatric unit for bulimia. She was a freshman at an Ivy League University and had always been a hard-working student who strove for excellence in her academic work. Her physical appearance was striking; many patients on the unit referred to her as the "beautiful" patient who "could be a model." The other patients could not understand why Carmella was in the hospital because she looked so "perfect."

On the unit, Carmella tried to be a peacekeeper; she avoided any expression of dissatisfaction or conflict with others and tried to please everyone — patients and staff. Carmella came from a very close and religious Italian family in which three generations lived together. On the third night of her hospitalization, Carmella's mother visited her. Carmella's primary nurse wanted to assess Carmella's responses after the visit, based on her awareness that family factors are often related to eating disorders. Five minutes after the visit, Carmella entered the kitchen, removed 2 gallons of ice cream from the refrigerator, and began binge eating. The nurse followed Carmella into the kitchen and asked her what she was feeling as she began binge eating. Carmella said she had felt "ready to explode" with anger at her mother during the visit but could not express it. This represented a breakthrough in Carmella's treatment because it was the *first time* Carmella made a connection between her feelings and her binge eating behaviors. The primary nurse, psychiatrist, and patient continued to explore this connection in treatment. A major goal was to help Carmella to develop new ways to express her anger, conflict, and disappointment in others. Family therapy, group therapy, and milieu therapy were used to address this goal.

Family Support: Psychoeducational Models

Family involvement in the care of clients with chronic mental illness results in better outcomes for the client. For example, family support of the patient has been shown to improve medication compliance in schizophrenic clients with severe and persistent mental illness (Mulaik, 1992). And enhanced family interaction has been related to a better quality of life in families with a schizophrenic member (Sullivan, Wells, & Leake, 1992). However, the burden of caring for a mentally ill family member is often overwhelming. Without adequate support, caregivers may become exhausted and relinquish their responsibilities. One of the most promising interventions to emerge in recent years is psychoeducation (Walsh, 1987). Psychoeducational programs target the family as a unit; the benefits may be experienced by both the chronically mentally ill member and the family caregivers.

The content of psychoeducational interventions varies with the treatment philosophy as well as the needs of the specific client and family. For example, one psychoeducational model called Behavioral Family Management (Falloon, Boyd, & McGill, 1984) involves training families in family communication and problem solving. Another approach called Supportive Family Management (Zastowny, Lehman, Cole, & Kane, 1992) provides clients and families with detailed information about the illness, treatment plan, and services. Supportive Family Management may also include information on the availability of community services, and advice on daily living and management of client symptoms and family issues. A study comparing these two psychoeducational interventions found similar clinical improvements with both approaches. Both interventions prevented frequent relapses and rehospitalization, decreased psychiatric symptoms, allowed a reduction in drug dosage, and improved the quality of life for patients and their families. The following case example illustrates the use of the Supportive Family Management approach for a client with chronic schizophrenia.

Case Study: Use of the Supportive Family Management Model

Walter J., aged 38 years, was first diagnosed with schizophrenia when he was 19 years old. He had not been able to work gainfully since his initial diagnosis and he remained at home with his mother Agnes J., aged 68 years, and her sister Grace W., aged 63 years. Walter's father died when Walter was 7 years old. Thus, Walter's mother had been his only caregiver for most of his life. Walter had had more than 20 hospitalizations over the course of his illness. Hospitalization was usually precipitated by Walter's refusal to take his medications regularly. During his brief hospitalizations, Walter was stabilized on his medication and then discharged back to the care of his mother. The only follow-up care that Walter received was monthly meetings with his psychiatrist for medication management. Walter rarely kept those appointments because, in his delusional thinking, he was convinced that his medications had caused him to have cancer. Walter's mother was afraid to push him too hard to take the medications because she feared it would cause his symptoms to worsen and Walter would become violent, as he had several times in the past.

During his most recent hospitalization, Walter was referred to the psychoeducational treatment planning team to begin Supportive Family Management. Once Walter was stabilized on his medication, Supportive Family Management focused on the following:

1. Education for the family about Walter's medications
2. Instruction on the signs and symptoms of acute exacerbations of schizophrenia
3. Instruction on behavior modification strategies to reinforce Walter's successful attendance in outpatient treatment and to reinforce compliance with medications
4. Information about the availability of public services to transport Walter to and from his outpatient appointments
5. Information for Mrs. J. about the local chapter of NAMI, a family support group designed to help families understand and cope with the serious mental illness of a member
6. Hot line phone numbers and local resources to help Mrs. J. if Walter became violent

A mental health nurse specialist visited the family's home weekly to determine how the family was managing, to offer advice and information as needed, and to provide Mrs. J. with support. Weekly visits continued for the first 3 months following discharge from the hospital. Eventually the visits were tapered to an as-needed basis. Walter was able to stay out of the hospital for 16 months following the implementation of Supportive Family Management. This was a dramatic change for the J. family, given Walter's history of frequent admissions to the hospital.

Although psychoeducational programs do not offer a cure for serious and persistent mental illness, they do assist clients to remain relatively free of the debilitating symptoms associated with the illness and they also provide support for family caregivers to allow them to continue in that role. Minimally, family intervention programs for the chronically mentally ill should include: (1) reduction of the stressful impact of the illness on the family; (2) information about the illness, patient abilities, and prognosis; (3) methods of stress reduction and problem solving; and (4) linkages to supplementary services to support the efforts of family members to maintain their patient in the community (Walsh & Anderson, 1987).

IMPLICATIONS FOR PRACTICE, EDUCATION, RESEARCH, AND HEALTH POLICY

It is exciting that the body of knowledge about family mental health nursing is expanding. As shown in the case examples in this chapter, nurses may apply this knowledge in many different settings — in inpatient psychiatric and nonpsychiatric settings, in outpatient psychiatric and nonpsychiatric settings, in other community settings, and in the home. The expanding knowledge also has clear and compelling implications for theory development, research, education, and health policy.

Conceptualizations of families are changing. Some family systems theories appear to emphasize the relationship between family interactions and illness in a unidirectional flow from family to illness (family $\longrightarrow$ illness). However, clinicians and researchers are now recognizing the reciprocal influences between the family and illness within a sociocultural context: illness in a family member influences the family and the family may influence the course of an illness. The challenge for mental health professionals is to integrate this view into research and care of individuals and families. Traditional theories may need to be expanded or modified to consider these reciprocal influences. It is not helpful to point a finger and blame individuals or families for illness. It is more helpful to engage the individual and family in a partnership for the benefit of both. It is also useful to draw on the patient's and family's resources in a collaborative process of goal setting and treatment. Those theories that are more resource-based need further development and testing. No matter what the debate about the etiologies of problems, it is clear that both individuals and families suffer with them, and both deserve our empathy and care.

In the current context for health care reform, increased emphasis must be placed on theory and research in the promotion of mental health in families, prevention of mental illness in families, and treatment of acute and chronic mental illness within families. Research on families is necessary to provide empirical support for funding family-based services. Most health care services in the United States are not organized around the family but around a health problem in the individual. Furthermore, reimbursement for health care is based on the individual; most third-party payers do not see the family as a client and do not accept family-level diagnoses. They provide coverage only for individual diagnoses included in the Diagnostic and Statistical Manual of Mental Disorders (4th ed.) (DSM–IV; APA, 1994), the diagnostic classification system for psychiatric illnesses.

Nursing education needs to incorporate a stronger family mental health focus in the curriculum, not only in mental health nursing, but also *in every clinical area* because nurses in every area encounter families confronting mental health issues. Undergraduate students need to learn how to assess the mental health of individuals and the family and how to intervene therapeutically with families in hospital, home, and clinic. Graduate students in psychiatric and mental health nursing need an in-depth understanding of family theories and clinical experience with family therapy in varied settings. As advanced practice nurses, they will be called on to perform comprehensive assessments and to intervene with families within shorter periods than in the past.

Education of the public is also critical; people need to become more aware of the role the family plays in its own health and in the health of its members. This is particularly important with the greater emphasis on preventative care.

As stated in *Nursing: Social Policy Statement*, "the family is the necessary unit of service" (ANA, 1980, p. 5). The challenge now is for mental health nurses to embrace this idea and make it a reality in their thinking, practice, and research.

STUDY QUESTIONS

1. Which of the following *recent* trends have influenced both the client's treatment needs and the system of care delivery in family mental health nursing?
   a. Freudian psychoanalytic movement, deinstitutionalization
   b. Downward turn in the economic market, consumer advocacy
   c. Health care reform, shortened length of hospital stay, more manageable medication protocols
   d. Freudian psychoanalytic movement, the medical model

2. A family mental health nurse who is using Structural Family Theory to guide his or her practice would assess which of the following areas in families?
   a. Differentiation of self, anxiety, and triangulation
   b. Power, subsystems, and boundaries
   c. Multigenerational trust, multigenerational loyalty, and other multigenerational family processes
   d. Disconfirmation, disqualification, and double-bind messages

3. A family mental health nurse who is using Bowen's Family Theory to guide his or her practice would assess which of the following areas in families?
   a. Differentiation of self, anxiety, and triangulation
   b. Power, subsystems, and boundaries
   c. Multigenerational trust, multigenerational loyalty, and other multigenerational family processes
   d. Disconfirmation, disqualification, and double-bind messages

4. A family mental health nurse who is using Contextual Family Theory to guide his or her practice would assess which of the following areas in families?
   a. Differentiation of self, anxiety, and triangulation
   b. Power, subsystems, and boundaries
   c. Multigenerational trust, multigenerational loyalty, and other multigenerational family processes
   d. Disconfirmation, disqualification, and double-bind messages

5. A family mental health nurse who is using Communication Theory to guide his or her practice would assess which of the following areas in families?
   a. Differentiation of self, anxiety, and triangulation
   b. Power, subsystems, and boundaries
   c. Multigenerational trust, multigenerational loyalty, and other multigenerational family processes
   d. Disconfirmation, disqualification, and double-bind messages

6. A family mental health nurse who is using a Multiple Systems View to guide his or her practice would assess which of the following areas in families?
   a. Family interactional patterns
   b. Biological factors
   c. Psychological factors
   d. Cultural, environmental, and spiritual factors
   e. All of the above

7. Nancy is an advanced practice nurse practicing family nursing in a community mental health center. She is developing a health promotion program for the community. Health promotion seeks to:
   a. Increase positive coping abilities and counteract harmful conditions that may produce disability
   b. Provide early diagnosis and treatment and prompt referral as necessary
   c. Assist the client and the family to resume the highest level of productivity in all aspects of daily living
   d. Assist the client and the family to cope with residual disability that warrants continued assistance

8. Following a potentially lethal suicide attempt by drinking rat poisoning, 33-year-old Maria was admitted to the intensive care unit for stabilization of her physical condition. The nurses sought a consultation from the mental health consultation liaison nurse. The role of the consultation liaison nurse in a medical treatment setting is to:
   a. Refer the client for inpatient psychiatric treatment
   b. Help the client and the family begin to understand the crisis that has just occurred and options for family treatment
   c. Provide intensive psychotherapy
   d. Focus on assisting the client and the family to open lines of direct communication

9. John has been suffering from the debilitating effects of schizophrenia for the past 10 years. Following his most recent discharge from the hospital, he was admitted to a psychoeducational program. A psychoeducational program might include all of the following elements *except*:
   a. Information about the availability of specific community services

b. Helping the family to understand how they caused John's illness
c. Detailed information about the illness, treatment plans, and medications
d. Home visits by a medical health nurse specialist

10. Melissa is a 19-year-old who has recently been diagnosed with bipolar disorder. She was admitted to an inpatient treatment setting that emphasizes family-focused treat-

ment. Family-focused treatment is likely to include:

a. Use of therapeutic leave of absences to provide a break from the demands of treatment
b. Custodial care and companionship from the nurses
c. Regular scheduled conferences that include the family in setting treatment goals
d. The use of psychopharmocological interventions only

REFERENCES

American Nurses Association Council on Psychiatric and Mental Health Nursing (1994). *Statement on Psychiatric-Mental Health Clinical Practice and Standards of Psychiatric-Mental Health Clinical Nursing Practice.* Washington, DC: ANA.

American Nurses Association Division on Psychiatric and Mental Health Nursing. (1976). *Statement on Psychiatric and Mental Health Nursing Practice.* Kansas City, MO: ANA.

American Nurses Association. (1980). *Nursing: Social policy statement.* Kansas City, MO: ANA.

American Psychiatric Association. (1994). *Diagnostic and statistical manual of mental disorders* (4th ed.). Washington, DC: APA.

Bachrach, L. (1991). The chronic patient: Community psychiatry's changing role. *Hospital and Community Psychiatry, 42,* 573–574.

Baker, A. F. (1989). Living with a chronic schizophrenic can place great stress on individual family members and the family unit: How families cope. *Journal of Psychosocial Nursing, 27,* 31–36.

Baker, A. F. (1993). Schizophrenia and the family. In C. S. Fawcett (Ed.), *Family psychiatric nursing* (pp. 342–355). St. Louis, MO: Mosby Year Book.

Bateson, G., Jackson, D., Haley, J., & Weakland, J. (1956). Toward a theory of schizophrenia, *Behavioral Science, 1* (19), 251–275.

Berkey, K. M., & Hanson, S. M. (1991). *Pocket guide to family assessment and intervention.* Philadelphia: Mosby Year Book.

Boszormenyi-Nagy, I., & Krasner, B. (1986). *Between give and take: A clinical guide to contextual theory.* New York: Brunner/Mazel.

Boszormenyi-Nagy, I., & Spark, G. (1973). *Invisible loyalties.* New York: Harper & Row.

Bowen, M. (1976). Theory in the practice of psychotherapy. In P. J. Guerin (Ed.), *Family therapy: Theory and practice* (pp. 42–90). New York: Gardner Press.

Bowen, J. (1978). *Family therapy in clinical practice.* New York: Jason Aronson.

Bowers, J., & McNally, K. (1983). Family-focused care in the psychiatric inpatient setting. *Image: The Journal of Nursing Scholarship, 15,* 26–31.

Brooker, C. & Butterworth, C. (1991). Working with families caring for a relative with schizophrenia: The evolving role of the community psychiatric nurse. *International Journal of Nursing Studies, 28,* 189–200.

Brown, F. H. (Ed.). (1991). *Reweaving the family tapestry.* New York: W. W. Norton.

Chafez, L., & Barns, L. (1989). Issues in psychiatric caregiving. *Archives of Psychiatric Nursing, 3*(2), 61–68.

Clements, I. W., & Roberts, F. B. (Eds.). (1983). *Family health: A theoretical approach to nursing care.* New York: Wiley & Sons.

Cotroneo, M. (1982). The role of forgiveness in family therapy. In A. Gurman (Ed.), *Questions and answers in family therapy: Vol. 2.* (pp. 241–244). New York: Brunner/Mazel.

Cotroneo, M. (1986). Families and abuse: A contextual approach. In M. Karpel (Ed.), *Family resources* (pp. 413–437). New York: Guilford Press.

Cotroneo, M., Hibbs, B. J., & Moriarty, H. (1992), Uses and implications of the contextual approach to child custody decisions. *Journal of Child and Adolescent Psychiatric and Mental Health Nursing, 5*(3), 13–26.

Cotroneo, M., & Moriarty, H. (1992). Intergenerational family processes in the treatment of incest. In A. Burgess (Ed.), *Child trauma: Issues and research* (pp. 293–305). New York: Garland.

Cotroneo, M., Moriarty, H., & Smith, E. (1992). Managing family loyalty conflicts in child custody disputes. *Journal of Family psychotherapy, 3*(2), 19–38.

Danielson, C. B., Hamel-Bissell, B., & Winstead-Fry, P. (1993). *Families, health, and illness: Perspectives on coping and intervention.* St. Louis, MO: Mosby Year Book.

Duffy, M. E. (1988). Health promotion in the family: Current findings and directives for nursing research. *Journal of Advanced Nursing, 13*, 109 – 117.

Emery, R. (1982). Interparental conflict and the children of discord and divorce. *Psychological Bulletin, 92*, 310 – 330.

Falloon, I. R. H., Boyd, J. L., & McGill, W. (1984). *Family care of schizophrenia.* New York: Guilford Press.

Fawcett, J., & Whall, A. (1991). *Family theory development in nursing: State of the science and the art.* Philadelphia: F.A. Davis.

Gillis, J. M. (1973). *Family therapy in clinical practice: An abstract.* Unpublished manuscript. University of Pennsylvania School of Nursing, Philadelphia.

Goren, S. (1992). Practicing in partnership with families in the inpatient setting. *Journal of Child and Adolescent Psychiatric and Mental Health Nursing, 5*(3), 43 – 46.

Haber, J., Hoskins, P. P., Leach, A. M., & Sideleau, B. F. (1987). *Comprehensive psychiatric nursing* (3rd ed.). New York: McGraw-Hill.

Haley, J. (1963). *Strategies of psychotherapy.* New York: Grune & Stratton.

Haley, J. (1976). *Problem-solving therapy.* San Francisco: Jossey-Bass.

Hare-Mustin, R. (1976). Paradoxical tasks in family therapy: Who can resist? *Psychotherapy: Theory, research and practice, 13*, 128 – 130.

Helzer, J. E., & Guze, S. B. (1986). *Psychoses, affective disorders, and dementia.* New York: J. B. Lippincott.

Herrick, C. A., & Goodkoontz, L. (1989). Neuman's systems model for nursing practice as a conceptual framework. *Journal of Child and Adolescent Psychiatric Nursing, 2*(2), 61 – 67.

Hetherington, E. (1981). Children and divorce. In R. Henderson (Ed.), *Parent-child interaction: Theory, research and practice* (pp. 35 – 58). New York: Academic Press.

Hetherington, E., Cox, M., & Cox, R. (1978). The aftermath of divorce. In J. Stevens & M. Mathews (Eds.), *Mother/child, father/child relationships* (pp. 149 – 176). Washington, DC: National Association for Education of Young Children.

Institute of Medicine. (1989). *Research on children and adolescents with mental, behavioral and developmental disorders.* Report of a study by a committee of the Institute of Medicine (Division of Mental Health and Behavioral Medicine), National Academy of Sciences. Washington, DC: National Academy Press.

Jackson, D. D. (1965a). Family rules: Marital quid pro quo. *Archives of General Psychiatry, 12,* 589 – 594.

Jackson, D. D. (1965b). The study of the family. *Family Process, 4*, 1 – 20.

Kerr, M. E., & Bowen, M. (1988). *Family evaluation.* New York: W. W. Norton.

Kneisl, C. R., & Riley, E. A. (1992). Suicide and self-destructive behavior. In H. S. Wilson and C. R. Kneisl (Eds.), *Psychiatric nursing* (4th ed.) (pp. 548 – 576). Menlo Park, CA: Addison-Wesley.

Lefley, H. (1990). Culture and chronic mental illness. *Hospital and Community Psychiatry, 41*, 277 – 286.

Lin, K. M., & Kleinman, A. M. (1988). Psychopathology and clinical course of schizophrenia: A cross-cultural perspective. *Schizophrenia Bulletin, 14*, 555 – 567.

Main, M. C., Gerace, L. M., & Camilleri, D. (1993). Information sharing concerning schizophrenia in a family member: Adult siblings' perspectives. *Archives of Psychiatric Nursing, 7*(3), 147 – 153.

Maurin, J. T., & Boyd, C. B. (1990). Burden of mental illness on the family: A critical review. *Archives of Psychiatric Nursing, 4*(2), 99 – 107

McBride, A. B. (1990). Psychiatric nursing in the 1990s. *Archives of Psychiatric Nursing, 4*, 21 – 28.

McKeon, K. L. (1990). Introduction: A future perspective on psychiatric mental health nursing. *Archives of Psychiatric Nursing, 4*, 19 – 20.

Minuchin, S. (1974). *Families and family therapy.* Cambridge, MA: Harvard University Press.

Minuchin, S., & Fishman, H. C. (1981). *Family therapy techniques.* Cambridge, MA: Harvard University Press.

Minuchin, S., Rosman, B. L., & Baker, L. (1978). *Psychosomatic families: Anorexia nervosa in context.* Cambridge, MA: Harvard University Press.

Moltz, D. A. (1993). Biopolar disorder and the family: An integrative model. *Family Process, 32*, 409 – 423.

Mulaik, J. S. (1992). Noncompliance with medication regimens in severely and persistently mentally ill schizophrenic patients. *Issues in Mental Health Nursing, 13*, 219 – 237.

Olds, D., Henderson, C., Chamberlin, R., & Tatelbaum, R. (1986). Preventing child abuse and neglect: A randomized trial of nurse home visitation. *Pediatrics, 78*, 65 – 78.

Peplau, H. E. (1993). Foreword. In C. S. Fawcett (Ed.), *Family psychiatric nursing* (pp. vii – ix). St. Louis, MO: Mosby Year Book.

Price-Hoskins, P. (1992). The chronic mentally ill. In J. Haber, A. L. McMahon, P. Price-Hoskins, & B. F. Sideleau (Eds.), *Comprehensive psychiatric nursing* (4th ed.) (pp. 751 – 772). St. Louis, MO: Mosby Year Book.

Ramshorn, M. T. (1978). Mental health services. In J. Haber, A. M. Leach, S. M. Schudy, & B. F. Sideleau (Eds.), *Comprehensive Psychiatric Nursing* (pp. 9 – 17). New York: McGraw-Hill.

Skultans, V. (1991). Women and affliction in Maharashtra: A hydraulic model of health and illness. *Culture, Medicine and Psychiatry, 15*, 321 – 359.

Stanton, M. D. (1981). Strategic approaches to family therapy. In A. Gurman & D. Kniskern (Eds.), *Handbook of family therapy.* New York: Brunner/Mazel.

Sullivan, G., Wells, K. B., & Leake, B. (1992). Clinical factors associated with better quality of life in a seriously mentally ill population. *Hospital and Community Psychiatry, 43,* 794–798.

Walsh, F. (1987). New perspectives on schizophrenia and families. In F. Walsh & C. M. Anderson (Eds.), *Chronic disorders and the family* (pp. 3–18). New York: Haworth Press.

Walsh, F., & Anderson, C. M. (1987). Chronic disorders and families: An overview. In F. Walsh & C. M. Anderson (Eds.), *Chronic disorders and the family* (pp. 3–18). New York: Haworth Press.

Walsh, F., & Anderson, C. (Eds.). (1987). *Chronic disorders and the family.* New York: Haworth Press.

Wallerstein, J., & Kelly, J. (1980). *Surviving the breakup.* New York: Basic Books.

Watzlawick, P., Beavin, J., & Jackson, D. (1967). *The pragmatics of human communication.* New York: Norton.

Watzlawick, P., Weakland, J. H., & Fisch, R. (1974). *Change: Principles of problem formation and problem resolution.* New York: W. W. Norton.

Weakland, J. H. (1976). Communication theory and clinical change. In P. J. Guerin, Jr. (Ed.), *Family theory: Theory and practice.* New York: Gardner Press.

Whall, A. L. (1991). Family system theory: Relationship to nursing conceptual models. In A. L. Whall & J. Fawcett (Eds.), *Family theory development in nursing: State of the science and art* (pp. 317–341). Philadelphia: F. A. Davis.

Zastowny, T. R., Lehman, A. F., Cole, R. E., & Kane, C. (1992). Family management of schizophrenia: A comparison of behavioral and supportive family treatment. *Psychiatric Quarterly, 63,* 159–186.

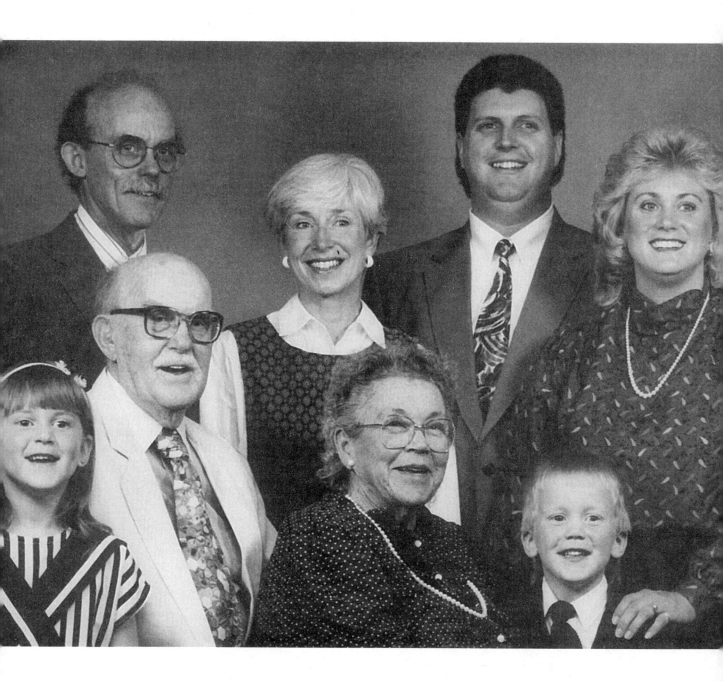

Gerontological Family Nursing

In our society, nearly every family is concerned with the well-being of at least one elderly member. Readers are urged to reflect on this statement and identify the elderly members of their own families. Because current health care delivery is oriented primarily toward meeting the needs of the individual, not the family unit, many families "go it alone" and seek professional help only during emergencies or periods of acute illness. The family is where members learn about health and illness and also where most care is given and received throughout life. Consequently, the family has great potential as an ally in maintaining and restoring the health of its members.

This chapter looks at intergenerational family caring. Although this practice has long been the established norm, it is not without negative consequences. Thoughtful, well-planned nursing interventions that recognize and use family strengths can promote the health of the members and prevent or alleviate many of the negative outcomes of illness. Using a holistic approach to working with families, nurses are uniquely able to exert a positive influence in the lives of older persons and their loved ones by assisting them both physically and psychologically.

The challenges, decisions, and transitions faced by many families as they move through later life are also examined in this chapter, as are the many facets of the nurse's role in working with the family to provide care and services to their older members.

CHAPTER 14

Gerontological Family Nursing

Beverly S. Richards, RN, DNS

OBJECTIVES   *Upon completion of this chapter, the reader will be able to:*
1. Describe the nature, scope, and goals of gerontological family nursing, including goals and implications for practice.
2. Discuss demographic and social trends that are influencing the dynamics and structure of the contemporary older family.
3. Describe the normative changes and non-normative events that challenge today's older families in relation to family functioning and caregiving.
4. Demonstrate the use of the Family Life Cycle Model and the Resiliency Model of Family Stress, Adjustment, and Adaptation as a basis for assessing the family and for formulating interventions within a family systems framework.
5. Provide guidelines and direction for the nurse to develop and maintain a therapeutic alliance with the family.
6. Present implications for future research and social policy.

THE NATURE OF GERONTOLOGICAL
FAMILY NURSING PRACTICE

Changing demographic and social trends make it imperative to respond to the complex, growing health care needs of our aging citizens and their families. Families vary greatly in their ethnicity, histories, structures, coping styles, values, resources, living circumstances, and needs. Likewise, older adults as individuals vary in their past life experiences as well as in their current physical, financial, and living circumstances. The goal of family gerontological nursing is to work in partnership with the family to maintain optimal functioning, restore health, and prevent and/or reduce the effects of illness in the older members. To accomplish this, the nurse must help families provide care to their older loved ones that promotes the optimal health and functioning of *all* members, regardless of age. The nurse must use skillful, thoughtful communication to assist family members to define and clarify problems, problem solve, set limits, and clarify boundaries and family roles. Sometimes when the demands of family caring exceed the family's resources and compromise their well-being, the nurse is called upon to help the family choose other forms of care. To be successful, the nurse must focus assessment, planning, management, intervention, and evaluation of care on the family as a unit. An extensive background in the biological sciences and the physical aspects of health and illness is important in working with older families because it allows the nurse to monitor physical symptoms and teach family members to carry out medical regimens and nursing care procedures.

Because the types and levels of care needed by older persons vary widely, gerontological family nurses practice in a variety of settings. For example, home health agencies such as visiting nurse services have special programs that provide various levels of care in the elderly person's home. Some general hospitals in urban areas provide follow-up care of older patients after hospitalization for acute illness. Gerontological family nurses also practice in long-term care facilities, mental health centers, inpatient psychiatric units, specialized clinics such as Alzheimer's centers or geriatric institutes, interdisciplinary group practices with primary care physicians, and nurse-managed clinics in the community.

By its very nature, gerontological family nursing challenges the nurse to assume a variety of roles that includes advocate, health care broker, liaison, health teacher, family counselor, consultant, and case manager. Because many conditions and illnesses in the elderly are chronic, the nurse's relationship with a family may extend over time. During periods of greatest need, the nurse may even be viewed as a part of the family.

THE EFFECTS OF DEMOGRAPHIC AND SOCIAL TRENDS
ON THE AGING FAMILY

The demographic realities of our aging society are having a profound effect on many institutions in America, but especially health care and the family. The number of persons over 65 has increased by 22% or 5.7 million since 1980, while the number of those under 65 has increased by 8%. The older population itself is getting older. The group over age 85, which has the greatest need for health care, is growing fastest. By the year 2030, when the "baby boomers" reach old age, there will be 66 million older persons, or two and a half times as many as in 1980 (American Association of Retired Persons [AARP], 1991).

Advances in biomedical science have reduced early deaths from acute diseases and prolonged life for those with chronic conditions like cancer and heart disease. Unfortunately, living longer also brings increased possibilities for debilitating illnesses and conditions such as Alzheimer's disease, diabetes, arthritis, and stroke. A national survey revealed that four out of five persons 65 years of age have at least one chronic condition, and the incidence of multiple conditions increases with age (Porterfield & St. Pierre, 1992). Because age is commonly accompanied by one or more chronic health problems an older person can be deprived of independence by limitations in the ability to function and carry out self-care activities. Help may be needed with at least one of the following daily activities: bathing, dressing, transfer, toileting, indoor mobility, and taking medications. Assistance may also be required with household tasks, meal preparation, shopping, transportation, and management of finances.

Many individuals who live to age 85 and older experience a period of dependence and need for care before reaching the end of life (Brody, 1985). These are called the "frail" or "fragile" elderly. More women than men are in need of help, because older women are more likely to be widowed and to live alone, they have less income than elderly men, and they have more chronic health problems such as arthritis, osteoporosis, and diabetes (AARP, 1991; Biegel, Shore, & Gordon, 1984).

In spite of these facts, only 5% of the population 65 years of age and over live in long-term care facilities. The majority of elderly persons who live in nursing homes are older, female, single, childless, and have multiple health problems. Over 50% of nursing home residents have some form of dementia (Katzman, 1986). It can thus be safely concluded that many older persons with chronic conditions are able to remain in the community with the care and assistance of family and friends.

Over the past few decades, an immense body of research has focused on the nature of family relationships, including the informal caregiving network within the aging family. (See Horowitz, 1985, and Given & Given, 1991, for comprehensive reviews). Approximately two thirds (67%) of older noninstitutionalized persons (81% of older men and 56% of older women) live in a family setting. The remaining 32% live alone. They represent nearly 42% of older women and 16% of older men. Also, eight out of ten noninstitutionalized older persons have at least one living child (AARP, 1991). Two thirds live within 30 minutes of a child. The majority (66%) had at least weekly visits with children and even more (76%) had weekly phone conversations. Studies have firmly established that aging is a family affair and elderly members continue as integral parts of their family networks until death (Aldous 1987; Cicirelli, 1983; Shanas, 1979). Reciprocal patterns of intergenerational support and care extend throughout the life cycle of the family, although they tend to shift as the older generation experiences more financial and health problems (Brody, 1985; Cantor, 1980; Kain, 1990; Lee & Ellithorpe, 1982; Townsend & Poulshock, 1986).

NATURE OF CAREGIVING IN OLDER FAMILIES

What Is the Extent?

The family, not the formal health care system, provides 80% to 90% of care to their elderly members, including medical and nursing care, personal services such as transportation, and help with household tasks and shopping (Brody, 1985). The family responds to emergencies, provides acute care and assistance, and initiates and maintains links with the formal care system as necessary. Also, the more frail an elder member becomes, the more responsibility for care the family assumes (Biegel & Blum, 1990; Stoller, 1983). Despite this evidence, there is a lingering myth among many nurses that family members — especially adult children — do not provide care for elderly family members when they need it but instead rely on formal services such as nursing homes. In truth, adult children are providing more assistance and more difficult care to their elderly parents than in the "good old days" (Brody, 1985; O'Neill & Sorenson, 1991). Further, the prospective payment system has shortened hospital stays, sending people home "quicker and sicker" and creating more pressure on the family to provide care for which they may be unprepared. Unfortunately, help in the form of community-based support services is sparse, poorly funded, uncoordinated, or absent altogether. This is especially true for families in rural areas (Henderson, 1992; Lee, 1993).

Who Provides the Care?

The support and care given by all family members are usually lumped together under the term "family caregiving." Closer examination reveals, however, that there is a customary sequence in who assumes the primary responsibility of caregiver and it usually is given by one member at a time (Johnson & Catalano, 1983). When the elderly person is married, the spouse is first in line. Adult children are usually less involved in the care of a married parent, relying instead on the other parent to provide the majority of care. This may work satisfactorily unless the caregiving parent's health is also declining. Unfortunately, many elderly couples do not receive the assistance they need because they hide the seriousness of the difficulties from the rest of the family until a crisis occurs.

When there is no spouse available, the children — usually a daughter or daughter-in-law — assume the caregiving role. If there are no children, another family member such as a sibling, niece, or nephew may step in to help provide care. These more distant relatives generally do not provide the intensity of care that spouses or children provide; instead, they serve more as intermediaries to obtain care from formal sources (Johnson & Catalano, 1981).

Women have always been the traditional caregivers and they continue to provide nearly three fourths (72%) of the family care given to older members. This figure remains constant, even though more women than ever are in the work force (the percentage of working women rose from 38% in 1960 to 55% in 1987 (Select Committee on Aging, 1987).

Daughters outnumber sons as caregivers by four to one (Brody, 1990). Also, women provide more hours of care and they are more likely to give assistance with personal hygiene, household tasks, and meal preparation. Men, on the other hand, more typically help with financial management, transportation, and home repairs (Dwyer & Coward, 1991; Horowitz, 1985; Stone, Cafferata, & Sangl, 1987). Although women provide the bulk of care, the contributions of men should not be overlooked. They frequently provide support and affection to the primary caregiver. Also, many elderly husbands assume the role of primary caregiver if their wives become ill or disabled, meeting both their personal care needs and taking over household tasks.

At What Price?

Research findings over the past several decades have consistently pointed to the key role that family relationships play in helping older members maintain their independence and health (Field, Minkler, Folk, & Leino, 1993; Fletcher & Winslow, 1991; Shanas, 1979; Stone, Cafferata, & Sangl, 1987), and indeed, the term "family caregiving" has become so common that its meaning is taken for granted. Providing informal assistance to family members is a normative and usual activity throughout life. When does it cross the bounds of what is expected and ordinary and become extraordinary care? Biegel, Sales, and Schulz (1991) point out that ". . . caring for a family member who has a chronic illness involves a significant expenditure of time and energy over potentially long periods of time, involves tasks that may be unpleasant and uncomfortable, is likely to be nonsymmetrical, and is often a role that had not been anticipated" (p. 17). Depending upon the type and stage of the illness, the tasks and responsibilities can vary greatly over time.

While family caregiving of elderly members will no doubt continue, researchers have raised questions about the capacity of family caregivers to provide the bulk of long-term care to the elderly (Baille, Norbeck, & Barnes, 1988; Brody, 1981, 1985; Brody, Litvin, Hoffman, & Kleban, 1992). Brody (1985) notes that ". . . parent care has become a normative but stressful experience for individuals and families and its nature, scope, and consequences are not yet fully understood" (p. 19).

Some of the negative consequences of caring for older loved ones, especially those with dementing illnesses such as Alzheimer's disease, are known. Those caregivers have been found to be at greater risk for physical and emotional illness — especially depression, greater social isolation and lack of social support, and an increase in financial burdens (Cattanach & Tebes, 1991; Cohen & Eisdorfer, 1988; Cohen et al., 1990; Gallagher, Wrabetz, Lovett, Del Maestro, & Rose, 1990; Haley, Levine, Brown, Berry, & Hughes, 1987; Neundorfer, 1991a, b; Robinson, 1989).

Recent studies have also linked long-term family care to increased potential for family aggression and violence and suggest that aggression among elderly caregiving families is a growing social problem (Paveza et al., 1992; Pillemer & Finkelhor, 1988, 1989; Sayles-Cross, 1993; Semple, 1992; Williams-Burgess & Kimball, 1990). Some of these studies not only reported mistreatment, neglect, and abuse of the elder member, but also found abuse of the caregiver by the elderly person (Anetzberger, 1987; Steinmetz, 1988). Family members caring for a person with Alzheimer's disease may be at higher risk for abuse, aggression, and injury than other elderly caregiving situations. There are reports that 57% to 65% of demented elders are aggressive toward family members at some time (Hamel et al., 1990; Ryden, 1988).

Other Pressures Facing Families

Conflicts between caregiving and other responsibilities can produce tremendous role strain and overload. These conflicts can strain the adult child's relationship with the elderly parent (Scharlach, 1987). Research findings suggest that the competing demands contribute to the most pervasive consequence of caregiving — emotional stress (Cantor, 1983; George & Gwyther, 1986). Two important sources of caregiver stress are competing familial obligations and conflict with work (Stone et al., 1987). One large study found that many women either quit their jobs or cut their hours in order to care for their elderly relative (Brody, 1985). However, this was not the case for men. Instead, men who were employed appeared to give less assistance, possibly indicating that men gave work priority over caregiving whereas women gave caring priority over work (Stoller, 1983). The conflicts between adult middle-aged women's filial responsibilities and other needs and obligations reflect society's unrealistic and contradictory expectations of middle-aged women (Brody, 1985).

Societal trends influence the structure of contemporary families and thus affect their caregiving capacity. The increasing divorce rate has brought about more single-parent families, most of them headed by working women. Also, the steadily decreasing birthrate since World War II means that as the need for caregivers increases there will be fewer family caregivers available. Many couples are postponing childbearing, which means that in the future they will be providing care to their elderly parents while they are still responsible for dependent children.

The demands on family caregivers will intensify as hospital stays become shorter and care shifts into the community. At the same time, more elderly are going to need more long-term care, which is rarely covered by insurance. These trends will create a dilemma for many older families. Faced with the need for expensive long-term care, many elderly couples are forced to "spend down" their assets in order to quality for Medicaid coverage. This may leave the healthier spouse with seriously reduced resources.

The fierce pride that many older people take in their independence and lifelong self-sufficiency means that they try to avoid accepting government assistance at any cost. In order to protect hard-earned assets, these older persons may attempt to get by, denying their need for formal care until a medical crisis occurs. This can place added stress on the entire family because they may be unaware of the seriousness of an elderly member's health problems until the crisis occurs. This situation can also place unanticipated demands on family members for immediate care and assistance for which they are unprepared.

Economic trends may be a major source of stress for families. Many young adult and middle-aged family members are facing increased economic pressures through unemployment, layoffs, forced early retirements, cuts in health care benefits, and the rising cost of living. As a result, some adult children are finding it necessary to move back into their parents' homes, at least temporarily. Also, a small but steadily growing number of grandparents are assuming responsibility for raising their grandchildren because of the financial or personal problems of their adult children (Kelley, 1993). These trends may affect traditional family caregiving patterns.

THEORETICAL PERSPECTIVES

Background

Families are like individuals in that each has a life cycle with predictable developmental stages and changes. The changes that families experience over time are like those in a kaleidoscope. The turn of events, whether an accumulation of small changes or the advent of a major stressor, results in the creation of a new pattern from the existing components of family life. While some changes are subtle, others are more dramatic, but the changing patterns unfold progressively and unidirectionally.

Until the occurrence of a stressor event or crisis that demands change, families maintain fairly stable patterns of interaction over time. Events that demand change take two forms — normative and non-normative. Normative changes or transitions are those expected, somewhat predictable maturational life events such as marriage, birth of the first child, retirement, and death of a spouse in old age. Although these are expected changes, a period of floundering or crisis may occur until adjustment is achieved. Non-normative crises, on the other hand, are not predicted or expected and may occur with little warning. Examples include the diagnosis of a serious, chronic illness, the accidental death of a family member, a job transfer, the unexpected unemployment of a primary breadwinner, or adult children having to move back home with parents. The suddenness of the event does not allow the family to plan or rehearse options, and there can be considerable family disequilibrium, confusion, and distress until new patterns in roles and responsibilities are established.

Neugarten (1968) pointed out in an earlier work that both biological and social clocks create a framework for change in individuals and families alike. As the family grows older, the health status of members may change as a result of natural aging or illness. At the same time, living arrangements, financial concerns, and alliances ebb and flow in response to marriages, deaths, divorces, remarriages, relocations, retirements, and illnesses. Parent-child relationships change as caregiving responsibilities shift. Changes may also result from social and environmental pressures that occur outside the family, such as bad economic times, an increase in crime, or natural disasters.

The ways in which families work together to meet these demands and changes, maintain equilibrium, and meet the needs of members have been studied extensively from the perspective of family systems theory. Two system-based models provide a framework for understanding and working effectively with aging families. The first is the Family Life Cycle Model, which provides a view of how families change over time (Aldous, 1978; Carter & McGoldrick, 1980; Duvall & Miller, 1985). It points out places in family development where changes in status and roles are likely to occur and it can be useful in predicting many facets of family behavior and vulnerability. The second model is the Resiliency Model of Family Stress, Adjustment, and Adaptation (McCubbin & McCubbin, 1993). This approach to the family is concerned with how families negotiate change and adapt to stressful life events over time, particularly to stressors such as illness. The approach is especially useful because it incorporates the characteristics of the individual members, the family system, and the community, all of which interact to shape the course of family behavior and adaptation. It also stresses the importance of family resilience and the natural healing qualities of family life.

Family Life Cycle as Related to Older Families

The family's life cycle includes the various stages of development of the family system over time. These stages are convenient divisions that help to study a process that, in real life, flows from one stage to another without a pause or break. The family's life cycle is in reality like a chain, with each stage beginning in a previous one and coming to fruition in a future one (Duvall & Miller, 1985).

Stages divide the lifetime of a family into distinctive periods that are marked by changes in status and roles. Stages are initiated by critical events that can originate either inside or outside the family system. Internal events in the older family include becoming a couple again after launching the last child, becoming grandparents, and experiencing the onset of physical or cognitive incapacity in a spouse or elderly parent, or the death of the spouse. Events originating outside the family may occur in connection with education or work life and include retirement or starting a second career.

As with the development of individuals, each stage requires the completion of certain tasks in order to move on to the next stage. Duvall and Miller (1985, p. 318) identify eight family developmental tasks of the aging couple:

1. Making satisfying living arrangements as aging progress
2. Adjusting to retirement income
3. Establishing comfortable routines
4. Safeguarding physical and mental health
5. Maintaining love, sex, and marital relations
6. Remaining in touch with other family members
7. Keeping active and involved
8. Finding meaning in life

As families move from one stage into the next, role transitions require changes in earlier interaction patterns and create a permanent change within the family system. Eventually all members are affected to some degree, because a change in roles and responsibilities of one member naturally influences the roles and responsibilities of the others. Even though critical role transitions are considered "points of no return," this does not mean they are dead ends; a family's life cycle is continuously evolving and developing over time (Aldous, 1978).

Brubaker (1983) identified four common events that initiate significant transitions in the careers of aging families. Each requires family members—either willingly or unwillingly—to participate in negotiating the change. These are (1) the empty nest, or launching of children into independence; (2) retirement of one or both spouses from employment; (3) an incapacitating illness that compromises independence or requires institutionalization; and (4) disruption of the family through death. A fifth event that is as an important transition in older families is need for relocation or change in living arrangements because of declining health or functional abilities.

Assessment of the Family Life Cycle

The family development model provides a framework from which to assess both existing and potential strengths and vulnerabilities in the family. The results of the assessment can be built into the plan of care using anticipatory guidance, education, and support. In the life cycle of the family, roles, responsibilities, individual developmental tasks, career demands, and resources are rarely synchronized. Therefore, understanding the timing and intersection of internal and external events is crucial in determining family vulnerability. It is especially important to examine critical role transitions within the family—recent, current, or anticipated—because some have greater potential than others for causing stress and vulnerability.

Transitions within older families occur when roles and responsibilities start to shift across the generations. Middle-aged children often find their aging parents coming to them for emotional support, advice, and other forms of help. This may occur at a time when their own children are leaving home, the family's financial resources are stretched to pay for college tuition, and the mother is returning full-time to the work force. For the older generation, the changes brought by retirement, possible loss of income, and physical decline may bring fear and trepidation. Reaching out to their children for help is often a disturbing and even humiliating experience. As much as they need the help, they may have great difficulty in asking for it.

As elderly members begin to develop signs of physical or cognitive decline that threaten their independence and capacity for self-care, several things are likely to happen. There may also be a shift in the traditional hierarchial structure as parental authority and influence decline, which brings shifts in roles, responsibilities, and boundaries. Adult children are confronted with the **filial crisis**, a concept introduced by Blenkner (1965) in an attempt to explain the experience of adult children when parent care becomes necessary. The children are forced to face the fact that their belief that their parents will "be there" forever is a fantasy. Instead of continuing to be the recipient of parental nurturance, they must become the nurturing ones—both to their parents and to the younger generation. Middle-aged children's sense of loss and distress may be intensified because they must admit to their own mortality as their aging parents must acknowledge their decline, need for help, and loss of independence (King, Bonnacci, & Wynne, 1990).

As the parents' need for care and assistance increases, the adult children—particularly adult daughters—may find themselves caught in the middle between the needs of the older and the younger generation, as illustrated in Figure 14–1. This group has been described as the **sandwich generation** (Brody, 1981; Hooyman & Lustbader, 1986). These family members are a vulnerable group because as the need to provide care for others increases, the caregivers often neglect their own needs (Cantor, 1983; Bunting, 1989).

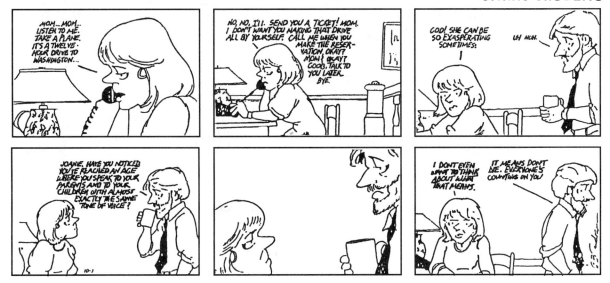

FIGURE 14–1
Contemporary illustration depicting the sandwich generation. (Doonesbury, Copyright G.B. Trudeau. Reprinted with permission of Universal Press Syndicate. All rights reserved.)

Resiliency Model of Family Stress, Adjustment, and Adaptation

The Resiliency Model of Family Stress, Adjustment, and Adaptation developed by McCubbin and McCubbin (1993) provides a framework for understanding a family's response, adjustment, and finally, adaptation to stress over time. These authors have worked extensively with families responding to a loved one's chronic illness or condition. Their framework is useful for understanding the demands and challenges that older families experience and allows for assessment and intervention at many points to promote adaptation. The resiliency model evolved form Hill's (1958) earlier formulation of family vulnerability to crisis events and, more recently, the Double ABCX Family Stress and Adaptation Model developed by McCubbin and Patterson (1983). The model is oriented toward adaptation, which is its central concept. Adaptation is the outcome of family efforts to bring a new level of balance, harmony, coherence, and functioning to a family crisis situation over time.

The model includes a number of interacting components that influence successful or unsuccessful family adjustment. These are illustrated in Figure 14–2.

The stressor (A) and its severity interact with the family's vulnerability (V). Vulnerability is influenced by the pileup, or number and timing, of other family stresses, transitions, and strains that occur along with the main stressor. Family vulnerability interacts with the family typology (T), that is, the patterns of family interaction that have been established over time. These components then interact with the family's resistance resources (B) and, in turn, interact with the family appraisal (C) of the stressor. Their appraisal interacts with the family's problem-solving and coping strategies (PSC) (McCubbin & McCubbin, 1993). All of these components work together to influence the family's adjustment.

The Stressor (A) and Its Severity

"A stressor is a demand placed on the family that produces, or has the potential of producing, changes in the family system" (McCubbin & McCubbin, 1993, p. 28). The event or demand can influence many aspects of family life including health, roles and responsibilities,

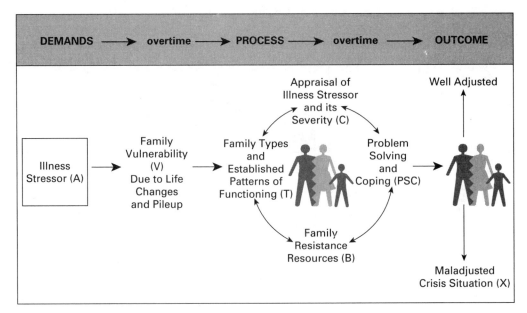

FIGURE 14–2
Adjustment phase of the resiliency model of family stress, adjustment, and adaptation. (From Danielson, CB, Hamel-Bissell, B, and Winston-Frey, P: Families, Health, and Illness: Perspectives on Coping and Interventions. CV Mosby, St. Louis, 1993, p. 67, with permission.)

and boundaries. Severity is determined by the degree to which the stressor threatens the stability of the family. In many older families, the stressor event is the onset, or recognition through diagnosis, of the deterioration in health of an older member.

Family Vulnerability (V): Pileup and Family Life Cycle Changes

Vulnerability is the degree of fragility in the interpersonal and organizational state of the family. It is influenced by the number of normative changes in the family's life cycle and by the accumulation or pileup of demands from inside or outside the family. The model outlines six categories of stresses and strains that contribute to a pileup of demands as a family attempts to adapt to a stressor such as illness:

1. The illness and related hardships over time
2. Normative transitions in individual family members and the family as a whole
3. Prior family strains accumulated over time
4. Situational demands and contextual difficulties
5. The consequences of family efforts to cope
6. Intrafamily and social ambiguity that provides inadequate guidelines on how families should act or cope effectively (McCubbin & McCubbin, 1993, p. 37)

Specific demands might include economic stress due to poor health, heavy health care expenses, need to relocate, death of a member, or adult children leaving or returning home.

Family Types (T): Profile of Family-Established Patterns of Functioning

The family type is characterized by fairly stable, observable patterns of functioning. Two family attributes that are important in helping families manage chronic illness are moderate degrees of cohesion and adaptability. This supports early findings by Pratt

(1976). From his research on family health behavior, he concluded that a fluid organization with flexible role relationships and shared power resulted in an "energized family" that promoted personal growth and individual member autonomy. This would lead to a spirit of cooperation, open communication, and negotiation as change becomes necessary.

Family Resistance Resources (B): Capabilities and Strengths

Resistance resources are capabilities and strengths that enable the family to manage the stressor and prevent major upheaval in their functioning. The following critical family resources have been identified by McCubbin and McCubbin (1993): economic stability, cohesiveness, flexibility, hardiness, shared spiritual beliefs, open communication, traditions, celebrations, routines, and organization.

Resources outside the family are also important to adaptation. These include the family's social support network of friends and neighbors, as well as community-based agencies such as day-care centers, respite programs, and self-help groups. Social support serves to protect and insulate the family from the effects of stress and promotes recovery from crisis. The elderly, especially the very old or those without available family, may have a limited social support network because of poor health, restricted mobility, limited finances, deaths of friends, and lack of transportation.

Family Appraisal of the Stressor (C)

Appraisal includes the family's perceptions and definition of the stressor and its accompanying hardships, as well as the family's perceptions of their available resources and the actions needed to meet the demands and regain family balance (Mays, 1988). If family members perceive the situation as hopeless or beyond their ability to manage, they may not be able to recognize and use available resources, or seek additional resources. Therefore, they will be at high risk for maladaptation. On the other hand, if they can accept the situation and see it as a challenge, they can deal with, they are more likely to engage in constructive efforts to manage the situation.

Family Problem Solving and Coping (PSC)

The model includes a consideration of the problem-solving skills and coping strategies the family uses in order to manage the demands created by the stressor. Steps in the problem-solving process include (1) organizing the stressor into manageable components, (2) identifying alternative management strategies, and (3) taking steps to resolve the problem. Coping includes family patterns and a wide range of efforts to maintain and strengthen the family, obtain family and community resources, and attend to the well-being and developmental needs of family members.

Family Response—Stress and Distress

When a stressor occurs that necessitates family management or change, it causes tension in the family. If this tension is not resolved or at least brought within manageable limits, it becomes stress. Stress occurs when there is a perceived imbalance between the demands on the family and its resources and capabilities. If balance is not restored, family distress may occur and the stress can even threaten the stability and integrity of the family system.

Together, the Family Life Cycle Model and the Resiliency Model of Family Stress, Adjustment, and Adaptation provide a comprehensive framework for assessing the aging family's strengths and areas of vulnerability in times of stress and change. This is a crucial aspect of assisting families to adapt positively to their changing lives.

In the following vignette, the Murphys, a fairly typical, contemporary, middle-class family illustrate a number of developmental transitions and changes faced by older adults and their families.

Case Study: The Murphy Family

Ten years ago Jim and Noreen Murphy moved from their family home in central Ohio to a retirement community in Arizona following his retirement from a large industrial firm. They have lived comfortably though not extravagantly, through careful management of their resources, which include social security, Jim's pension from the company, and some modest investments. Noreen was always a full-time homemaker and did not work outside the home during their marriage. Jim always handled the family's finances and Noreen took care of their home. Jim is now 75 years of age and Noreen is 72 years of age. They recently celebrated their 50th anniversary. They have two children — a son Bob, age 43 years, and a daughter Doris, age 48 years. Bob, an attorney, lives in Alabama with his two daughters, ages 11 and 14 years. His wife died of cancer 2 months ago. Doris lives in Ohio with Ed, her husband of 24 years. They have three children — a 16-year-old son in high school, a 19-year-old son, and a 21-year-old daughter, the latter two both away at college. The daughter recently announced her engagement and plans a big summer wedding following graduation. Doris and Ed are both employed. He is an architect and she is a self-employed interior designer. For the past several months, Ed's company has experienced a slowdown. Recently he was assigned to a large out-of-state project and he is now home only on weekends.

Over the years, as the children were growing up, Doris worked only part-time in order to devote her attention to the family. Last year, when the youngest son, a junior in high school, began driving, she decided to return to work full-time. She took a calculated risk and opened a small studio. After several months of uncertainty, her business is now growing.

Recently, Noreen has been calling Doris with growing concerns about Jim, Doris's father. He is having noticeable problems with his short-term memory and they are getting progressively worse. He is having difficulty handling the finances and last week he got lost while driving only three blocks from home. The calls are coming more frequently and her mother is hinting that Doris should come and spend 3 or 4 weeks to help them "get things straightened out." Doris fears that her father may have Alzheimer's disease because it was suspected that both his mother and his uncle had the disease. So far, Doris has been able to reassure and give suggestions to her mother over the phone, but she is coming to the realization that she may soon need to go to Arizona to help her aging parents.

This vignette illustrates critical role transitions within a typical middle-class aging family. These expected transitions can produce stress, disequilibrium, and the need for change within the family. The addition of an unexpected event, that is, the possibility of Alzheimer's disease in an otherwise healthy parent who lives several thousand miles away, increases family stress and creates a need for renegotiation of roles and responsibilities among the family members.

PRACTICE CONSIDERATIONS OF GERONTOLOGICAL FAMILY NURSING

The role of the gerontological family nurse includes teaching, giving advice, providing encouragement and support, and advocating for the family within the health care delivery system. The first step is to establish a therapeutic alliance with the elderly members and the rest of their family. To do this successfully, it is necessary to view the family as a system, not as individual victims who need to be rescued. It is important to recognize that adult children often experience powerful feelings of abandonment, anger, and guilt when their parents' health fails. These emotions may alternate with denial of the seriousness of the health problems. Older spouses may also experience these feelings, especially when the healthier spouse has always been dependent on the person who is declining. Frequently, it is the nurse in the home, hospital, or clinic who first notices the frustration and tension in family caregivers. The family's negative or angry feelings may be temporarily displaced onto the nurse or other professional caregivers and mistakenly interpreted as hostility or treatment resistance. In reality, these are a natural response to a tragic, sad, irreversible situation (King et al., 1990). It is often helpful at this point to explain to the family that these are normal reactions and help them explore their perceptions of the situation and its meaning for them. In situations that involve long-term caregiving, it may be useful to refer family members to support groups or teach them stress management techniques (Dellasega, 1990).

It should be noted that, in addition to *working* with families, nurses *belong* to families. Working intensively with families who are under stress has the potential to evoke powerful feelings in the nurse. Awareness of the developmental stage of the nurse's own family, along with its accompanying emotions and challenges, can help the nurse understand the client family's responses to the decisions and changes they are facing. On occasion, when the nurse has experienced a similar situation, some self-disclosure can be helpful and reassuring to the family.

Families may differ culturally, ethnically, and racially from the gerontological family nurse. Sometimes health professionals stereotype or show bias toward families that do not share their personal values and views of effective family functioning (Danielson, Hamel-Bissell, & Winstead-Fry, 1993). To avoid bias, it is crucial that the nurse be open and sensitive to the family's beliefs, values, and practices in relation to health and family functioning. Families must never be stereotyped: each family is unique and families vary widely even within identified ethnic and racial groups.

Goals and Intervention Strategies

The nurse's initial contact with the older person occurs when help is sought for an acute or worsening health problem. Following the medical evaluation, the family nurse should set up a conference that includes the patient and all other family members who may be involved in providing care and assistance. The physician and other members of the health care team, such as the social worker, visiting nurse, and physical therapist, are to be included as needed. The first step is to establish a working partnership with the family so that they are comfortable in expressing their feelings, ideas, and concerns. Inform them that the goal is to provide support and information, and also to help them set realistic goals by clarifying what needs to be done, establishing a plan of action, and determining the best way to carry it out.

Start by obtaining a picture of the family using the concepts from the Family Life Cycle Model and Resiliency Model of Family Stress, Adjustment, and Adaptation described earlier. First explore their perceptions of the current stressor—the elderly member's illness or condition. Do they understand the diagnosis? What do they believe that it will mean in terms of changes or demands on the family? How are they defining the situation in relation to themselves, to a spouse, or to a parent? What resources are available to them personally, within the family, and in the community? How do they perceive those resources? What other stressful events and transitions are occurring, for example, health problems, job stress, or other family disruptions? How have they coped with other stressful events or periods in the past? Did they pull together (cohesion) and make adjustments (flexibility) or did they freeze and pull apart?

Next, the family's priorities—both as individuals and as a group—should be brought into the open and discussed. Priorities include both what they hope to accomplish in their elderly member's care as well as their individual personal goals. Financial concerns, time constraints, and generational responsibilities should be discussed openly. The elderly member's wishes, priorities, and expectations *must* be included in order for an plan to be successful.

The next step is to help the family establish caregiving goals that are realistic and acceptable (Kashner, Magaziner, & Pruitt, 1990). Some elderly members' desire to remain in their own home may be so strong that rather than leave they would accept mediocre care or no care at all. They may also have an unspoken expectation that the adult children will "pitch in" and help. This may create increasing tension and stress in the family because the adult children, while wanting their loved one to have the best care possible, may be unaware of this expectation or be unable to deliver the assistance needed because of other demands.

It may also be helpful to inquire whether any family members have ever promised the elderly member that "I will never put you in a nursing home. I will always take care of you, no matter what happens." Many family members—especially wives and daughters—make this well-meaning but unrealistic commitment either under duress, as a result of guilt or denial, or as a form of reassurance to an aging relative. It can, however, have a profoundly negative effect on the family when they face difficult caregiving decisions. Through open, guided discussion, the nurse can help them see the situation realistically so that they can face appropriate alternatives when necessary.

After all family members have had an opportunity to express their priorities and goals for caregiving, role clarification needs to occur. At this point, the nurse should help the family evaluate how they plan to work together to meet not only the needs of the elderly member, but also those of the other members, as the effects of the illness require inevitable role and structural changes in the family. The day-to-day care expectations need to be made explicit, including the responsibilities of individual members and the plan for emergencies and other contingencies such as illness or vacations.

Whatever their role in caregiving, *all* family members should be taught about the illness or condition, including the actual caregiving activities and the resources required. Then both the designated caregiver and those less directly involved in day-to-day care will know the actual requirements for care and the resources necessary. This can prevent conflict and misunderstanding between family members at a later time.

The nurse must ensure that decisions are made with the full participation of the elderly person whenever possible, even if the person has an early dementing disorder. It is also necessary to help the family coordinate their caregiving activities over time. The nurse can lay the groundwork for formal assistance by connecting the family with appropriate community resources, such as adult day care, respite care, in-home health services, support groups, and family workshops or classes.

It is highly desirable, whenever possible, to visit the elderly person at home with family caregivers present. This is a useful strategy because visiting on family's "turf" tends to strengthen the nurse's therapeutic alliance with the family; at the same time it is possible to see their usual patterns of interaction and evaluate the home in terms of safety and available resources.

Legal counsel is an important aspect of caregiving that is often overlooked until a crisis occurs. Not only do families need to know about the benefits of their elderly members, including health care insurance, Medicare, pensions, and social security, but they also need to know about advance directives, living wills, health care representatives, and estate planning. With progressive dementing disorders it is particularly important to plan for the time when the person is no longer competent to handle legal or financial matters. Many families are hesitant to discuss these matters and need encouragement and assistance to do so.

Yet such planning assures that the elderly person's wishes are known and honored and may prevent later family guesswork, hassles, and conflicts.

The older members' spiritual needs must not be overlooked (Reed, 1991). Religious affiliation and spiritual beliefs have an important place in many older persons' lives. Also, the church, parish, synagogue, temple, etc. is often a great source of formal and informal support to its elderly members. The gerontological family nurse helps the family identify, coordinate, and use all their available resources to facilitate continuing family functioning and adaptation.

Case Study: The Murphy Family Revisited

Let us revisit the Murphy family 2 months later.

Doris and Ed rearranged their schedules so that Doris could visit her parents for 2 weeks. Their 16-year-old son and Ed managed the household and handled her client messages. Doris's brother was unable to go to Arizona with Doris but indicated that he would help his parents with financial management and legal advice when needed. Upon arriving in Tuscon, Doris saw that her father's cognitive ability was very impaired. While he recognized her, he had a great deal of difficulty remembering recent events and continually repeated the same questions over and over. She arranged an appointment for a diagnostic evaluation at a nearby geriatric clinic. Their worst fears were confirmed when he was diagnosed with moderate to severe cognitive impairment due to probable Alzheimer's disease. The nurse in the clinic brought the family together in a conference to explore the family's perceptions and feelings about the diagnosis and to discuss the available options. Several decisions would need to be made about the couple's living arrangements and future care for Doris's father. The nurse made sure that Bob was able to participate in the meeting by telephone conference call. The physician had given the family members a full and detailed report of the test results. Because of the family history of the disease, they had some idea of what to expect. This knowledge was both a stressor and a resource. After many tears and much family discussion, they decided that with Doris and Ed's help, Jim and Noreen would move back to Ohio into a retirement center near Doris and her family. The center, which is affiliated with the church that they belonged to for years, provides a continuum of living arrangements from independent to skilled care. It employs two gerontological family nurses and is also creating a special care unit for older persons with cognitive impairment; this means that appropriate care will be available for Ed when it becomes necessary. Bob offered to fly out to help his parents put their finances in order, sell their condominium, and begin estate planning. The nurse, with Jim and Noreen's permission, communicated her assessment and recommendations to the nurse in the retirement center. The nurse also scheduled a follow-up home visit with Jim and Noreen in 2 weeks to provide support and help them plan their relocation.

At first glance this vignette appears somewhat idealistic, because this family seemed to have little difficulty accepting the diagnosis and reaching a logical and reasonable solution. However, the nurse must realize that this is the beginning, not the end of the Murphys' story. The major stressor for the entire family is the diagnosis of Alzheimer's disease in their father-husband. Jim and Noreen are facing the meaning of the diagnosis for their future, the loss of independence, relocation, loss of their social network, and major reallocation of roles and responsibilities. Doris, Ed, and Bob will now have to face additional filial responsibilities, the increasing dependence of parents, their own family transitions, and the loss of their father and father-in-law as they knew him in earlier days. The grandchildren will also be affected by the changes. Redefining and renegotiating both family roles and responsibilities and patterns of communication while maintaining multigenerational responsibilities will be a challenge for all family members. This family has resources to help them adjust and make changes — strong family bonds, adequate financial resources, and flexibility. The gerontological family nurse needs the knowledge and skills necessary to assist them with these adjustments and facilitate their adaptation over time.

SOCIAL POLICY CONSIDERATIONS FOR OLDER FAMILIES

Given current social and demographic trends, it is certain that the future will bring increasing demands for family caregiving of elderly members. At a time when biomedical breakthroughs are succeeding in slowing or halting chronic conditions, health care reform is moving more care into the community and placing even greater responsibility for care on family members. The difficulty of caring for an elderly family member is compounded by economic pressures and additional demands at work and at home. While elderly husbands and wives care for one another as long as possible, this responsibility is often assumed by an adult daughter or daughter-in-law when one parent dies or either of them becomes disabled (Stone et al., 1987). The strain experienced by these adult daughter caregivers has been well documented (Brody, 1990; Horowitz, 1985).

As the population continues to age, more adult daughters will be widowed or divorced. This is because women outlive men and also tend to have a lower remarriage rate than men after divorce or death of their husbands. Recently, caregiving daughters without husbands have been shown to be at higher risk for mental health problems than those with husbands. They are also less well off economically than their married sisters (Brody et al., 1992). The Family Leave Act will not solve the dilemma of caregivers who cannot afford to take leaves without pay. For such families a tax credit similar to the Child and Dependent Care Tax Credit needs to be explored (Stone et al., 1987).

The vulnerability of the growing group of caregivers must be addressed. Failure to do so will result in increased mental and physical health problems for overburdened family members, and ultimately, increased costs to society. The informal family caring system is a national resource that must be protected and supported, not overwhelmed. No institution can replace the support and care given by family members; rather, elderly persons' needs for care are best served by a combination of formal and informal services. This requires the development of affordable support services in the community that supplement family caregiving, such as respite care, homemaker services, adult day-care centers, and neighborhood wellness clinics. The challenge is to provide appropriate, accessible forms of tangible assistance with caregiving, and not simply view family members as unpaid workers who need to be "cheered on" in their caregiving work (Brody, 1985).

IMPLICATIONS FOR FUTURE RESEARCH IN GERONTOLOGICAL FAMILY NURSING

The challenges facing the aging family are complex. In order to meet the needs of our noninstitutionalized elderly, we need answers to many questions. For example, what functions do formal and informal care systems perform best? What balance of formal and informal services is needed to meet the care needs of the elderly? How can caregivers balance competing family and work demands, and what interventions are effective in reducing caregiver distress (Knight, Lutzky, & Macofsky-Urban, 1993)? Only recently has it been recognized that abuse and violence are serious problems in older caregiving families. What are the factors that contribute to the aggression and violence, and under what conditions do they occur?

Studies of interventions for elders with various illnesses and chronic conditions need to be conducted with family caregivers in the home, to test the effectiveness of approaches to specific care situations. Finally, further research is needed to determine the best ways to reach older families of various ethnic and racial backgrounds and develop care options that they will accept.

SUMMARY   Our society is aging rapidly. While this demographic shift is influencing every institution in our society, none are more affected than the family and health care. With increasing longevity, there is an increase in chronic, incapacitating conditions. At the same time, as efforts to contain health care costs intensify, more and more responsibility for care and assistance is being shifted into the community. The family is the single most important resource to elderly persons, but the burdens of responsibility for caregiving are compounded by increasing demands at work and home. Some family researchers have raised questions about the family's capacity to continue to assume increasing responsibility for informal care. Gerontological family nurses are in an excellent position to understand the challenges facing older families, the dynamics of family caregiving, and the stress it produces; they can work with families to lighten their load. To do so, however, the nurse must build an effective partnership with the family to maximize their capabilities, minimize their vulnerabilities, and serve as a bridge to the formal care system.

STUDY QUESTIONS

1. Which of the following statements are true?
   a. Adult children should be discouraged from talking to their elderly parents about their benefits and finances.
   b. Older families, like older people, seem more alike than different.
   c. Families provide the bulk of health care to older people.
   d. Sons and daughters share the care of elderly parents equally.

2. List and describe three common, normative events that can trigger significant transitions in older families.

3. Social support outside the family is important in helping older individuals remain independent and functioning in the community. Name four factors or conditions that may hinder or limit the availability of social support.

4. A major goal of gerontological family nursing is:
   a. To help the family system restore and maintain the functioning and health of its older members

   b. To assist the family in making health care placement decisions for its older members
   c. To set appropriate caregiving goals for the family
   d. To help the family avoid the need for institutionalization of elderly members

5. List and discuss three potential stressors that are commonly experienced by the "sandwich generation." How might these affect their coping and adaptation to a decline in health of aging parents?

6. Which of the following are true statements?
   a. Most older persons tend to rely heavily on the formal health care system to meet their needs.
   b. The formal health care system is set up to meet the needs of the family.
   c. Older people tend to rely on family assistance and "make do" until a crisis occurs.
   d. Families caring for an elderly member with a dementing illness are at greater risk for poor health and/or elder mistreatment.

REFERENCES

Aldous, J. (1978). *Family careers: Developmental change in families*. New York: John Wiley & Sons.

Aldous, J. (1987). New views on the family life of the elderly and the near-elderly. *Journal of Marriage and the Family, 49,* 277-234.

Anetzberger, G. J. (1987). *The etiology of elder abuse by adult offspring*. Springfield, IL: Charles C. Thomas.

American Association of Retired Persons (AARP). (1991). *A profile of older Americans*. Washington, DC: American Association of Retired Persons and the Administration of Aging, US Department of Health and Human Services.

Baille, V., Norbeck, J. S., & Barnes, L. E. A. (1988). Stress, social support, and psychological distress of family caregivers of the elderly. *Nursing Research, 37,* 217-222.

Biegel, D. E., & Blum, A. (1990). *Aging and caregiving: Theory, research, and policy*. Newberry Park, CA: Sage Publications.

Biegel, D., Sales, E., & Schulz, R. (1991). *Family caregiving in chronic illness*. Newberry Park, CA: Sage Publications.

Biegel, D. E., Shore, B., & Gordon, E. (1984). *Building support networks for the elderly: Theory and applications*. Beverly Hills, CA: Sage Publications.

Blenkner, M. (1965). Social work and family relationships in later life with some thoughts on filial maturity. In E. Shanas & G. J. Streib (Eds.), *Social structure and the family: Generational relations*. Englewood Cliffs, NJ: Prentice-Hall.

Brody, E. M. (1981). Women in the middle and family help to older people. *Gerontologist, 25,* 19-29.

Brody, E. M. (1985). Parent care as a normative family stress. *Gerontologist, 25,* 19-29.

Brody, E. M. (1990). *Women in the middle: Their parent care years*. New York: Springer.

Brody, E. M., Litvin, S. J., Hoffman, C., & Kleban, M. H. (1992). Differential effects of daughters' marital status on their parent care experiences. *Gerontologist, 32,* 58-67.

Brubaker, T. H. (Ed.) (1983). *Family relationships in later life*. Newberry Park, CA: Sage Publications.

Bunting, S. (1989). Stress on caregivers of the elderly. *Advances in Nursing Science, 11,* 63-73.

Cantor, M. J. (1980). The informal support system: Its relevance in the lives of the elderly. In E. Borgatta & N. McCloskey (Eds.), *Aging and society*. Beverly Hills: Sage Publications.

Cantor, M. J. (1983). Strain among caregivers: A study of experience in the United States. *Gerontologist, 25,* 597-604.

Carter, G. A., & McGoldrick, M. (1980). *The family lifecycle: A framework for family therapy*. New York: Family Press.

Cattanach, L., & Tebes, J. K. (1991). The nature of elder impairment and its impact on family caregivers' health and psychosocial functioning. *Gerontologist, 31,* 246-255.

Cicirelli, V. G. (1983). A comparison of helping behavior to elderly parents of adult children with intact and disrupted marriages. *Gerontologist, 23,* 619-625.

Cohen, D., & Eisdorfer, C. (1988). Depression in a family member caring for a relative with Alzheimer's disease. *Journal of the American Geriatrics Society, 36,* 885-889.

Cohen, D., Luchins, D., Eisdorfer, C., Paveza, G., Ashford, J. W., Gorelick, P., Hirschman, R., Freels, S., Levy, P., Semla, T., & Shaw, H. (1990). Caring for relatives with Alzheimer's disease: The mental health risks to spouses, adult, children and other family caregivers. *Behavior, Health, and Aging, 1,* 171-182.

Danielson, C. B., Hamel-Bissell, B., & Winstead-Fry. P. (Eds.). (1993). *Families, health, & illness: Perspectives on coping and interventions*. St. Louis, MO: C. V. Mosby.

Dellasega, C. (1990). Coping with caregiving: Stress management for caregivers of the elderly. *Journal of Psychosocial Nursing, 28,* 15-22.

Duvall, E. M., & Miller, B. C. (1985). *Marriage and family development* (6th ed.). New York: Harper & Row.

Dwyer, J. W., & Coward, R. T. (1991). A multivariate comparison of the involvement of adult sons versus daughters in the care of impaired parents. *Journal of Gerontology, 46,* S259-269.

Field, D., Minkler, M., Folk, R. F., & Leino, E. V. (1993). The influence of health on family contacts and family feelings in advanced old age: A longitudinal study. *Journal of Gerontology: Psychosocial Sciences, 48,* P18-28.

Fletcher, K. R., & Winslow, S. A. (1991). Informal caregivers: A composite and review of needs and community resources. *Family Community Health, 14*(2), 59-67.

Gallagher, D., Wrabetz, A., Lovett, S., Del Maestro, S., & Rose, J. (1990). Depression and other negative affects in family caregivers. In E. Light & D. Lebwitz (Eds.), *Alzheimer's disease treatment and family stress: Directions for research* (pp. 218-244). New York: Hemisphere.

George, L. K., & Gwyther, L. P. (1986). Caregiver well-being: A multidimensional examination of family caregivers of demented adults. *Gerontologist, 26,* 259-259.

Given, B. A., & Given, C. W. (1991). Family caregivers for the elderly. In J. J. Fitzpatrick, R. L., Taunton, & A. K. Jacox (Eds.). *Annual review of nursing research, Vol. 9* (pp. 77-101). New York: Springer.

Haley, W. E., Levin, E. G., Brown, S. L., Berry, J. W., & Hughes, G. H. (1987). Psychological, social, and health consequences of caring for a relative with senile dementia. *Journal of the American Geriatrics Society, 35,* 405–411.

Hamel, M., Gold, D. P., Andress, D., Reis, M., Dastoor, D., Graur, H., & Bergman, H. (1990). Predictors and consequences of aggressive behavior by community-based dementia patients. *Gerontologist, 30,* 206–211.

Henderson, M. C. (1992). Families in transition: Caring for the rural elderly. *Family Community Health, 14*(4), 61–70.

Hill, R. (1958). Generic features of families under stress. *Social Casework, 49,* 139–150.

Hooyman, N. R., & Lustbader, W. (1986). *Taking care: Supporting older people and their families.* New York: Free Press.

Horowitz, A. (1985). Family caregiving to the frail elderly. In C. Eisdorder, M. P. Lawton, & G. L. Maddox (Eds.), *Annual Review of Gerontology and Geriatrics, Vol. 5* (pp. 194–246). New York: Springer.

Johnson, C. L., & Catalano, D. J. (1981). Childless elderly and their family supports. *Gerontologist, 21,* 610–618.

Johnson, C. L., & Catalano, D. J. (1983). A longitudinal study of family supports to impaired elderly. *Gerontologist, 23,* 612–618.

Kain, J. (1990). *The myth of family decline.* New York: W. W. Norton.

Kashner, T. M., Magaziner, J., & Pruitt, S. (1990). Family size and caregiving of aged patients with hip fractures. In D. E. Biegel & A. Blum (Eds.). *Aging and caregiving: Theory, research, and policy* (pp. 184–203). Newberry Park, CA: Sage Publications.

Katzman, R. (1986). Alzheimer's disease. *New England Journal of Medicine, 314,* 964–973.

Kelley, S. K. (1993). Caregiver stress in grandparents raising grandchildren. *Image: Journal of Nursing Scholarship, 25,* 331–338.

King, D. A., Bonacci, D. D., & Wynne, L. C. (1990). Families of cognitively impaired elders: Helping adult children confront the filial crisis. *Clinical Gerontologist, 10,* 3–15.

Knight, B. G., Lutzky, S. M., & Macofsky-Urban, F. (1993). A meta-analytic review of interventions for caregiver distress: Recommendations for future research. *Gerontologist, 33,* 240–248.

Lee, G. R., & Ellithorpe, E. (1982). Intergenerational exchange and subjective well-being among the elderly. *Journal of Marriage and the Family, 44,* 217–224.

Lee, H. J. (1993). Health perceptions of middle, "new middle," and older rural adults. *Family Community Health, 16,* 19–27.

Mays, R. M. (1988). Family stress and adaptation. *Nurse Practitioner, 13*(8), 52–56.

McCubbin, H. I., & McCubbin, M. A. (1993). Families coping with illness: The resiliency model of family stress, adjustment, and adaptation. In C. B. Danielson, B. Hamel-Bissel, & P. Winstead-Fry (Eds.), *Families, health and illness: Perspectives on coping and intervention* (pp. 21–63). St. Louis, MO: C. V. Mosby.

McCubbin, H. I., & Patterson, J. M. (1983). Family Transitions: Adaptation to Stress. In H. I. McCubbin & C. R. Figley (Eds.), *Stress and the family, Vol I. Coping with normative transitions* (pp. 5–25). New York: Brunner/Mazel

Neugarten, B. L. (1968). Adult personality — toward a psychology of the life cycle. In B. L. Neugarten (Ed.), *Middle age and aging* (pp. 137–147). Chicago: University of Chicago Press.

Neundorfer, M. M. (1991a). Coping and health outcomes in spouse caregivers of persons with dementia. *Nursing Research, 40,* 261–265.

Neundorfer, M. M. (1991b). Family caregivers of the frail elderly: Impact of caregiving on their health and implications for interventions. *Family Community Health, 14,* 48–58.

O'Neill, C., & Sorenson, E. S. (1991). Home care of the elderly: A family perspective. *Advances in Nursing Science, 13*(4), 28–37.

Paveza, G. J., Cohen, D., Eisdorder, C., Freels, S., Semla, T., Ashford, J. W., Gorelick, P., Hirschman, R., Luchins, D., & Levy, P. (1992). Severe family violence and Alzheimer's disease: Prevalence and risk factors. *Gerontologist, 32,* 493–497.

Pillemer, K., & Finkelhor, D. (1988). The prevalence of elder abuse: A random sample survey. *Gerontologist, 28,* 51–57.

Pillemer, K., & Finkelhor, D. (1989). Causes of elder abuse: Caregiver stress versus problem relatives. *American Journal of Orthopsychiatry, 59,* 179–187.

Porterfield, J. D., & St. Pierre, R. (1992). *Healthful aging.* Guilford, CT: Dushkin Publishing Group.

Pratt, C. C., Schmall, V. L., Wright, S., & Cleland, M. (1985). Burden and coping strategies of caregivers to Alzheimer's patients. *Family Relations, 34,* 27–33.

Reed, P. G. (1991). Self transcendence and mental health in the oldest-old adult. *Nursing Research, 11,* 143–163.

Robinson, K. M. (1989). Aggressive behavior in persons with dementia living in the community. *Alzheimer's Disease and Associated Disorders International Journal, 2*(4), 342–355.

Ryden, M. (1988). Aggressive behavior in persons with dementia living in the community. *Alzheimer's Disease and Associated Disorders International Journal, 2*(4), 342–355.

Sayles-Cross, S. (1993). Perceptions of familial caregivers of elder adults. *Image: Journal of Nursing Scholarship, 25*(2), 88–92.

Scharlalch, A. E. (1987). Role strain in mother-daughter relationships in later life. *Gerontologist, 27*(5), 627 – 631.

Select Committee on Aging, US House of Representatives. (1987). *Exploding the myths: Caregiving in America.* Committee Publication No. 99 – 611. Washington, DC: US Government Printing Office.

Semple, S. H. (1992). Conflict in Alzheimer's caregiving families: Its dimensions and consequences. *Gerontologist, 32,* 648 – 655.

Shanas, E. (1979). The family as a social support system in old age. *Gerontologist, 19,* 3 – 9.

Steinmetz, S. K. (1988). *Duty bound: Elder abuse and family care.* Newbury Park, CA: Sage Publications.

Stoller, E. P. (1983). Parental caregiving by adult children. *Journal of Marriage and the Family, 45,* 851 – 858.

Stone, R., Cafferata, G. L., & Sangl, J. (1987). Caregivers of the frail elderly: A national profile. *Gerontologist, 27,* 616 – 626.

Townsend, A. L., & Poulshock, S. W. (1986). Intergenerational perspectives on impaired elders' support networks. *Journal of Gerontolgoy, 41,* 101 – 109.

Williams-Burgess C., & Kimball, M. J. (1990). The neglected elder: A family systems approach. *Journal of Psychosocial Nursing, 30*(10), 21 – 25.

BIBLIOGRAPHY

Archbold, P. G. (1983). The impact of parent-caring on women. *Family Relations, 32,* 39 – 45.

Cicirelli, V. G. (1981). *Helping elderly parents: The role of adult children.* Boston: Auburn.

Cohen, D., & Eisdorfer, C. (1986). *The loss of self: A family resource for the care of Alzheimer's and related disorders.* New York: W. W. Norton.

Dillehey, R. C., & Sandys, M. R. (1990). Caregivers for Alzheimer's patients: What we are learning from research. *International Journal of Aging and Human Development, 30,* 263 – 285.

Given, C. W., Collins, C. E., & Given, B. A. (1988). Sources of stress among families caring for relatives with Alzheimer's disease. *Nursing Clinics of North America, 23,* 69 – 83.

Hogstel, M. O. (1990). *Geropsychiatric nursing.* St. Louis, MO: C. V. Mosby.

Pratt, C. C., Schmall, V. L., Wright, S., & Cleland, M. (1985). Burden and coping strategies of caregivers to Alzheimer's patients. *Family Relations, 34,* 27 – 33.

Pruchno, R. A., & Potashnik, S. L. (1989). Caregiving spouses: Physical and mental health in perspective. *Journal of the American Geriatric Society, 37,* 697 – 705.

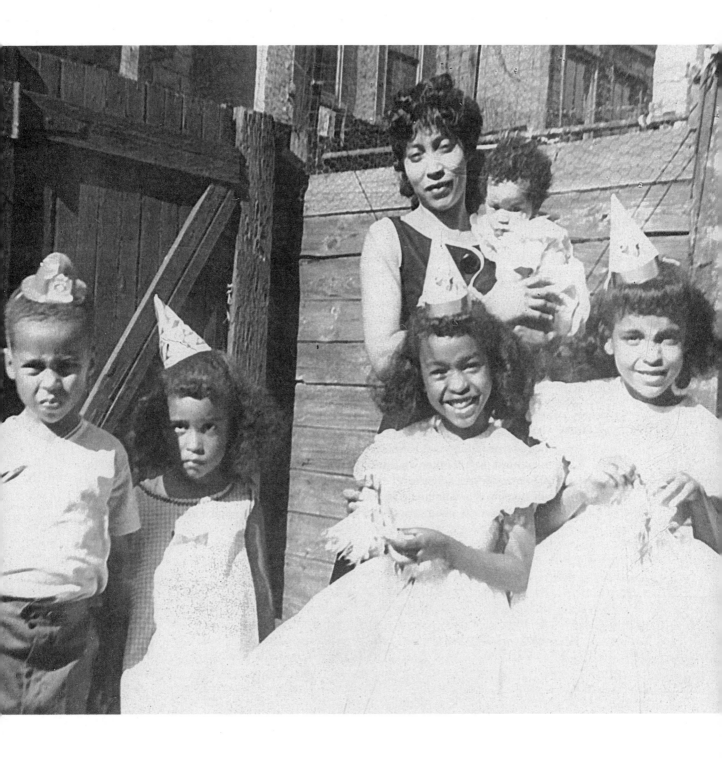

Families and Community Health Nursing

In this last clinical chapter, students have an opportunity to explore the commonalties and linkages between family nursing and community health nursing. The complementary principles of each of these practice areas are carefully described. Historical roots of the connections between family and community are explained, and their continued importance to practice is emphasized as changes in health care delivery move services out of institutions and into the community.

This chapter discusses models that provide a perspective for viewing the family as the client within the community setting. Through the use of examples, students are helped to understand these models and their usefulness to practice. The importance of prevention-focused frameworks of community health and community interventions is explored in a similar fashion.

Students are reminded that community health nurses working for public health agencies or private home health agencies, and family nurses in clinics and acute care settings, must use their knowledge of both families and communities to provide nursing care. To practice at a single level excludes a large and important area of nursing practice. Family nursing is in a unique position to bridge the gap between the individual and community and has significant contributions to make in assuring a healthy population.

CHAPTER 15

Families and Community Health Nursing

Cecelia Capuzzi, RN, PhD

OUTLINE

WHAT IS COMMUNITY HEALTH NURSING
    Community Health Nursing Roles

HISTORICAL ROOTS OF THE CARE OF FAMILIES IN COMMUNITY SETTINGS
    Community Health Nursing Today

THEORETICAL PERSPECTIVES IN FAMILY AND COMMUNITY HEALTH NURSING
    Nursing Models with the Family as the Unit of Care and the Community as Context
    Nursing Models with the Community as the Unit of Care

COMMUNITY HEALTH CONCEPTS BASIC TO THE NURSING CARE OF
FAMILIES IN THE COMMUNITY
    Strategies for Health Promotion and Disease Prevention for Families in the Community
    The Family as Client in the Community Setting
    Community as Client and Nursing Care of Families
    Acute and Chronic Illness Care for Families in the Community
    Secondary and Tertiary Prevention in Families with Acute and Chronic Illness
    Nursing Interventions for Acute and Chronic Illness When the Community Is Client

IMPLICATIONS OF COMMUNITY HEALTH NURSING FOR PRACTICE, EDUCATION,
RESEARCH, AND HEALTH CARE POLICY
    Practice
    Education
    Research
    Policy

CASE STUDY: THE YORKE FAMILY

OBJECTIVES

Upon completion of this chapter, the reader will be able to:

1. Describe the practice of community health nursing.
2. Understand the historical antecedents of family and community health nursing.
3. Understand the interface between the practices of family and community health nursing.
4. Describe selected theoretical models that guide the practice of community health family nursing.
5. Describe selected concepts from community health nursing and their application to family health.
6. Apply the concept of "levels of prevention" to family and community health.
7. Identify community health nursing interventions that promote health and that provide care for acute and chronic illnesses in families.
8. Discuss the implications of community health nursing for family nursing practice, research, education, and social policy.

Community health nurses have a long history of working with families, and they recognize that the health of individuals is intertwined with the health of families and the community. Families have a major impact on the health of individuals; for example, the family provides social support, which is both health-promoting and restoring. Likewise, the health of the family is important to the community's well-being. In fact, the health of a community is measured by the collective health of its individuals and families (e.g., the rate of low-birth-weight infants born to single mothers in a community). Lastly, the character of the community and its ability to deal with health issues influences the well-being of all who live there. This chapter describes how the principles and practice of family nursing and community health nursing are integrated to yield what might be called family-centered community nursing.

WHAT IS COMMUNITY HEALTH NURSING

The term **community** has various meanings. One meaning of the term is a geographic location such as a neighborhood, a city, or a state. "Community" can also mean an **aggregate** of people with similar characteristics, such as all people infected with HIV. The term "community" also describes groups who have a specific function — for example, a group of families with disabled children who lobby for better health services (Clark, 1992). The use of the term community in this chapter reflects all these definitions.

The practice of community health nursing includes caring for the community as a whole in addition to caring for individuals and families within the community. Community health nursing practice is:

> a synthesis of nursing practice and public health practice applied to promoting and preserving the health of populations. The practice is general and comprehensive. It is not limited to a particular age group or diagnosis and is continuing, not episodic. The dominant responsibility is to the population as a whole; nursing directed to individuals, families, or groups contributes to the health of the total population. Health promotion, health maintenance, health education and management, coordination, and continuity of care are utilized in a holistic approach to the management of the health care of individuals, families, and groups in a community (American Nurses Association, 1980, p. 2).

This definition of community health nursing suggests that the target of care is the community; the community is the client receiving care. Individuals, families, and groups are subunits of the community. It also suggests, however, that the community is a setting and that any nurse working outside an inpatient health care facility is thus a community health nurse. Nurses working in community settings direct care toward individuals, families, and groups, and the community serves as the context within which care is given. Both types of community health nursing are important to the health of families.

Community Health Nursing Roles

Working with individuals and families in the context of the community involves one set of nursing roles and interventions, while working directly with the community as a client involves others. Clark (1992) categorizes these nursing roles as (1) client-oriented, (2) delivery-oriented, and (3) group-oriented. Client-oriented roles are directed toward providing of services to clients, and they include the roles of caregiver, educator, counselor, referral source, role model, advocate, primary care provider, and case manager. Delivery-oriented roles are directed toward facilitating the operation of the health care delivery system; they indirectly enhance the care of clients. These roles include those of coordinator, collaborator, liaison, and discharge planner. Lastly, group-oriented roles are directed toward promoting the health of the population of a community, and they include the roles of case finder, leader, change agent, community care agent, and researcher. Client-oriented and delivery-oriented roles are used most frequently when providing care to individuals, families, and groups in community settings, while group-oriented roles are used when care is directed toward the community.

Not all community health nurses perform all of these roles. Often the setting and employing agency determine which roles are utilized. Nurses with baccalaureate degrees are more likely to focus on the care of individuals, families, and groups (client-oriented and delivery-oriented roles); advanced practitioners in community health nursing are more apt to focus on group-oriented roles.

HISTORICAL ROOTS OF THE CARE OF FAMILIES IN COMMUNITY SETTINGS

Initially, the focus of care in the community was on individual patients; the family was a source of care for the sick household member. Usually care was provided in the patient's home and the nurse was called a "visiting nurse." Visiting nurses were described as early as the pre-Christian eras in India, Egypt, Greece, and Rome (Gardner, 1928). Visiting nursing is documented from the eleventh to sixteenth centuries in Europe, with both secular and religious orders providing care (Rue, 1944).

In the mid-1800s, the importance of health promotion and disease prevention began to be recognized. Community health nurses, or visiting nurses, then expanded their roles to include health education as well as sick care, and in order to function effectively, they directed their care not only to the individual, but also to the family (Gardner, 1928; Rue, 1944). Recognizing that the nurse was more effective when care involved all family members, Lillian Wald, who established a home visiting service in the early 1900s, developed guidelines for nursing the family in the home (Rue, 1944; Whall, 1986).

In the early 1900s, subspecialties in community health nursing developed. Some nurses cared for mothers and infants, others cared for those with communicable diseases, and still others worked with the mentally ill. Also, community health nurses began seeing individuals in other settings besides the home, including clinics, tenements, day nurseries, schools, and industries (Spradley, 1985). In each instance, the importance of the family was recognized.

In 1912, the National Organization for Public Health Nursing (NOPHN) recommended a curriculum for community health nursing that included family nutrition and budgeting (Gardner, 1928). Later, in 1934, NOPHN reported a national survey indicating that family care was an integral component of public health nursing (Rue, 1944).

Despite these early trends, community health nurses did not fully direct their practice to the family as a unit of care until the 1950s. The family as a unit of care remained the orienting perspective for community health nurses until the 1970s (Spradley, 1985).

Community Health Nursing Today

Over the past 20 years, community health nursing has undergone a major shift, in part due to societal developments beginning in the late 1960s. First, nurses began to recognize that the entire community needs health services, not just the sick poor. Second, other nursing specialists such as home health nurses began practicing outside the hospital setting, and some of these stated that the family was their focus of practice. Third, changes in the health care delivery system began to blurr the distinctions between private, public, and nonprofit services. All of these developments led community health nurses to re-examine their scope of practice (Spradley, 1985).

Some community health nurses have redirected their care toward the **community as client**, with the family as an important subunit; others have continued to emphasize the family as the unit of service. Despite the differing viewpoints of community health nurses, knowledge about families remains an important component of community health nursing today.

THEORETICAL PERSPECTIVES IN FAMILY AND COMMUNITY HEALTH NURSING

Many theoretical perspectives on the family are available to guide community health nursing practice. Among the nursing models for families, some are based on the view that the family is the unit of care and the community is context, while others focus on the community as client and view the family as a subunit.

Nursing Models with the Family as the Unit of Care and the Community as Context

Most early nursing models focused on the individual as the recipient of care. Both family nurses and community health nurses criticized these models because they did not represent the perspective of their practice. In addition, community health nurses criticized these early models for directing care primarily toward the restoration of health rather than toward maintaining wellness. The models either did not mention the community, or they considered it part of the environment.

More recently, several of these earlier, individually focused models (e.g., those of Roy, Levine, Orem, Johnson, Rodgers, King, and Neuman) have been adapted to view the family as the unit of care and the community as context. Community health nurses working in roles that are family-oriented and who view community as context use these models.

One recent model that views the family as client in the community setting is Zerwekh's (1991) Family Caregiving Model for Public Health Nursing. This model was created on the basis of descriptions, by expert community health nurses, of home visiting activities that made a difference in the outcomes for maternal-child clients. From these descriptions, 16 competencies were identified and a model of their relationships was developed (Fig. 15–1). The center of this model is the family. The nurse's actions are aimed at encouraging family self-help through believing in the family's ability to make choices and aiding them to believe in themselves, listening to the family's needs, expanding the family's vision of choices, and feeding back reality so that the family can see patterns in their lives and the consequences of their decisions.

The first three competencies establish the foundation for family caregiving: (1) locating the family, (2) building trust, and (3) building strength. After this foundation is laid, eight encouraging self-help competencies are employed when working with families:

1. Being available
2. Mobilizing resources
3. Collaborating with other professionals
4. Resolving problems
5. Resolving crises
6. Working through emotions

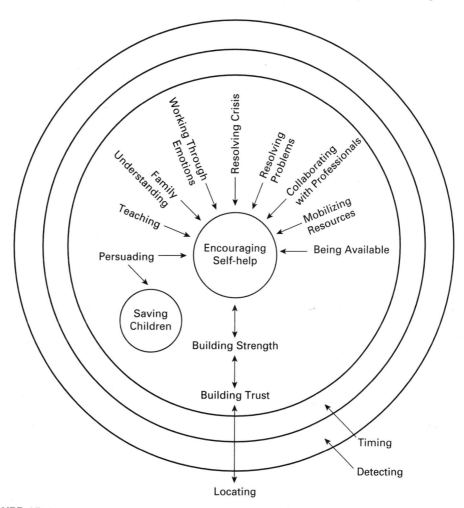

FIGURE 15–1
Zerwekh's family caregiving model for public health nursing. (From Zerwekh, JV: A family caregiving model. Nursing Outlook 1991, 39:214, with permission.)

7. Fostering family understanding

8. Teaching

Three of these competencies help to foster community: being available, mobilizing resources, and collaborating with other professionals. Thus, the model acknowledges that the community is the context for family care.

If **family self-help** cannot be achieved and the nurse finds a family member is still at risk, two additional forceful competencies are employed: (1) persuading, which includes the use of reasoning, confronting, and threatening action (for example, calling child protective services); and (2) saving the children. In these at-risk situations, the nurse's responsibility for the child (or individual at risk) becomes primary.

Two competencies are used simultaneously with the other competencies and are ongoing during the care of the family. These are called encompassing competencies. The first of these, timing, relates to the speed of introducing an intervention and has three dimensions: (1) detecting the right time to initiate the action, (2) persisting in implementing the intervention, and (3) futuring, whereby the nurse considers the present action based on a view of the future (e.g., the child's development). The second encompassing competency, detecting, uses comprehensive assessment to identify potential and actual health problems. Although Zerwekh's (1991) model needs further testing, it is an important step in providing an original model of family nursing care in the community setting.

Nursing Models with the Community as the Unit of Care

While few nursing models have been developed to describe the practice of community health nursing in which the family is the focus of care, fewer still have focused on the community as client. Several of the nursing models that have been adapted to view the family as the client also have been modified to focus on the community as client (e.g., those of Roy, Levine, Orem, Johnson, Rodgers, and King). Some community health nurses believe that the adaption of individually or family-focused nursing models is a "forced fit" and that such adaptations miss the essence of community health nursing's conceptualization of community as client (Butterfield, 1993). More consistent with the conceptualization of community as client is an approach where society is the focus of change and the improved health of families is a major outcome.

One early model that took a community health nursing perspective was created by Ruth Freeman (1970). This model has three of the basic elements thought essential in a model of community health nursing today: areas of interaction, process, and areas of responsibility (Anderson & McFarlane, 1988). Areas of interaction include the family, special populations, and the community; the process is a problem-solving method analogous to the nursing process; and areas of responsibility include nursing, public health, and health-related roles (Fig. 15–2). This model acknowledges the perspectives in which the family is client and those in which the community is client.

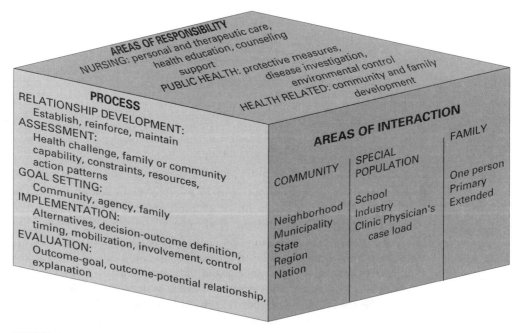

FIGURE 15–2
Freeman's model for community health nursing. (From Freeman, RB: Community Health Nursing. W.B. Saunders, Philadelphia, 1970, p. 32, with permission.)

A more recent model of community health nursing is White's (1982) Public Health Nursing Conceptual Model (Fig. 15–3). This model also includes three elements, with scope of practice being a continuum extending from individuals through families, groups, and communities. The process of public health nursing dynamics includes the nursing process and the valuing process. Practice priorities include prevention, protection, and promotion. Interventions include education, engineering, and enforcement. White's (1982) model also includes a fourth element, the determinants of health (human/biological, social, environmental, and medical/technological/organizational), which were developed by Dever (1980). **Human biology** includes physiological function, genetics, and maturational factors. The **environment** is the physical, psychological, and social context that affects health. **Lifestyle** factors include consumption, leisure, and employment. **Health-care system** factors include the availability, accessibility, and utilization of health services. Like

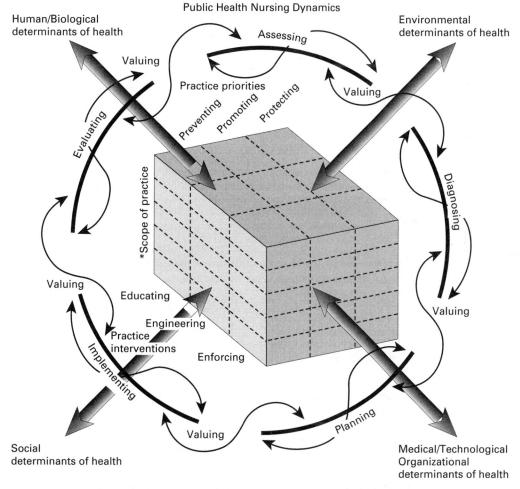

*The scope of practice is an open-ended continuum extending from individuals through such aggregates as groups, communities, and entire populations to include the entire globe.

FIGURE 15–3
White's public health nursing conceptual model. (From White, MS: Construct for public health nursing. Nursing Outlook 1982, 30:529, with permission.)

Freeman's conceptualization of community health nursing, White's model includes a focus both on the family and on the community as client.

One area in which models for community health nursing agree is that the family is important, regardless of whether the family is viewed as the client or as a subunit of the community. They also agree that the goal of community health nursing is to promote the health of all clients.

COMMUNITY HEALTH CONCEPTS BASIC TO THE NURSING CARE OF FAMILIES IN THE COMMUNITY

Several concepts basic to community health nursing have set the direction for care provided to individuals, families, groups, and communities. First, there is the concept of **health promotion**, which includes activities that improve the well-being of people (Albrecht & Swanson, 1993; Clark, 1992). An exercise class is an example of a health promotion activity (Clark, 1992). Second is **disease prevention**, which includes those activities that protect the population from diseases and disabilities and their consequences (Albrecht & Swanson, 1993; Clark, 1992). Water fluoridation and accident control programs are examples of preventive activity (Clark, 1992; Spradley, 1985).

Disease prevention occurs at three different levels: primary, secondary, and tertiary (Leavell & Clark, 1958). **Primary prevention** focuses on preventing the occurrence of health problems (e.g., through immunizations). **Secondary prevention** activities are designed to identify and treat health problems early (e.g., hypertension) and are carried out during the early stage of an acute or chronic illness. **Tertiary prevention** is aimed at correcting health problems and preventing further deterioration (e.g., by teaching diet management to diabetics) and is used with both acute or chronic illnesses.

Community health nurses use concepts from **epidemiology** to promote health and prevent disease. Epidemiology is "the study of the distribution of various states of health within the population. . ." (Clark, 1992, p. 102). An important epidemiological concept is **risk**, which refers to the probability that individuals in a community will be affected by a health problem. Community health nurses attempt to identify those individuals, families, and populations at risk for health problems using **case-finding** methods that include review of health statistics, screening programs, and contact tracing (Freeman & Heinrich, 1981).

These concepts are useful both when the family is the focus of care and when the community is client. Likewise, while the major focus of community health nursing is on health promotion and disease prevention, these concepts are applicable during the various phases of the health – illness trajectory.

Strategies for Health Promotion and Disease Prevention for Families in the Community

Many health promotion and disease prevention strategies are directed at both the family and the community. Clark (1992) outlines five categories of health promotion and disease prevention strategies: (1) health appraisal, (2) health education, (3) lifestyle modification, (4) provision of a healthy environment, and (5) development of effective coping skills. In addition, *Promoting Health/Preventing Disease: Objectives for the Nation* (US Department of Health and Human Services, 1980) suggests that (1) planning and providing health services (e.g., family planning clinics), (2) instituting health legislation and regulations, (3) offering economic incentives, and (4) developing health technology (e.g., condoms) are additional measures to promote health. While community health nurses are not usually involved in technology development, they frequently use all the other measures in the care of the family as client in the community setting and in the care of community as client (of which families are considered subunits). These strategies also can be employed in a variety of community settings (e.g., the family's home, schools, clinics).

The Family as Client in the Community Setting

An initial health-promoting and disease-preventing strategy is to conduct a health appraisal of the family and its environment to identify strengths and potential risks to health. Dever's (1980) four **determinants of health** (i.e., human biology, lifestyle, environment, and health system) provide a useful framework for systematically assessing these real and potential health risks. For example, a health history assesses aspects of human biology and lifestyles of individual family members and families as a whole. Additionally, families should be asked about their use of health care services to identify real and potential problems such as limited access to care. Increasing numbers of people are not covered by health insurance, or they are excluded from coverage because of pre-existing conditions; for these people the cost of a visit to a health professional can be a major factor limiting access to health care.

Appraisal of the family's environment is often a unique function of community health nursing. If the community health nurse is able to make a home visit, that environment can be directly observed. Likewise, the community health nurse who works in a school or occupational setting can directly appraise the effects of these environments.

An environmental appraisal includes assessment of physical, psychological, and social environments. Assessment of the physical environment of the home includes examination of safety hazards (e.g., loose rugs, absence of fire extinguishers, dangerous playground equipment), facilities for hygiene (e.g., running water, indoor plumbing), items to meet basic needs (e.g., heating, cooking facilities, refrigeration), and objects that promote social, emotional, and physical development (e.g., toys, books). A similar assessment can be applied to other settings. The neighborhood also should be assessed for safety hazards, availability of transportation, access to needed goods and services, access to recreational facilities, and the presence of environmental pollutants (Clark, 1992).

The community health nurse also appraises the family's psychological and social environment. In the home, family communication patterns, role relationships, family dynamics, emotional strengths, coping strategies, and childrearing and discipline practices can be assessed directly. Likewise, the effects of the social environment (e.g., religious practices, culture, social class, economic status, and social support system) on health can be assessed. Specific methods of assessing factors in the psychological and social environment are discussed in Chapter 4 through 7. In settings other than the home, factors that promote the psychological and social growth of individual family members also should be assessed. Texts on school health and occupational health nursing frequently contain guides for assessing these aspects of the environment.

A second community health nursing strategy to promote health and prevent disease in families is health teaching and information giving. After completing the health appraisal, the community health nurse reinforces those behaviors that are health promoting and provides health information and teaching in areas identified as risky. Again, the four determinants of health provide a useful framework for developing a health teaching plan. For example, topics such as child development and childrearing are based on normal human development (human biology).

The community health nurse uses a variety of strategies to modify risky lifestyles identified in the health appraisal. Teaching and health information can be used to discuss immunizations, nutrition, rest, exercise, use of seat belts, and abuse of harmful substances such as alcohol and drugs. The community health nurse may also refer the family to programs and resources that assist in lifestyle modifications (e.g., smoking cessation classes, exercise programs). Furthermore, the community health nurse might also promote a healthy lifestyle and influence lifestyle changes as a counselor and role model.

A fourth health promotion strategy is to provide a healthy environment. Health teaching based on appraisal of the physical environment might include information on child safety and prevention of falls. Other teaching might focus on psychological or social environmental problems such as family communications or how to deal with peer pressure. In some situations, the community health nurse promotes a healthy environment by providing information to community members outside the family. For example, community health nurses working in schools might need to inform officials about playground hazards or poor food-handling practices.

Helping families develop effective strategies for coping with stress is another health promotion strategy. The chapter on family mental health nursing discusses the effects of stress and provides detailed information on how to assist families in coping with stress. Health education, referral to community agencies, counseling, and role modeling are among the strategies used by community health nurses.

Finally, a major health promotion strategy is ensuring access to health promotion and prevention services, including immunizations, family planning, prenatal care, well-child care, nutrition, exercise classes, and dental hygiene. These services may be provided directly by the community health nurse in the home or in clinics, schools, or work settings. In some cases, the community health nurse facilitates access to these services through referrals, case management, discharge planning, advocacy, liaison, coordination, and collaboration.

Community as Client and Nursing Care of Families

When nursing care focuses on the community with the goal of promoting health and preventing disease, nurses use strategies and interventions similar to those used with families, but the strategies are refocused toward the community (e.g., health appraisal, health education). Nurses also use some additional strategies (e.g., program planning and policy development).

One strategy for promoting the health of families when the community is client is to conduct a **community assessment** (i.e., health appraisal of a community) to identify potential and actual health risks to all individuals and families living in the community. After these potential health risks are identified, the community health nurse intervenes to reduce these risk factors.

A community assessment involves collecting health and social data about the population, the social institutions (e.g., health and social services, economics, education, safety and transportation, recreation, politics and government, and communication), and the environment (physical, psychological, and social). Demographic information about the **population** provides information regarding possible health problems. For example, a community with a large population under 5 years of age might benefit from strategies aimed at increasing competence in parenting and increasing immunizations. Information on social institutions is helpful in assessing the adequacy of the community's resources. Such information can indicate whether there are enough pediatricians, whether municipal transportation is available to go to hospitals and clinics, and whether fire and emergency services are staffed for immediate response. Assessment of the environment includes evaluating the types and adequacy of sewage and water treatment, and investigating for the presence of disease-bearing insects such as the ticks that cause Lyme disease.

Methods of gathering data for a community assessment include windshield surveys, interviews with key informants, analysis of secondary data gathered by health departments such as morbidity and mortality rates, and large population surveys. A windshield survey is the motorized equivalent of simple observation. Through an automobile windshield many dimensions of a community's life and environment are carefully observed (Stanhope & Lancaster, 1984). Often the data are about families in the community—for example, the proportion of single-parent families or the number of day-care facilities. A detailed description of community assessment is beyond the the scope of this chapter. However, most community health nursing texts provide guidance for implementing a community assessment.

Once data has been collected, it is analyzed to identify the community's health problems, that is, to make "community diagnoses." An example of a **community diagnosis** is, "The children are at risk for lead poisoning due to the amount of old housing stock in the community." After community diagnoses are made, goals are developed to correct the problems and plans are made to intervene.

Thus, a second strategy for promoting the health of families in communities is **program planning** to develop needed health services identified in the community assessment. Program planning includes:

Identification of potential solutions to the problem
Analysis and comparison of alternative solutions
Selection of one program and/or solution
Development of program goals and objectives
Identification of resources
Development of the specific activities of the program
Development of methods to evaluate the program

Usually program planning involves multidisciplinary teams of health and nonhealth professionals. The community and its families also should be involved in the planning and implementation to assure that the program meets their needs. During these situations, community health nurses employ the group-oriented roles of community care agent, leader, and change agent.

Awareness of the need to design community health programs with a family-centered approach is growing. For example, in 1986, Congress passed PL 99-457, the Education for All Handicapped Children Act and mandated that services be provided to the families of children with developmental disabilities as well as to the child (Shelton, Jeppson, & Johnson, 1987). Since then, the Association for the Care of Children's Health (ACCH) has developed a definition of **family-centered care** that many other groups working with families have adapted (Korteland & Cornwell, 1991, p. 57). Figure 15-4 lists the elements of family-centered care. Community health nurses can facilitate development of health programs that are supportive to families by using these elements during program planning and implementation.

Once health programs are developed, individuals and families who can use the services need to be identified and made aware of the services. Information about health risks and preventive services can be disseminated through pamphlets, notices on community bulletin boards, and in the media.

Another intervention strategy at the community level involves health teaching and providing information to promote the health of families. Educational programs can be developed to reach large groups or even entire communities. The community assessment will provide topics for health teaching. For example, if the community assessment indi-

1. Recognition that the family is the constant in the child's life whereas service systems and personnel within those systems fluctuate.

2. Facilitation of parent-professional collaboration at all levels of health care.

3. Sharing of unbiased and complete information with parents about their child's care on an ongoing basis in an appropriate and supportive manner.

4. Implementation of appropriate policies and programs that are comprehensive and provide emotional and financial support to meet the needs of families.

5. Recognition of family strengths and individuality and respect for different methods of coping.

6. Understanding and incorporation of the developmental and emotional needs of infants, children, and adolescents and their families in health care delivery systems.

7. Encouragement and facilitation of parent-to-parent support.

8. Assurance that the design of health care delivery systems is flexible, accessible, and responsive to family needs.

9. Respect for the racial, ethnic, cultural, and socioeconomic diversity of families.

FIGURE 15–4

Elements of family-centered care. (From Korteland, C and Cornwell, JR: Evaluating family-centered programs in neonatal intensive care. Children's Health Care 1991, 20:56–61, with permission.)

cates that substance abuse is a major problem, health education about the effects of substance abuse is needed. The media and other information technologies frequently are used to provide health education at the community level. For example, local television and radio stations might broadcast educational information on substance abuse.

One final strategy for promoting health and preventing disease in communities is policy development and implementation. Community health nurses frequently interact in local and state policy arenas by alerting policy makers about the health problems in their communities. Nurses can give direct accounts of the effects these health problems have on families in the community. They can write letters, make telephone calls, testify before committees, and take part in other political activities to create awareness of the health problem. Nurses also sit on advisory boards and task forces at all levels: community, city, county, state, and national. In these positions nurses can directly influence policy to promote health and prevent disease.

Once a health problem is recognized, community health nurses work with others to propose and shape policy solutions. The community health nurse's perspective on a proposed policy's effect on families is important to the development of health proposals. Lastly, community health nurses often implement these policies to ensure optimum results for family health.

Acute and Chronic Illness Care for Families in the Community

Nursing care for families in the community who have either an acute or chronic illness involves secondary and tertiary prevention. Secondary prevention strategies include (1) early detection of health problems in families and communities, (2) **referral** for further evaluation and treatment, and (3) health teaching about the potential illness and the need for follow-up.

Tertiary prevention focuses on (1) monitoring the health problem, (2) providing treatments, (3) providing health education, and (4) promoting adjustment to the illness. Additionally, community assessment, program planning and implementation, case finding, community education, and health policy development are secondary and tertiary prevention measures. These strategies, in relation to the care of the family as client, can be carried out in a variety of community settings.

Secondary and Tertiary Prevention in Families with Acute and Chronic Illness

One secondary prevention strategy is early detection of acute or chronic illnesses. **Screening** for detection of illness is a major function of community health nurses and is accomplished through health appraisals, as described previously in this chapter, and by using screening tools and methods. Many screening procedures are available for detecting health problems in family members of all ages and in the family as a whole; these procedures and instruments are discussed in other chapters in this text.

Once community health nurses detect a health problem, they initiate appropriate nursing care and/or make referrals to nurse practitioners or physicians for medical evaluation of the condition and treatment. The community health nurse is responsible for assuring that the patient receives the needed health care.

The referral process includes identifying the need for referral, identifying appropriate health resources, preparing the client for the referral, communicating with the referral agency, and evaluating the outcome of the referral for the client (Clark, 1992). During this time, the community health nurse also provides health education and information about the significance of positive screening results and the need for follow-up and treatment of the condition. Patients vary in their ability to find and use health care resources. Clemen-Stone, Eigisti, and McGuire (1991) suggest that there are three levels of nursing intervention in the referral process. Level I patients are dependent on the nurse to identify needed health care resources, coordinate referrals, and assist the patient to use the referral services. Level II patients are moderately independent. They seek information from the nurse and may need some help in identifying resources and in completing the referral process. Level III patients are independent; after they are given information about health resources, they can complete the referral process.

One tertiary prevention strategy is to monitor the individual's physical condition. Follow-up health appraisals provide information that can be compared to the initial health appraisal data to chart progress. For example, the nurse monitors the diabetic client's blood glucose levels to determine whether the treatment is effective. Another tertiary prevention strategy is to provide nursing treatments to correct the illness and prevent further health problems. In these instances, the community health nurse provides direct patient care such as dressing changes, medication administration, and range of motion. In some communities, home health nurses employed by private agencies provide these treatments; in other communities, community health nurses from public health departments provide this care. Home health nursing is a subspecialty of community health nursing; however, home health nurses in private agencies tend to provide more intensive technological nursing care. School nurses and occupational health nurses also provide direct nursing interventions.

A third tertiary prevention strategy is to provide health teaching to the patient and the family to help them carry out prescribed treatments. The nurse also provides information about the disease and ways to prevent further problems.

A fourth tertiary prevention strategy is to assist the patient and family in coping with the illness through counseling, or to help mobilize other support resources within the family and the family's extended network, or in the community.

Nursing Interventions for Acute and Chronic Illness When the Community Is Client

Care for families with acute and chronic illnesses at the community level involves using (1) community assessment to identify significant acute and chronic health problems in the community; (2) planning and providing screening and treatment services, (3) identifying those at risk for particular acute and chronic illnesses, (4) providing community educational programs; and, in some instances, (5) developing health policy. These strategies focus on acute and chronic health problems in the community.

IMPLICATIONS OF COMMUNITY HEALTH NURSING FOR PRACTICE, EDUCATION, RESEARCH, AND HEALTH CARE POLICY

Practice

Although nurses have focused on the family unit in the community for many years, there are still many obstacles to family-centered care. First of all, nurses must have access to families in order to provide care; thus care needs to be provided in settings where families commonly reside. These include homes, the schools where younger family members spend a large portion of their day, the occupational settings where adult members are easily located, and sites where the elderly congregate.

Also, barriers to care of families in the community need to be removed. Most health agencies, even those that espouse a family focus, in reality direct care to the individual. Patient records usually contain only data about the individual. Thus family members have separate records; either family assessment data are only in one family member's record or they are duplicated in all records; or more commonly, they are not recorded at all. This fragmentation makes it difficult to view the family as a unit. In the past, there were legal constraints to recording one individual's assessment information in another's record because of confidentiality. Some agencies have not found ways to overcome this legal barrier.

Education

Nursing education needs to include a strong family orientation and a strong community orientation to enable students to understand the interplay between the health of the community and the health of families. Undergraduate students need to learn community-focused interventions that can promote the health of families; graduate students specializing in family and community health nursing need to study the theoretical perspectives of community-focused and family-focused interventions.

Research

Research is needed to identify common family health problems in the community, resources to meet family needs, and effective organization of services to promote family health and coping. Some health agencies are beginning to develop such frameworks for planning (Vahldieck, Reeves, & Schmelzer, 1989).

Research is also needed to determine which intervention strategies are most effective in promoting family health and preventing family illness. Research on the effects of home visiting on individual health problems needs to be broadened to include the effect on family problems. Moreover, specific health programs need to be evaluated to determine when these services are effective and for what types of health problems. There is little research on the effect of community-focused interventions on the health of families.

Policy

Policy-level barriers to providing family-centered care in the community include the current organization of health services and reimbursement for health care. Health services in the community frequently are not family focused but are arranged according to specific health problems (e.g., sexually transmitted diseases) or by age and/or life stage (e.g., prenatal care, teenage clinics). This occurs because funding is allocated for specific services. Such arrangements preclude the health provider from focusing on the family as a unit and force, instead, a focus on the specific health problem or life stage of the individual.

Reimbursement for health care also promotes an individual focus. Only specific health conditions or treatments are reimbursable, and furthermore, reimbursement is paid for the individual presenting the problem; most insurance does not recognize the family as a client or accept family health diagnoses. Lastly, it frequently happens that not all family members are covered by health insurance and that reimbursement is thus limited to those who are covered. To remove these barriers, there need to be health policy changes; and to effect these changes, there must be a strong nursing voice.

Case Study: The Yorke Family

The following case study describes a typical community health nursing role. The scope of activities and breadth of responsibility described here are common to many community health nurses. As you read through the case, consider the following:

What nursing models are helpful in understanding the Yorkes' situation and planning for care?

How would the care given by Catherine Parker be different if she had an individual rather than a family focus?

How do the geography of the community and the availability of resources influence the Yorkes' health?

What types of prevention strategies is Catherine Parker using in caring for the Yorkes?

Are there other strategies that would be helpful?

What actions should Catherine Parker take at the community level to improve the Yorkes' health?

Catherine Parker, RN, is a community health nurse for Monroe County Health District. She has a caseload of 50 families who live in the northwest section of the county. The health department sponsors 15 clinics a week, including clinics for prenatal care, well-child, family planning, immunizations, sexually transmitted diseases, and hypertension. Catherine works Tuesday and Thursday mornings in the prenatal care and well-child clinics. She also works with the city hospital's discharge coordinator to identify patients who need community services after leaving the hospital. Monroe County Health District's Nursing Department is responsible for providing school health services to the county's three elementary schools, two middle schools, and one high school; Catherine spends one afternoon a week at the high school. Recently, Catherine was asked to be on a task force to develop protocols for working with mothers with substance abuse; this group meets monthly. Also, the State Health Department is planning to implement a child health information tracking system and has directed each county to conduct a feasibility study. Catherine is surveying the young families in her caseload for their views on having their child's health information available to multiple health providers.

Last week when Catherine was doing discharge planning at the County Hospital, she realized that the Yorke family could use additional services and arranged a postpartum home visit. Gina Yorke, aged 23 years, delivered her fourth child 1 week ago and is now at home. Gina's husband, Rob Yorke, aged 24 years, is an unemployed logger receiving job retraining at the local community college. The other three children are aged 13 months, and 2 and 3 years old. Rob's parents live nearby. The Yorkes recently moved to Monroe and live in a rural part of the county. Gina received late prenatal care at the Monroe Health Clinic. The family lives in a rented, two-bedroom house 15 miles from town. Rob uses the only car for transportation to classes.

The Yorkes are just one of many families who live in the rural part of the county. There is no public transportation. Most families that live in this area rent their homes because it is less expensive than buying. The median family income of the people residing in this area is $12,120 a year. The mean age of the residents in this area is 25 years. Most houses have indoor plumbing with running water; the water comes from the county system. All houses have septic tanks. In the past year, three methamphetamine labs have been discovered in the area; adolescent substance abuse is a problem.

Catherine returns to visit the Yorke family for a 6-week postpartum follow-up. She weighs and measures the new baby and measures the infant's head circumference. The baby is gaining weight adequately and appears to be healthy. Gina Yorke also is feeling well and has had her 6-week checkup with the nurse midwife at the health department.

Gina mentions that the 2-year-old is not feeling well. He feels hot and has a rash on his chest. Catherine takes the child's temperature and it is 101°F. He has a runny nose and congestion in his chest. The rash on his trunk has vesicles; Catherine determines that he has varicella (chickenpox). None of the other children have had chickenpox, nor do they have any symptoms yet.

Catherine teaches Gina to take the child's temperature and discusses skin care and hygiene. She also emphasizes the importance of giving the child fluids and makes suggestions for diet. Catherine tells Gina that the child should be kept isolated from people outside the household until the vesicles are dried. If the child becomes more ill, Gina should call the doctor at the health clinic. Catherine asks Gina if any of her family can help her with the care and Gina indicates that Rob's mother is available. Catherine returns in a week to find that the family is coping well, although the other children now have caught varicella.

County health statistics indicate that there is a high incidence of lead poisoning in young children, particularly children in rural areas. It is possible that the source of lead is the water pipes since older homes have plumbing that used to be soldered with lead; also, many of these older homes were painted with lead-based paints. Nearby, there also is a factory that makes lead pipe fittings; this factory has been cited by the Environment Protection Agency for high levels of toxic waste emission.

While working in the well-child clinic Catherine Parker screens all children for high lead blood levels. Gina Yorke brings her children to this clinic for preventive care, and when the children are tested, all are found to have lead in their blood.

SUMMARY

In summary, community health nurses are concerned with the health of families and the community. The settings in which community health nurses work varies and includes public and private health agencies, schools, and occupational sites. Community health nurses utilize concepts from public health including epidemiology and prevention. Community health nurses employ a large repertoire of roles that include those that are client-oriented, delivery-oriented, and group-oriented. These roles vary according to whether the nurse is focusing on the family as the unit of care in the context of the community or focusing on the health of the community with families being a subunit. Health intervention strategies used by community health nurses include individual and family health appraisals, community assessment, health education, referral to community resources, monitoring health problems, providing treatments, coordinating care, planning and providing health services, and instituting health legislation and regulations.

STUDY QUESTIONS

1. A historical antecedent of community health nursing is:
   a. Visiting nursing
   b. Family nursing
   c. Communicable disease nursing
   d. Maternal-child nursing

2. Care of families is an important aspect of community health nursing because:
   a. It is easier to visit families in the community.
   b. The health of the family affects the health of the community.
   c. The basis for reimbursement of public health services is the family unit.
   d. Health departments are organized to provide care to the family as a unit.

3. Community health nursing models with the greatest applicability to the care of the family are those that:
   a. View the individual as a component of the family
   b. Focus on the restoration of the health of the family
   c. Focus on the development of health services to families
   d. View the interaction between the individual and family and the environment

4. A group of families living in Stanton County best describes which definition of the term "community?"

   a. An aggregate of individuals with a common function
   b. An aggregate of individuals with common characteristics
   c. A geographic setting
   d. An aggregate of individuals with a feeling of intimacy

5. The term "primary prevention" refers to those activities that:
   a. Identify early health problems and provide immediate interventions
   b. Provide illness management and prevent further disability
   c. Prevent the occurrence of health problems
   d. Improve the health of populations

6. The term "epidemiology" is defined as:
   a. The study of communicable diseases in a population, and of the environmental conditions, lifestyles, or other circumstances associated with those diseases
   b. The study of the environment and its effects on the lifestyles and the health of populations
   c. The study of the causes of illness in a population, and the means for preventing such conditions
   d. The study of the distribution of various states of health within a population, and the environmental conditions, lifestyles, or other circumstances associated with those states of health

7. Which of the following community health nursing interventions is most appropriate when viewing the community as client and the family as a subunit of the community?
   a. Educating the family about the need for immunizations
   b. Referring family members to the health department for immunizations
   c. Planning an immunization clinic for all families in the community
   d. Providing immunizations directly to all family members

REFERENCES

Albrecht, M, & Swanson, J. M. (1993). Health: A community view. In J. M. Swanson & M. Albrecht (Eds.) *Community health nursing, promoting the health of aggregates* (pp. 3–12). Philadelphia: W. B. Saunders.

American Nurses Association. (1980). *A conceptual model of community health nursing.* ANA Publication No. CH-10. Kansas City, MO: ANA

Anderson, E. T., & McFarlane, J. M. (1988). *Community as client, application of the nursing process.* Philadelphia: J. B. Lippincott.

Butterfield, P. (1993). Thinking upstream: Conceptualizing health from a population perspective. In J. M. Swanson & M. Albrecht (Eds.) *Community health nursing, promoting the health of aggregates* (pp. 68–80). Philadelphia: W. B. Saunders.

Clark, M. J. (1992). *Nursing in the community.* Norwalk, CT: Appleton & Lange.

Clemen-Stone, S., Eigisti, D. G., & McGuire, S. L. (1991). *Comprehensive family and community health nursing* (3rd ed.). St. Louis. MO: C.V. Mosby.

Cottrell, L. S. (1976). The competent community. In B. H. Kaplan, R. H. Wilson, & A. H. Leighton (Eds.). *Further explorations in social psychiatry* (pp. 195–209). New York: Basic Books.

Dever, G. E. A. (1980). *Community health analysis.* Germantown, MD: Aspen.

Freeman, R. B. (1970). *Community health nursing practice.* Philadelphia: W. B. Saunders.

Freeman, R. B., & Heinrich, J. (1981). *Community health nursing practice* (2nd ed.). Philadelphia: W. B. Saunders.

Gardner, M. S. (1928). *Public health nursing.* New York: Macmillian.

Korteland, C., & Cornwell, J. R. (1991). Evaluating family-centered programs in neonatal intensive care. *Children's Health Care, 20*(1), 56–61.

Leavell, H. R., & Clark, E. G. (1958). *Preventive medicine for the doctor in his community.* New York: McGraw-Hill.

Rue, C. B. (1944). *The public health nurse in the community.* Philadelphia: W. B. Saunders.

Shelton, T., Jeppson, E., & Johnson, B. (1987). *Family-centered care for children with special health care needs.* Washington, DC: Association for the Care of Children's Health.

Spradley, B. W. (1985). *Community health nursing, concepts and practice* (2nd ed.). Boston: Little, Brown.

Stanhope, M., & Lancaster, J. (1984). *Community Health Nursing, Process and Practice for Promoting Health.* St. Louis: Mosby.

US Department of Health and Human Services. (1980). *Promoting health/preventing disease: Objectives for the nation.* Washington, DC: Government Printing Office.

Vahldieck, R. K., Reeves, S. R., & Schmelzer, M. (1989). A framework for planning public health nursing services to families. *Public Health Nursing, 6*(2), 102–107.

Whall, A. L. (1986). The family as the unit of care in nursing: A historical review. *Public Health Nursing, 3*(4), 240–249.

White, M. S. (1982). Construct for public health nursing. *Nursing Outlook, 30*(9), 527–530.

Zerwekh, J. V. (1991). A Family Caregiving Model for Public Health Nursing. *Nursing Outlook, 39*(5), 213–217.

BIBLIOGRAPHY

Anderson, E. T., & McFarlane, J. M. (1988). *Community as client, application of the nursing process.* Philadelphia: J. B. Lippincott.

Buchanan, B. F. (1987). Human-environment interaction: A modification of the Neuman systems model for aggregates, families, and the community. *Public Health Nursing, 4*(1), 52–64.

Clark, M. J. (1992). *Nursing in the community.* Norwalk, CT: Appleton & Lange.

Lancaster, J., Lowry, L., & Lee, G. (1993). Conceptual models for community health nursing. In M. Stanhope & J. Lancaster (Eds.). *Community health nursing, process and practice for promoting health* (3rd ed., pp. 129–150). St. Louis MO: C.V. Mosby.

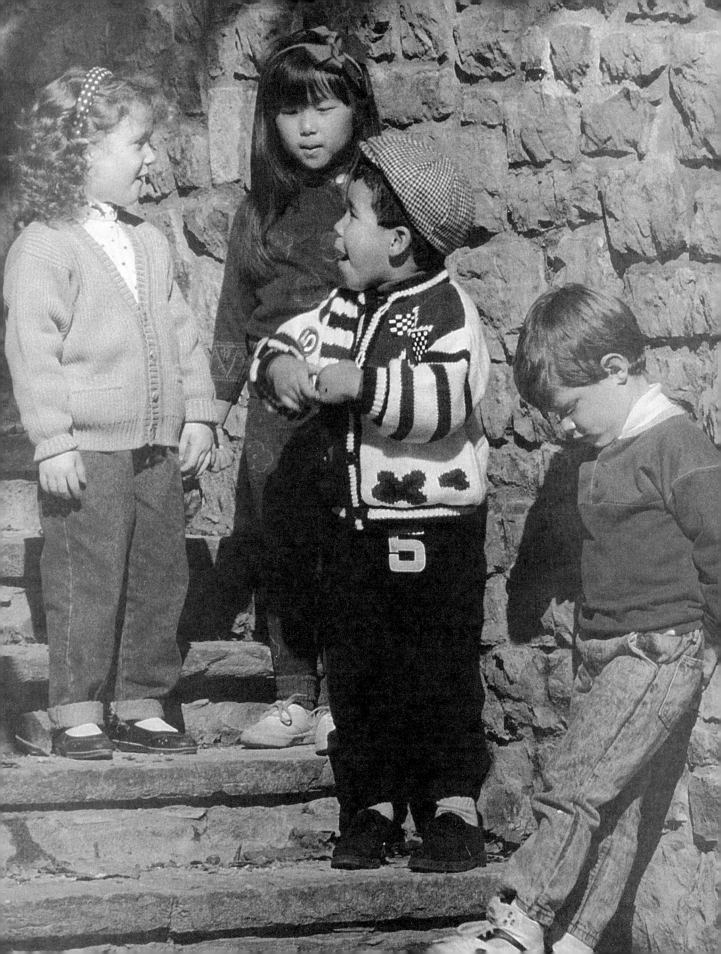

Family Nursing Practice in the Twenty-First Century

This is the final chapter in your journey into family nursing. You have become acquainted with the origins and development of family nursing, learned about the sociocultural influences on the family, and been provided with a clear discussion of the theoretical foundations of family nursing practice. The "big picture" to which you were introduced in Chapter 1 was illuminated considerably as you completed the important first section of this textbook.

The intricacies of family nursing practice in different settings became clearer as you began the second part of this text. Here the special roles of family nurses were identified and you learned about the practice of family nurses throughout the life span and in the community.

This final chapter turns to developments of the past two decades, when family nursing has emerged as a major focus of contemporary nursing practice. In the past, nursing education emphasized care of the individual; while that is still an important aspect of nursing, today an emphasis is also placed on the entire family unit, as client and as the context for care of the individual.

The development of family nursing is based on the continuing importance of families in society today and on the expectation that this role will be maintained in the future as well. The chapter and textbook close with an exploration of the future of the American family and the effects on the family of societal changes, technological advances, and changes in health care delivery systems.

CHAPTER 16

Family Nursing Practice in the Twenty-First Century

Sheryl Thalman Boyd, RN, PhD, FAAN ■
Shirley May Harmon Hanson, RN, PMHNP, PhD, FAAN

OUTLINE

THE CHANGING FAMILY
    General Characteristics of the Changing Family
    Demographic Characteristics of the Changing Family
    Social Factors Influencing the Family
    Health Care Technology
    Health Care Reform

THE FUTURE OF THEORY, PRACTICE, AND RESEARCH IN FAMILY NURSING

OBJECTIVES

Upon completion of this chapter, the reader will be able to:
1. Provide a brief overview of the social history of the American Family.
2. Describe projected demographic trends in the American family.
3. Discuss how health care reform will influence the practice of family nursing.
4. Discuss the impact of health care technology on family nursing practice.
5. Describe the impact of the changing family and social environment on the practice of family nursing, family nursing research, and theory development.

THE CHANGING FAMILY

American families have changed dramatically during the twentieth century. The nuclear family consisting of mother, father, and their children together is no longer the principal family structure; it is now just one of a multitude of well-recognized family forms that have been discussed throughout this book. Indeed, Spanier (1989) claims that "no normative family structural form exists in contemporary society . . . the dominance of a traditional familial structure has been a fictional notion throughout most of American history" (p. 4). Today we recognize that there are a variety of family forms, each of which is tenable and each of which has its own set of characteristics and qualities. As family structures have become more diverse, the education and training required for health care providers to give family care has become more complex.

General Characteristics of the Changing Family

Some believe that the family as a unit is in jeopardy. Others see the changes as part of an evolutionary process. At times, the American family has been romanticized as the unequaled foundation of positive emotional relationships and security. However, Calhoun (1960), in a classic description of the social history of the American family, provides another view, describing the eighteenth-century family as characterized by the economic and social subjugation of women, the selling of wives, the oppression of individual needs, and even infanticide. Cootz (1992) reminds us that families have always been in a state of "flux and often in crisis" (p. 2) and notes that idealizing families of previous decades discounts the strengths that families have developed in coping with a changing society. In contrast, however, Popenoe (1988; 1993) asserts that the American family is in decline and that action must be taken immediately to strengthen the institution of the family.

Whitehead (1992) and Doherty (1992), who both provide broad overviews of where family life has been and may be going, believe that American family life over the last 50 years can be divided into three distinct cultural periods. The first was called **Traditional Familism** by Whitehead and the **Institutional Family** by Doherty. This period extended from the mid-1940s to the mid-1960s and was characterized by the dominance of married couples with children, a high birthrate, a low divorce rate, and a high degree of marital stability. The period was marked by a robust economy, a rising standard of living, and an expanding middle class. Culturally, it was defined by conformity to social norms, the ideology of separate spheres for men and women, and idealization of family life. Younger adults in the postwar period tended to have strong identities and small egos. The television emblem of postwar family life was, and still is, the television show *Ozzie and Harriet*. The chief family value for this period was responsibility.

The second period was called the period of **Individualism** or the **Psychological Family**. This period extended from the mid-1960s to the mid-1980s and was characterized by greater demographic diversity, a decline in the birthrate, an accelerating divorce rate, individual and social experimentation, the breakdown of the separate spheres ideology, the creation of a singles "lifestyle," idealization of career and work life, and the search for meaning in life through self-expression. Younger adults in this period could be said to have big egos and weak identities. The emblematic television shows of this period were *The Mary Tyler Moore Show* in the 1970s and *LA Law* in the 1980s. Both programs treated work relationships and the workplace as the primary realm of intimacy, nurturing, and fulfillment. Unlike the 1940s, young children were no longer found in the work place, but instead there was a greater emphasis on their education. The chief family value for this period was satisfaction.

The third period, which we have not entered, may be termed the period of **New Familism** or the **Pluralistic Family** and has resulted largely from the fact that the baby boomers have reached adulthood and parenthood. The 1990s are characterized by a leveling off of the divorce rate, a leveling off of participation in the work force by women, and the highest number of births since 1964. Socially, it is less uptight than the first period but more uptight than the second period. It appears to be shifting away from expressive individualism and a fascination with self toward a greater attachment to family and commitment to others. We are beginning to see couples place happiness and well-being of the family above their individual desires or ambitions. A growing number of men and women are cutting back on work to devote more time to children. Women's career plans are including the time to actively participate in raising young children. These parents, who are of the baby-boom generation, have greatly influenced the media culture, reflecting new values and behaviors through television programs such as *Murphy Brown*, *Thirtysomething*, and *Life Goes On*. Flexibility and diversity are the hallmarks of this new period.

If a new family ethos is emerging, it is good news for children. There are many positive aspects to the social and cultural changes of the past 25 years: greater choice for adults, greater freedom and opportunities for women, and greater tolerance for difference and diversity. The period of the "me generation" was not altogether positive for children or families, however. The quality of the family of the future depends on whether a family ethic and family policies can be established that will help develop and maintain healthy bonds between family members in different living arrangements and between families and their communities. For example, it is critical that families in transition due to divorce are able to work through this period in such a manner as to sustain positive relationships between both parents and their children. And thus, the healthy development of the children will influence their ability to contribute to society.

Demographic Characteristics of the Changing Family

As noted in Chapter 1, the statistical profile of the American family has changed drastically over the past 20 years. If current trends endure, by the year 2000 the overall population of the United States will have grown about 7% to nearly 270 million people. By 2000, the population will increase by 6 million persons through immigration alone, with cities and states on the East and West Coasts receiving a disproportionate share of those immigrants. Average household size will decline from 2.69 in 1985 to 2.48 in 2000. The population will be older, with the median age above 37. People over age 85 years will represent about 13% of the population and the "oldest old" or the frail elderly (over 85 years of age) will have increased by about 30%. The number of children under age 5 will decline from 18 million to 17 million. By 2000, economic expansion will create 18 million new jobs. Women of all racial and ethnic groups will be the major new entrants into the job market, with women making up 47% of the workforce by 2000. Already it is estimated that nearly 65% of preschool children and 80% of school-age children have mothers who work. The occupations most likely to grow include service, professional, technical, sales, and executive and management positions (Children's Defense Fund, 1990; Public Health Service, 1990).

These changing demographics mean that a greater percentage of families will be diverse in structure and in their functioning, making it critical for the nurse to be sensitive and responsive to each unique family. For example, it has not been possible for a long time to depend on interventions which presume that two parents are in the home. Instead, the nurse must assess the structure and function of each family and adapt various approaches to family care, based on the specific and unique characteristics of the individual family. Nurses must recognize that certain family types or specific situations require greater attention because they make families more vulnerable. For example, when working with a family in which marital conflict, separation, or divorce is occurring, the nurse needs to pay special attention to parenting and the needs of the children, and to respond so as to minimize the effects of the marital problems or dissolution.

The complexity of families today and in the future demands greater collaboration among health care providers and between health care providers and other disciplines. Knowledge of resources in the community that can be drawn upon to meet the needs of families is essential. With the aging of the population, there will be greater demands on adult children to provide care to the elderly family members, and these children will have fewer siblings with whom they can share the caregiving role. The adult male within the family appears to be participating more in child care and household chores, yet women continue to have major responsibility for these roles. At the same time, more women are entering the work force and their multiple roles are often a source of stress within the family, especially for women. The role conflict and strain that result may also affect the marital relationship. Other changes in society are also putting greater demands and stresses on families. The increases in child abuse and domestic violence are symptoms of these stresses, which require broader social action and policy changes to promote the health of individuals and families.

The decline in the economic status of the family is another demographic change that gives reason for concern. According to a recent study by the US Department of Commerce, the official definition of poverty in 1992 was an income of less than $14,428 a year for a family of four (US Bureau of the Census, 1994); yet 18% of individuals with full-time jobs earned less than $13,091 in 1992. According to these figures trying to support a family on this wage is to live in poverty and thus affects health because of the difficulty of obtaining resources to meet health care needs. In addition to low wage earners, the unemployed, the uninsured or underinsured, minorities, the homeless, and undocumented individuals (those individuals who are not legally residing in the United States) are at risk for poor health care. Planning health care for these groups will continue to be a challenge in the twenty-first century. Family nurses will have the challenge of promoting health in families where health care is a scarce resource. Health care reform that will insure access to care for these populations is a significant need to which nursing must respond with active participation.

The changing ethnic makeup of the American population also creates greater challenges in promoting health in families. As Wisensale (1992) notes, "the United States is evolving into a multiracial, multicultural, and multilingual society. . . . In short, we as a nation are changing color" (p. 420). By 2000, it is estimated that the proportion of Caucasians in the total population will decrease from 76% to 72%. The proportion of Hispanics, African-Americans, American Indian and Alaska Natives, and Asians and Pacific Islanders will increase (Public Health Service, 1990). Minority families tend to be economically disadvantaged and have less access to health care. This is evident in many health outcomes related to prevention, such as teenage pregnancy rates, low-birth-weight newborns, high incidence of alcohol and drug abuse, and high incidence of family violence.

Orthner (1991) points out that many family trends are not evenly dispersed throughout society. The majority of first marriages do not end in divorce, the vast majority of families do not experience child abuse or domestic violence; and most teenage girls do not get pregnant. It is important to recognize that certain families are more vulnerable than others and their health care needs may be greater. Nurses need to target interventions to those families and individuals who are at high risk, and better assessment of families is a major step in identification of families at risk.

Social Factors Influencing the Family

Religious institutions have a major impact on families and the health practices of families. Many of the traditions of family life are closely tied with religious ceremonies, including weddings, births, passing into adulthood, and healing rituals. Families have passed these practices on from generation to generation. Also, many families find spiritual sources of strength, meaning, and assistance when they are experiencing hardship and are helped by using such strategies as prayer, becoming more involved in religious activities, and developing greater faith (Burr, Day, & Bahr, 1993). Further, religion has been recognized as playing an important role in the mental health of individuals and families, in their outlook on life, and in their lifestyle (Fong & Sandhu, 1993). Family nurses need to be aware of families' religious practices. Because of the diversity of such practices within even small communities today, nurses will encounter various religious or spiritual customs that may influence families' responses to health care practices.

The change in sexual moves is another element affecting the family today. With the sexual revolution of the late 1960s and 1970s, brought about by the development of the birth control pill, premarital sexual behavior became more common and cohabitation became an accepted form of family life. Births to unmarried women have increased over the past decade. For example, the percentage of births to unmarried women between the ages of 15 and 44 increased from 18.4% of all births in 1980 to 24.5% in 1987 (US Bureau of the Census, 1990).

Today, the threat of acquired immunodeficiency syndrome (AIDS) has heightened awareness of the danger of random sexual activity. However, it is too early to analyze the effects of AIDS on the sexual expression of Americans or to say whether the sexual revolution is truly over.

Health Care Technology

The complexity of health care practice has increased significantly in the past two decades as a result of advances in technology. With ongoing technological development, health care will continue to see rapid changes. It will be the challenge of family nurses to continue providing personalized care with high-touch delivery to family members as a balance to the dehumanization that can occur with highly technical patient care.

Changes in technology have not only increased the complexity of health care, but have also changed the nature of nursing practice in acute care settings and in the home. Patients today stay in the hospital for much shorter periods of time and return to their homes while still requiring care. Thus the family must either provide the care or ensure that appropriate providers come into the home for follow-up care. Practice is also changing due to the use of computers. For example, the creation of minimum data sets, which include data on assessments, interventions, referrals, follow-up, and so forth can be used in tracking the delivery of care and thus, planning effective health care to families.

The use of videotechnology and satellite telecommunication systems is relatively new. One of the major uses today is for health education, both basic education and continuing education. Nurses in rural areas are receiving continuing education or are able to pursue advanced degrees via educational video networks. Patient care via telecommunications systems is becoming more common, primarily through consultation with experts via interactive video.

Health Care Reform

Health care reform is a major issue in America today. Many questions are being asked: Does every person have the right to health care? What does universal access really mean? How will individuals pay for their health insurance? If the individual does not pay, who should pay for health care? Should there be a standard-benefit health insurance package to which every individual has a right? The rising cost of health care has made it impossible to ignore these issues any longer. Nearly all the states, as well as the federal government, are examining the funding and delivery of health care. Already we are beginning to see the emergence of managed care as a primary mode of organizing health care delivery. In a managed care system, insurance companies contract with selected health care providers to furnish a comprehensive set of health care services to individuals who are enrolled in an insurance program with a predetermined monthly premium (Iglehart, 1992). Participants in managed care systems generally have a primary care provider, and there are financial incentives for patients to use the providers and facilities associated with the plan in which they are enrolled. As managed care plans are emerging, variations in the mode of operation are developing, such as the health care providers to be included and the services to be covered. The role of public health departments, which have been the primary providers of health care to poor families in many areas of the country, is also changing. In some instances, public clinics are becoming part of managed care health plans. Many of these decisions regarding the delivery and funding of health care are being made at the community level. It is critical that nurses participate in the decision making and advocate the role of nursing in future health care systems.

Nurses who receive third-party reimbursement must continue to be visionary in guiding their practice to insure that they are included in managed care plans. As primary care providers, nurses who practice from a family nursing perspective will have an advantage in managing the health care of their patients. Understanding the dynamics of families and involving all family members in health care will be an advantage. Although the numbers of nurses graduating with advanced degrees have increased markedly during the past 20 years, there are still insufficient numbers of primary care nurses and of nurses with a sound foundation in family nursing practice.

In order to have an impact on health care delivery, nurses need to become active at every level of the political system and to advocate for family issues. Voting is no longer enough. Nurses must get to know the political candidates and elected officials in their cities, districts, and states, attend campaign events, write letters on health care issues from a nursing perspective, offer assistance in analyzing issues related to health care reform, and volunteer to serve on local or state commissions or boards related to health.

The challenge today is to establish health care systems in which these are opportunities for nurses to work with families as well as individuals. With the rising cost of health care and attempts to get these cost under control, budgets are under constant scrutiny. It is essential that family nurses demonstrate through practice and research the benefits of family health care. Vosburgh and Simpson (1993) have reported that families respond positively to nurses practicing with a family nurse perspective. Additional studies are needed to examine the effectiveness of family nursing practice.

Nurses must help families meet the developmental and situational transitions in life. One aim for the future must be to develop "family hardiness," or the ability to internalize a sense of control, a sense of meaningfulness in life, and a commitment to explore new challenges (McCubbin, McCubbin, & Thompson, 1987). Nurses must not only provide the physical care that individual family members need but also incorporate counseling and health promotion and prevention at every contact with the client. In the twenty-first century, we can no longer afford to overlook the family's role in health protection and promotion. The health care system must view the family as a significant influence on health care outcomes.

The changes in health care that are on the horizon mean that families must become better educated with regard to health care services in order to understand their rights and the options available to them. More than ever, families will need to become adept at participating in the decisions that will affect their health. For their part, nurses need to acquire the knowledge and skills to empower families, including the ability to participate in community organizing, coalition building, and other political activities (Williams, 1989).

THE FUTURE OF THEORY, PRACTICE, AND RESEARCH IN FAMILY NURSING

The vast changes occurring within health care today make it essential to integrate theory, practice, and research in family health care. Research must expand the knowledge base of family nursing practice and clinical decision making. Also, practice models need to be continually tested in order to improve family health care. Models of practice need to be adaptable to variations in family forms and to diverse family cultures and ethnic backgrounds. The definition of family is critical in this. For example, the definition of the family affects health insurance coverage, access to children's school and medical records, and eligibility for public assistance programs.

Most existing theoretical and conceptual models do not provide insight into cultural differences (Dilworth-Anderson, Burton, & Turner, 1993), so that a major challenge in developing models for family nursing practice is becoming more sensitive to and more knowledgeable concerning cultural and ethnic factors. This will require family nursing researchers to become more aware of their own values and to see how these affect their conceptualization and design of research.

Family nursing practice has evolved along with the changes in families and in society. Understanding the strengths and weaknesses of families in today's society will help the nurse to assess and intervene with families. Fine (1992) has identified the strengths and weaknesses of families today (Table 16–1): families are more diverse and have become more durable and resilient; yet the speed and extent of change have also left families confused about their roles and less prepared to socialize their children. As nurses work with families, awareness of social trends and their impact on the family is critical in helping families as they interact within society.

In addition to improving practice, an aim of nursing research is to influence policy development that will affect the health care of families. Zimmerman (1992) believes that family policy must take into consideration factors that influence outcomes, such as race and social class, in order to "make the playing field more even so that all families, regardless of type and however defined, have a chance to acquire their fair share of well-being" (p. 429). It is also important to take into consideration the similarities of families. As Fine (1993) notes, "Without examining such similarities, we may erroneously conclude that different types of families are more distinct than they actually are" (p. 236). In addition, research must identify and examine major social trends and thereby lead to specific policy recommendations to address those trends (Wisensale, 1992). Studies must be designed to include those issues which are of significance to decision makers. For example, the results of an intervention study will be much more relevant to a legislator if cost analysis is included in the design of the study.

Family nursing research needs to continue utilizing a variety of approaches as researchers add to the scientific knowledge base of family nursing. A variety of both qualitative and quantitative research methods are needed to examine family relationships and

TABLE 16–1

STRENGTHS AND WEAKNESSES OF FAMILY LIFE IN THE UNITED STATES

Strengths	Weaknesses
Durability	Socialization role of children
Diversity	Role confusion
Resilience	Individualism
	Lack of paternal involvement

SOURCE: Adapted from "Families in the United States: Their Current Status and Future Prospects," by M. A. Fine, 1992, *Family Relations*, 41.

family interactions with the health care system. Research that uses multiple methods of studying specific family variables is needed to gain a better understanding of the family and of health care interventions with families. As the family changes in structure and function, so changes the conceptualization of the family within nursing research.

Family nursing research is still in its infancy. Additional experimentation with research methods and approaches is needed — including methods such as observation and self-reporting, quantitative and qualitative studies, retrospective and prospective studies, case studies, and group sampling. Use of a variety of analysis techniques is also imperative if we are to build a strong foundation for family nursing science. When studies are consistent in their findings, using a variety of designs and methodologies, the results develop greater meaning and become more widely accepted.

Dissemination of research findings has long been an integral part of the nursing research process. However, nurses have generally taken this to mean simply publication in a professional journal. The future of family nursing research calls for an additional step. Research needs to be interpreted for policy-making bodies and the lay public. A vital role for the family nurses of the future is to communicate directly with the lay public on family health promotion. The future of family nursing depends on well-educated and dedicated nurses who are committed to providing nursing care that considers the family as a primary factor in health care.

STUDY QUESTIONS

1. What do you see as the future for the family? Describe the rationale for your response.

2. Match the cultural periods of the modern American family with its typical characteristics.

   a. Traditional Family
   b. Individualism
   c. New Familism

   1. Leveling off of divorce
   2. High birthrates
   3. High degree of marital stability
   4. Decline in birthrates
   5. Increased flexibility

3. Discuss the relationship between economic status and health care.

4. Describe the health care reform efforts within the state in which you are living.

5. Identify three ways in which a family nurse can affect health care policy.

6. Managed care implies that:
   a. All individuals will receive health care
   b. Individuals will not be able to choose their health care provider
   c. There are financial incentives for the patient to use specific facilities
   d. None of the above

7. Identify three ways in which technology has affected the practice of nursing.

8. Current trends indicate that families of the future will be:
   a. More diverse

b. Angrier due to change

c. Less prepared to cope with change

d. More prepared in the socialization role of their children

REFERENCES

Burr, W. A., Day, R. D., & Bahr, K. S. (1993). *Family Science*. Pacific Grove, CA: Brooks/Cole Publishing Company.

Calhoun, A. W. (1960). *A social history of the American family*. New York: Barnes & Noble.

Children's Defense Fund. (1990). *Children 1990: A report card, briefing book and action primer*. Washington, DC: Children's Defense Fund.

Coontz, S. (1992). *The way we never were: American families and the nostalgia trap*. New York: Basic Books.

Dilworth-Anderson, P., Burton, L. M., & Turner, W. L. (1993). The importance of values in the study of culturally diverse families. *Family Relations, 42,* 238–242.

Doherty, W. J. (1992). Private lives, public values: The new pluralism. *Psychology Today, 25*(3), 32–37, 82.

Ferketich, S. L., & Mercer, R. T. (1992). Focus on psychometrics: Aggregating family data. *Research in Nursing and Health,* 313–317.

Fine, M. A. (1992). Families in the United States: Their current status and future prospects. *Family Relations, 41,* 430–435.

Fine, M. A. (1993). Current approaches to understanding family diversity. *Family Relations, 42,* 235–237.

Fong, L., & Sandhu, D. (1993). Religion and the family in a global context. In K. Altergott (Ed.), *One world, many families*. Minneapolis, MN: National Council on Family Relations, 56–60.

Iglehart, J. K. (1992). The American health care system: Managed care. *New England Journal of Medicine, 327,* 742–747.

McCubbin, H. I., McCubbin, M. A., & Thompson, A. (1987). FHI: The Family Hardiness Index. In H. I. McCubbin & A. Thompson (Eds.), *Family assessment inventories for research and practice*. Madison: University of Wisconsin Press.

Orthner, D. (1991). The family in transition. In D. Blankenhorn, S. Bayme, & J. Elshtain (Eds.), *Rebuilding the nest: A new commitment to the American family* (pp. 93–118). Milwaukee, WI: Family Service America.

Popenoe, D. (1988). *Disturbing the nest: Family change and decline in modern societies*. New York: Aldine de Gruyter.

Popenoe, D. (1993). American family decline, 1960–1990: A review and appraisal. *Journal of Marriage and the Family, 55,* 527–555.

Spanier, G. B. (1989). Bequeathing family continuity. *Journal of Marriage and the Family, 51,* 3–13.

US Bureau of the Census. (1990). *Statistical abstracts of the United States, 1990*. Washington, DC: US Government Printing Office.

US Bureau of the Census. (1994). *The earnings ladder*. Washington, DC: US Department of Commerce.

US Public Health Service, US Department of Health and Human Services. (1990). *Healthy people 2000: National health promotion and disease prevention objectives* (DHHS Pub. No. [PHS]91-50212). Washington, DC: US Government Printing Office.

Vosburgh, D., & Simpson, P. (1993). Linking family theory and practice: A family nursing program. *Image: Journal of Nursing Scholarship. 25(3),* 231–235.

Whitehead, B. D. (1992). A New familism? *Family Affairs, 5*(1–2), 1–5.

Williams, D. M. (1989). Political theory and individualistic health promotion. *Advances in Nursing Science, 12,* 14–25.

Wisensale, S. K. (1992). Toward the 21st century: Family change and public policy. *Family Relations, 41,* 417–422.

Zimmerman, S.L. (1992). Family trends: What implications for family policy? *Family Relations, 41,* 423–429.

BIBLIOGRAPHY

American Nurses Association Cabinet on Nursing Research. (1985). *Directions for nursing research: Toward the twenty-first century*. St. Louis, MO: American Nurses Association.

Altergott, K. (Ed.). *One world, many families*. Minneapolis, MN: National Council of Family Relations.

Aydelotte, M. K. (1987). Nursing's preferred future. *Nursing Outlook, 35,* 114–120.

Barnum, B. (Ed.). (1989). Trends in the nineties. *Nursing and Health Care, 10,* 1–50.

Bender, D. L., & Leone, B. (Eds.). *The family in America: Opposing viewpoints*. San Diego, CA: Greenhaven Press.

Dail, P. W., & Jewson, R. H. (Eds.) (1986). *In praise of fifty years: The Groves Conference on the Conservation of Marriage and Family*. Lake Hills, IA: Graphic Publishing.

Glick., P. C. (1988). Fifty years of family demography: A record of social change. *Journal of Marriage and the Family, 50,* 861 - 873.

Hareven, T. (1982). American families in transition: Historical perspectives on change. In F. Walsh (Ed.), *Normal family process* (pp. 446 - 465). New York: Guilford.

Kirkendall, L. A., & Gravatt, A. E. (Eds.). (1984). *Marriage and the family in the year 2020.* New York: Prometheus Books.

Levine, M. O., Carey, W. B., Crocker, A. L., & Gross, R. T. (1983). Traditional and alternative family life styles. In M. O. Levine, W. B. Carey, A. L. Crocker, & R. T. Gross (Eds.), *Developmental behavioral pediatrics* (pp. 193 - 208). Philadelphia: W. B. Saunders.

Norton, A. J., & Moorman, J. E. (1987). Current trends in marriage and divorce among American women. *Journal of Marriage and the Family, 49,* 483 - 497.

Popenoe, D. (1989). The family transformed. *Family Affairs, 2* (2 - 3), 1 - 15.

Price, S., & Elliott, B. (Eds.). *Vision 2010: Families & health care.* Minneapolis, MN: National Council on Family Relations.

Scanzoni, J. (1983). *Shaping tomorrow's family: Theory and policy for the 21st century.* Beverly Hills, CA: Sage Publications.

Schneider, J. A. (1986). Rewriting the SES: Demographic patterns and divorcing families. *Social Science and Medicine, 23,* 211 - 222.

Sprey, J. (1988). Current theorizing on the family: An appraisal. *Journal of Marriage and the Family, 50,* 875 - 890.

US Bureau of the Census. (1987). Monthly vital statistics report. *Advance report of final divorce statistics, 1985.* Washington, DC: US Government Printing Office.

US Bureau of the Census. (1988). Current population reports, Series p-70, No. 13. *Who's helping out: Support work among American families.* Washington, DC: US Government Printing Office.

US Bureau of the Census. (1989). Current population reports, Series p-25, No. 1018. *Projections of the population of the United States by age, sex, and race: 1988 to 2080.* Washington, DC: US Government Printing Office.

US Bureau of the Census. (1989). Current population reports, Series p-60, No. 163. *Poverty in the United States: 1987 and earlier.* Washington, DC: US Government Printing Office.

US Bureau of the Census. (1989). Current population reports, Series p-23, No. 162. *Studies in marriage and the family.* Washington, DC: US Government Printing Office.

US Bureau of the Census. (1989). Current population reports, Series p-20, No. 445. *Marital status and living arrangements: March 1989.* Washington, DC: US Government Printing Office.

US Bureau of the Census. (1991). Current population reports, Series p-60, No. 173. *Child support and alimony: 1989.* Washington, DC: US Government Printing Office.

US Bureau of the Census. (1991). Current population reports, Series p-20, No. 461. *Marital status and living arrangements: March 1991.* Washington, DC: US Government Printing Office.

US Bureau of the Census. (1992). Current population reports, Series p-20, No. 458. *Household and family characteristics: 1991.* Washington, DC: US Government Printing Office.

Zigler, E., & Black, K. B. (1989). America's family support movement: Strengths and limitations. *American Journal of Orthopsychiatry, 59,* 6 - 19.

National Resource List for Family Nursing

Academy of Family Mediators
P.O. Box 10501
Eugene, OR 97440-2507

Active Parenting
810 Franklin Court, Suite B
Marietta, GA 30067

Administration on Aging
330 Independence Avenue SW
Washington, DC 20201

Adoptive Families of America
3333 Highway 100 N
Minneapolis, MN 55422

Age Base Directory of Health Promotion Programs for Older Adults
Brookdale Foundation Group
126 East 56th Street, 10th Floor
New York, NY 10022

AIDS Hotline
For information about AIDS or about caring for a person with AIDS. 1-800-342-AIDS. The Spanish hotline is 1-800-344-7432. The deaf access hotline is 1-800-AIDS-TTY.

AIDS Public Education Program
1730 E Street NW
Washington, DC 20006

Al-Anon/Alateen
1372 Broadway
New York, NY 10018

Alcoholics Anonymous
P.O. Box 459
Grand Central Station
New York, NY 10163

Alliance of Information and Referral Systems
P.O. Box 3546
Joliet, IL 60434

Alliance for Justice
600 New Jersey Avenue NW
Washington, DC 20001

Alzheimer's Association
70 East Lake Street, Suite 600
Chicago, IL 60601

America Responds to AIDS
P.O. Box 69003
Rockville, MD 20850

American Academy of Pediatrics
P.O. Box 927
141 Northwest Point Boulevard
Elk Grove Village, IL 60009-0927

American Association for Geriatric Psychiatry
P.O. Box 376-A
Greenbelt, MD 20768

American Association of Homes for the Aging
1129 20th Street NW, Suite 400
Washington, DC 20036

American Association for Protecting Children
c/o American Humane Association
9725 East Hampton Avenue
Denver, CO 80231

American Association of Retired Persons
601 E Street NW
Washington, DC 20049

American Association of Suicidology
Central Office
2459 South Ash Street
Denver, CO 80222

American Bar Association
Division for Communications and Public Affairs
750 Lake Shore Drive, 8th Floor
Chicago, IL 60611

American Bar Association
Division on the Mentally Disabled
1800 M Street NW, Suite 200
Washington, DC, 20036

American Cancer Society
1599 Clifton Road
Atlanta, GA 30329-4251

American Civil Liberties Union
1232 West 43rd Street
New York, NY 10036

American Diabetes Association
P.O. Box 25757
1660 Duke Street
Alexandria, VA 22314

American Divorce Association for Men
1008 White Oak Street
Arlington Heights, IL 60005

American Family Society
P.O. Box 80
Rockville, MD 20851

American Geriatric Society
770 Lexington Avenue, Suite 400
New York, NY 10021

American Guidance Service
P.O. Box 99
4201 Woodland Road
Circle Pines, MN 55014-1796

American Health Care Association
1201 L Street NW
Washington, DC 20005

American Heart Association
7272 Greenville Avenue
Dallas, TX 75231

American Lung Association
1740 Broadway
New York, NY 10019

American Society on Aging
833 Market Street, Suite 512
San Francisco, CA 94103

Arthritis Foundation
1314 Spring Street NW
Atlanta, GA 30309

Association of African American People's Legal Council
P.O. Box 20053
Detroit, MI 48220

Association for the Care of Children's Health (ACCH)
7910 Woodmont Avenue
Suite 300
Bethesda, MD 20814

Association for Couples in Marriage Enrichment
P.O. Box 10596
Winston-Salem, NC 27108

Association for Retarded Citizens
P.O. Box 6109
Arlington, TX 76005

Association of Trial Lawyers of America
1050 31st Street NW
Washington, DC 20007

Association of Women's Health, Obstetric, and Neonatal Nurses (AWHONN)
700 14th Street NW
Washington, DC 20005-2019

Candlelighters Childhood Cancer Foundation
7910 Woodmont Avenue, Suite 460
Bethesda, MD 20814

Center for Constitutional Rights
666 Broadway, 7th Floor
New York, NY 10012

Center for Family Resources
384 Clinton Street
Hempstead, NY 11550

Center on Human Policy
724 Comstock Avenue
Syracuse, NY 13244-4230

Center for Public Representation
520 University Avenue
Madison, WI 53703

Child Care Law Center
22 Second Street, 5th Floor
San Francisco, CA 94105

Children's Defense Fund
122 C Street NW
Washington, DC 20001

Children's Healthcare Is a Legal Duty (CHILD)
P.O. Box 2604
Sioux City, IA 51106

Clearinghouse on Child Abuse and Neglect Information
P.O. Box 1182
Washington, DC 20013

Commission on Legal Problems of the Elderly
1800 M Street NW
Washington, DC 20036

Compassionate Friends
P.O. Box 3696
Oak Brook, IL 60522-3696

Council for Exceptional Children
1920 Association Drive
Reston, VA 22091

Cystic Fibrosis Foundation
6931 Arlington Road
Bethesda, MD 20814

Directory of Aging Resources
951 Pershing Drive
Silver Springs, MD 20910-4464

Epilepsy Foundation of America
4351 Garden City Drive
Landover, MD 20785

**Familial Alzheimer's Disease
  Research Foundation**
8177 South Harvard, Suite 114
Tulsa, OK 74137

Family Resource Coalition
200 South Michigan Avenue, Suite 1520
Chicago, IL 60604

Family Service America
11700 West Lake Park Drive
Milwaukee, WI 53224

Foundation for Critical Care
P.O. Box 65955
Washington, DC 20035

Foundation for Hospice and Homecare
519 C Street NW, Suite 350
Washington, DC 20005

Gates Family Support
2377 O'Brien SW
Grand Rapids, MI 49504

**Grandparents United for Children's
  Rights**
Executive Headquarters
137 Larkin Street
Madison, WI 53705

Gray Panthers
311 South Juniper Street, Suite 601
Philadelphia, PA 19107

Health Ministries Association
2427 Country Lane
Poland, OH 44514

Health Resources for Older Women
National Institute on Aging
9000 Rockville Drive
Bethesda, MD 20489

Help for Incontinent People
P.O. Box 544
Union, SC 29379

**Helping Other Parents in Normal Grieving
  (HOPING)**
Edward Sparrow Hospital
1215 East Michigan Avenue
Lansing, MI 48909

Huntington's Disease Society of America
140 West 22nd Street, 6th Floor
New York, NY 10011

**Information Center for Individuals
  with Disabilities**
20 Park Plaza, Room 330
Boston, MA 02116

**International Childbirth Education
  Association (ICEA)**
P.O. Box 20048
Minneapolis, MN 55420

International Marriage Encounter
955 Lake Drive
St. Paul, MN 55120

Interpersonal Communications Programs
7201 South Broadway
Littleton, CO

Juvenile Diabetes Foundation
432 Park Avenue
New York, NY 10016

Legal Advocates for Women
320 Clement Street
San Francisco, CA 94118

Make-A-Wish Foundation of America
2600 North Central Avenue, Suite 936
Phoenix, AZ 85004

**March of Dimes Birth Defects
  Foundation**
1275 Mamaroneck Avenue
White Plains, NY 10605

**Maternal and Child Health Bureau (1992,
  March).**
  *MCH program interchange: Focus on
school health.* Washington, DC: National Center
for Education in Maternal and Child Health.

Mended Hearts
7320 Greenville Avenue
Dallas, TX 75231

Mental Health Directory
Older Adult Services
Indiana Mental Health Division
402 Washington
Indianapolis, IN 46204-3647

Military Family Clearinghouse
4015 Wilson Boulevard, Suite 903
Arlington, VA 22203-5190

Mothers Against Drunk Driving
511 East John Carpenter Freeway, Suite 700
Irving, TX 75062

Mothers of AIDS Patients
c/o Barbara Peabody
3403 E Street
San Diego, CA 92102

Muscular Dystrophy Association
810 Seventh Avenue
New York, NY 10019

Narcotics Anonymous
NA World Service Office
P.O. Box 622
Sun Valley, CA 91352

National Alliance for the Mentally Ill
1901 Fort Meyer Drive, Suite 500
Arlington, VA 22209

National Association of Anorexia Nervosa and Associated Disorders
P.O. Box 7
Highland Park, IL 60035

National Association for the Education of Young Children (NAEYC)
1509 16th Street NW
Washington, DC 20036-1426

National Association for Home Care
519 C Street NE
Stanton Park
Washington, DC 20002

National Association of Private Geriatric Care Managers
P.O. Box 6920
Yorkville Station
New York, NY 10128

National Black Child Development Institute
1023 15th Street NW, Suite 600
Washington, DC 20005

National Child Abuse Hotline
800 – 422 – 4453

National Citizens Coalition for Nursing Home Reform
1424 16th Street NW, Suite L2
Washington, DC 20036

National Clearinghouse on Marital and Date Rape
2325 Oak Street
Berkeley, CA 94708

National Coalition on AIDS and Families
c/o Marriage and Family Therapy Program
008 Slocum Hall
Syracuse University
Syracuse, NY 13244-1250

National Committee for Prevention of Child Abuse
332 South Michigan Avenue, Suite 950
Chicago, IL 60604-4357

National Council on Aging
600 Maryland Avenue SW
West Wing, Suite 100
Washington, DC 20036

National Council for Children's Rights
2001 O Street NW
Washington, DC 20036

National Council on Family Relations (NCFR)
3989 Central Avenue NE, Suite 550
Minneapolis, MN 55421

National Directory for Eldercare Information and Referral
National Association of Area Agencies on Aging
1112 16th Street NW, Suite 100
Washington, DC 20036

National Down Syndrome Congress
1605 Chantilly Dr.
Suite 250
Atlanta, GA 30324

National Down Syndrome Society
141 Fifth Avenue
New York, NY 10010

National Easter Seal Society
2023 West Ogden Avenue
Chicago, IL 60612

National Hospice Organization
1901 North Moore Drive, Suite 901
Arlington, VA 22209

National Information Center for Children and Youth With Disabilities
P.O. Box 1492
Washington, DC 20013-1492

National Institute on Aging
National Institutes of Health
7550 Wisconsin Avenue, Room 618
Bethesda, MD 20892

National Institute of Mental Health
Mental Disorders of Aging Branch
5600 Fishers Lane, Room 11C-03
Rockville, MD 20857

National Institute of Neurological Disorders and Stroke
Office of Scientific and Health Reports
National Institutes of Health
Building 31, Room 8A-06
Bethesda, MD 20892

National Kidney Foundation
30 East Third Street
New York, NY 10016

National Mental Health Association
1021 Prince Street
Alexandria, VA 22314-2971

National Parish Nurse Resource Center
1800 Dempster Street
Park Ridge, IL 61068

National Self-Help Clearinghouse
25 West 43rd Street, Room 620
New York, NY 10036

National Senior Citizens Law Center
2025 M Street NW, Suite 400
Washington, DC 20036

National Stroke Association
300 East Hampden Avenue, Suite 240
Englewood, CO 80110-2622

Native American Community Board
P.O. Box 572
Lake Andes, SD 57356-0572

North American Council on Adoptable Children
1821 University Avenue, Suite N-498
St. Paul, MN 55104

Older Women's League
720 11th Street NW, Suite
Washington, DC 20001

Parents Anonymous
520 South LaFayette Park Place, Suite 316
Los Angeles, CA 90057

Parents of Murdered Children
100 East Eighth Street, Suite B-41
Cincinnati, OH 45202

Parents United
P.O. Box 952
San Jose, CA 95108

Parents Without Partners
8807 Colesville Road
Silver Springs, MD 20910

Pritchet & Hull Associates
3440 Oakcliff Road NE, Suite 110
Atlanta, GA 30340-3079

The Samaritans
500 Commonwealth Avenue
Boston, MA 02215

School-Age Child Care Project
Wellesley College
Center for Research on Women
Wellesley, MA 02181

SHARE
St. Elizabeth's Hospital
21 South Third Street
Belleville, IL 62222

Stepfamily Association of America
215 Centennial Mall S, Suite 212
Lincoln, NE 68508

Stepfamily Association of America
602 East Joppa Road
Baltimore, MD 21204

Sudden Infant Death Syndrome Alliance
10500 Little Patuxent Parkway, Suite 420
Columbia, MD 21044

United Cerebral Palsy Association
66 East 34th Street
New York, NY 10016

US Commission on Civil Rights
1121 Vermont Avenue NW
Washington, DC 20425

**US Department of Health and
Human Services**
Administration for Children, Youth, and Families
Office of Public Information and Education
P.O. Box 1182
Washington, DC 20013

US Department of Justice
Community Relations Service
5550 Friendship Boulevard, Suite 330
Chevy Chase, MD 20815

Veterans Administration (VA)
810 Vermont Avenue NW
Washington, DC 20005

Women's Legal Defense Fund
2000 P Street NW
Washington, DC 20036

Work and Family Information Center
The Conference Board
845 Third Avenue
New York, NY 10022

Working with Families Institute
Department of Family and Community
Medicine
444 Yonge Street, 2nd Floor
Toronto, Ontario M5B 2H4

Worldwide Marriage Encounter
1908 East Highland Avenue, #A
San Bernadino, CA 92404

Glossary

Acculturation: A process in which gradual changes are produced by the influence of one culture on another so that the two cultures become more similar.

Acute Illness: The sudden onset of signs and symptoms in such conditions as injuries, communicable diseases, or appendicitis. Treatment can usually restore affected individuals and their families to the predisease state.

Adaptation: The process of change and adjustment in response to a stressor. For example, adaptation to childbearing involves responding to new stressors during the time of pregnancy, birth, and the postpartum period and a return to a state of homeostasis that takes into account the new changes in physical functioning, family configuration, and interactions brought about by pregnancy and birth.

Affirming Family Communication: A supportive style of talking and discussing issues within the family to resolve problems and difficulties.

Aggregate: A group of individuals who share a common characteristic such as age, gender, or health problem.

Analysis: A critical review of collected data to identify and remedy gaps and inconsistencies, and the compilation of that data in an organized manner to determine those concerns or problems with which the client needs assistance or guidance. The analysis phase ends with the identification of the pertinent nursing diagnoses.

Assessment: The first step of the nursing process. Assessment is a continuously evolving process of data collection where the nurse, drawing on the past and the present, is able to predict or plan the future. It involves the gathering of complete and accurate data through reviewing the human situation and the physical, emotional, and social status of the client in order to determine needs for care. Typically it is followed by diagnosis, planning, intervention, and evaluation.

Attachment: An enduring emotional tie that develops and grows over time and is not transient or easily abandoned. Attachment is specific and unique to the involved individuals. It implies love, tenderness, and affection. Involved individuals seek proximity to each other and yearn to be in each other's presence. Attachment relationships can withstand anger, frustration, and periods of separation.

Case Finding: Identification of individuals at risk for a health problem through a review of health statistics, screening of populations, and contact tracing.

Childbearing Cycle: The period that begins with the preconceptual period, when a parent considers getting pregnant, and concludes with the end of the 6-week postpartum interval needed for involutional changes to return the woman's body to the normal prepregnancy physiological state. It includes pregnancy, labor, and birth.

Chronic Illness: Ongoing, repeated relapses of incurable but manageable disease/condition, such as juvenile arthritis, diabetes, cerebral palsy, mental retardation, and alcoholism.

Community: A geographical location, an aggregate of people with similar characteristics, or a group of individuals who are interdependent and function to meet each other's needs.

Community Assessment: The collection of data to identify the strengths and health problems in a community.

Community Diagnosis: A statement that defines a health problem in a community and its related cause(s).

Community as Client: The perspective that the community is the recipient of nursing interventions.

Community as Setting: The perspective that the community is the context for the individuals, families, and groups who receive nursing interventions.

Confluence: The process of completing two or more activities at the same time. In families this promotes togetherness.

Contract: A binding agreement between two or more parties.

    Contingency Contract: A contract that includes the process of setting a goal and determining the costs and rewards of attainment. The purpose of the contingency contract is to reinforce behaviors needed to reach a goal.

    Nurse-Client Contract: An agreement between the health professional and client (family) to work together to achieve a goal or goals identified by the client.

    Self-Care Contract: A contract that develops independent of a health professional. It is between two individuals for the purpose of making changes in health behavior(s).

Culture: Sets of shared world views and adaptive behaviors derived from simultaneous membership in a variety of contexts, such as ecological setting (rural, urban, suburban), religious background, nationality and ethnicity, social class, gender-related experiences, minority status, occupation, political leanings, migratory patterns and stage of acculturation, or values derived from belonging to the same generation, partaking of a single historical moment, or holding a particular ideology.

Determinants of Health: Those factors that influence the health of individuals (e.g., human biology, environment, lifestyle, and health system).

Developmental Perspective: A view of the changes that occur in families and individuals over time.

Developmental Task: Psychological and social tasks associated with growth, change, and transition. For instance, the developmental tasks of pregnancy are those associated with transition to parenthood and the assimilation of the expected baby into the life of the mother and father.

Disease and Injury Patterns: Pathology of physical, mental, or family processes.

Disease Prevention: Those activities that protect the population from diseases and disabilities, and their consequences.

Durable Power of Attorney for Health Care: A legal instrument appointing a proxy — usually a relative or trusted friend — to make medical decisions on behalf of the patient when he or she is not capable of making them.

Empowerment: The process of providing information and resources to help others attain their goals.

Environment: A determinant of health that includes physical, psychological, and social contexts that affect health.

Epidemiology: The study of the distribution of various states of health within the population and the environmental conditions, lifestyles, or other circumstances associated with those states of health.

Ethclass: The intersection of social class and ethnicity. This intersection produces identifiable dispositions and behavioral patterns in families.

Ethnicity: A group's sense of "peoplehood" based on a combination of race, religion, ancestral history, and nationality.

Evaluation: The fifth step of the nursing process. Evaluation is the appraisal of those changes brought about by the nurse and experienced by the client in achieving goals and realizing expected behavioral outcomes.

Expressive Behaviors: Actions designed to provide affective support.

Family: Refers to two or more individuals who depend on one another for emotional, physical, and/or economical support. The members of the family are self-defined.

Family Adaptation: The outcome of family efforts to manage family life events and changes in which a good fit is obtained at two levels: between the individual and the family system, and between the family system and the community. It indicates that changes have been made in the way the family typically operates and how family members behave.

Family Adjustment: The outcome of family efforts to manage family life events and transitions when no major changes are made in the way the family typically operates and family members behave. It is viewed as a short-term response by the family to events that bring only minimal disruption to the family or last for only a brief period.

Family Appraisal: How the family views the stressors and changes they face and perceives the impact these have on the family, the family's ability to manage the situation, and the way it alters their world view and long-term goals, expectations, and priorities.

Family Career: The dynamic process of change that occurs in the family during its life span. Family career includes family stages and transitions.

Family Child Health Nursing: Nursing care that focuses on the relationship between family life and children's health.

Family as the Client: Focus of assessment and intervention is on all individual family members. The family is in the foreground and the individuals are in the background. The family is the sum of individual family members.

Family as a Component of Society: Focus of assessment and intervention is on the family as an institution in society. The family as a whole interacts with other institutions (educational, religious, economic, health, etc.) to receive, exchange, or give communication and services.

Family as the Context: Focus of assessment and intervention is on the individual client. The individual is in the foreground and the family is in the background. The family is the context for the individual as either a resource or a stressor to their health and illness.

Family Coping: The family's affective, behavioral, and cognitive efforts to strengthen the family as a unit, maintain the well-being of its members, and use family and community resources to manage stress and hardships.

Family Crisis: A period of disorganization experienced by the family. It indicates a need for change in how the family operates and manages a given situation.

Family Cycle of Health and Illness: Seven phases that the family experiences during health, illness, and recovery and/or death.

Family Function: The purpose that the family serves for (1) its members and (2) the society in which it exists.

Family Hardiness: Internal strengths and durability of the family characterized by an ability to work together to solve problems and difficulties, by a view of change as beneficial and growth-producing, by an active rather than passive way of responding to changes, and by a sense of control over the outcomes of life events and changes.

Family Health: A dynamic changing relative state of well-being that includes the biological, psychological, spiritual, sociological, and cultural factors of the family system.

Family Health Care Nursing: The process of providing for the health care needs of families that are within the scope of nursing practice. Family health care nursing can be aimed at the family as context, the family as a whole, the family as a system, or the family as a component of society.

Family Health Promotion: The activities of the family directed toward achieving and maintaining optimal family wellness.

Family Interaction Model: Derived from the assumptions of symbolic interaction and developmental theory, the model has three concepts: family career, individual development, and patterns of health, disease, and illness.

Family Policy: Actions and strategies by governments that directly or indirectly affect families.

Family Process: The ongoing interaction between family members through which they accomplish their instrumental and expressive tasks.

Family Self-Help: The personal capability of family members to take charge of their lives and make their own choices.

Family Stages: Periods or phases in the development of the family: married couples without children, childbearing families, families with preschool children, families with school children, families with adolescents, families launching young adults (first child gone to last child's leaving home), middle-aged parents (empty nest to retirement), and aging family members (retirement to death of both parents).

Family Structure: The ordered set of relationships among the parts of the family and between the family and other social systems.

Family as a System: Focus of assessment and intervention is on the interactions between family members. The family is viewed as an interactional system whereby the whole is more than the sum of its parts. The focus is on the individual and family simultaneously.

Family Tasks: Activities that the family needs to perform: to provide economic resources that secure shelter, food, and clothing; to develop emotionally healthy individuals who can manage crisis and experience nonmonetary achievement; to assure each member's adaptation to social needs in school, work, spiritual, and community life; to connect to the next generation by giving birth, adopting a child, or contributing to society; and to provide care and promote health for members experiencing injury, disease, and illness.

Family Transitions: Events, both developmental and situational, that signal a reorganization of family roles and tasks. Family developmental transitions are predictable changes that occur in an expected time line congruent with movement through family stages. Family situational transitions include changes in personal relationships, roles and status, environment, physical and mental capabilities, and possessions.

Family Typology: A grouping of families based on certain characteristics that describe and explain how the family typically operates and behaves.

Regenerative Family Type: A pattern of family functioning characterized by family hardiness and coherence.

Resilient Family Type: A pattern of family functioning characterized by family bonding and flexibility.

Rhythmic Family Type: A pattern of family functioning characterized by valuing and use of family time and routines.

Family Values: A family's system of ideas, attitudes, and beliefs about the worth or priority of entities, or ideas that bind together the members of a family in a common culture.

Family Well-Being: A state of balance in which families have resources to meet their needs and are satisfied with their life situation.

Family-Centered Care: A philosophy of care that recognizes and respects the pivotal role of the family in the lives of its members by directing care to the intact family. It involves collaboration by families, nurses, and other health professionals to deliver safe, quality health care. Its characteristics are (1) recognizing that the family is "the constant" in its members' lives, while personnel in the health care system fluctuate; (2) openly sharing information about alternative treatments, ethical concerns, and uncertainties about health care treatments; (3) forming partnerships between families and health professionals in deciding what is important for families; (4) respecting the ethnic, cultural, and socioeconomic diversity of families and their ways of coping; and (5) supporting and strengthening families' abilities to grow and develop.

Filial Crisis: The realization by adult children that they must become the nurturing adults on whom both their parents and their children depend, that they can no longer be dependent on their parents, and that they must face the reality that their parents will not "always be there."

Health Care System: A determinant of health that includes the availability, accessibility, and utilization of health services.

Health Patterns: Interactive individual and family understandings and behaviors associated with optimal physical, mental, and social well-being, not merely with the absence of disease and incapacitation.

Health Promotion: Those activities that improve the well-being of people.

Homeostasis: A state of balance in the family system achieved by control over inputs and outputs so as to allow the family to function in its usual way.

Human Biology: A determinant of health that includes physiological function, genetics, and maturational factors.

Illness Patterns: Processes used by families to manage disease or injury treatments that have become a part of their daily lives. Patterns of illness include activities associated with the acute, chronic, and life-threatening aspects of pathology.

Implementation: The fourth step of the nursing process. It involves carrying out or putting into effect the care plan developed during the planning phase.

Incendiary Family Communication: A pattern of talking and discussing issues within the family that tends to make matters worse and exacerbates conflict rather than resolving issues.

Individual Development: A family member's developmental tasks and interactions across the life span.

Individuation: The time provided for each family member to be alone to develop a sense of self and spirituality.

Instrumental Behaviors: Actions designed to complete a task.

Life-Threatening Illness: A serious situation with an acute or chronic injury or disease that is characterized by hospitalization, threat of death, and uncertainty.

Lifestyle: A determinant of health that includes consumption patterns, leisure activities, and employment factors.

Living Will: A legal document stating what medical treatment a patient chooses to omit or refuse in the event he or she is terminally ill and is unable to make those decisions for him- or herself.

Measurement: The process of using an instrument to measure particular attributes, assign numbers to the attributes, and statistically analyze the data. Measurement can be part of the assessment process.

Nursing Diagnosis: A clinical judgment about individual family or community response to actual and potential health problems and/or life processes. Nursing diagnoses provide the basis for selecting nursing interventions to achieve outcomes for which the nurse is accountable.

Nursing Process: A systematic manner of determining a client's problems, making plans to solve them, initiating the plan of care or assigning others to implement it, and evaluating the extent to which the plan was effective in resolving the problems identified.

Organ Procurement Organization (OPO): An organization that coordinates, procures, and distributes organs and tissues for and within its service area.

Parenting: Activities that nurture and socialize children to be healthy, responsible adults. Parents' tasks include promoting health, preventing disease, and coping with illness in their children.

Permeability of Family Boundaries: The status of a family boundary that allows access or admittance to some influences while excluding others. Totally closed boundaries do not allow outside forces to influence the family system, while totally open boundaries allow all influences to affect the family. Boundaries of the family are healthy to the extent that their permeability allows needed influences to be admitted while screening out destructive influences.

Planning: The third step of the nursing diagnosis. It involves the selection or design of nursing interventions, in consultation and collaboration with the client, that will facilitate the achievement of the desired objectives. It is the process by which objectives are determined, interventions chosen, and the care plan is written.

Policy: A set of choices or decisions that is selected in order to reach a particular goal.

Population: A collection of individuals who share one or more personal or environmental characteristics.

Postpartum Period: The 6-week period during which the mother's body returns to the prepregnant physiological state. Psychological changes may take longer.

Prenatal (Antenatal) Period: The period between conception of the baby and birth.

Primary Prevention: Those activities that focus on preventing the occurrence of health problems.

Program Planning: The process of anticipating and making decisions about a set of activities occurring within the health care system.

Prospective Payment System: A system of payment in accord with prearranged policies that are negotiated before services are provided.

Qualitative Data: Data derived from family assessment that describe the family's characteristics or qualities. The characteristics or attributes of a family are usually derived from open-ended questions and summarized in narrative form.

Quantitative Data: Data derived from family assessment that measures, counts, or compares properties or aspects of the family. This information is usually derived from closed questions that assign a value to the answers. These are then submitted to analysis and expressed as descriptive or inferential statistics.

Referral: An action that guides clients toward and helps them to use available resources to resolve their problems.

Religion: A set of beliefs and values relating to a superhuman power. These beliefs and values guide actions and aid in evaluating the actions of others.

Religiousness: Adherence to the beliefs and practices of a specific, organized religious group or faith.

Risk: The probability that individuals in a community will be affected by a health problem.

Role Delineation: The identification of the behavioral expectations associated with a role.

Role Enactment: The actual behavior demonstrated by a person in the performance of a role.

Sandwich Generation: Those middle-aged individuals (more often women than men) who still have responsibilities for dependent children and are, at the same time, assuming more and more of the burden of caring for and assisting elderly parents.

Screening: Efforts to detect unrecognized or preclinical illnesses through testing of large groups of asymptomatic individuals.

Secondary Prevention: Those activities that focus on early identification and treatment of health problems.

Social Class: A large group of people with relatively similar incomes, amount of wealth, life conditions, life chances, and lifestyles. Synonymous terms are "socioeconomic status" and "social status."

Social Support: A person's social network that provides help, the amount of help actually received, and the satisfaction with that help. The help received may be in the form of instrumental or physical aid, information, emotional support, or the appraisal of one's role performance.

Sociocultural Dimensions: The socioeconomic status and cultural background of an individual or family.

Spiritual Well-Being: A sense of inner peace, contentment, compassion, purpose in life, a realistic view of hardships and loss, and a relationship with God or a higher spiritual power.

Spirituality: A sense of relatedness or connectedness within oneself, with others, and with a higher power or unseen God.

Stress: The state of disequilibrium created when a stressor challenges the usual coping behaviors of a family.

Stressor: An event or change experienced by the family that creates a state of tension or distress.

Symbolic Interaction Theory: A perspective that explores how individuals learn meanings and gestures through social and family interactions.

Tertiary Prevention: Those activities that correct health problems and prevent further deterioration.

Unacculturated Families: Families that have not integrated dominant American core values and practices into their lives.

Underclass: The poorest families, those who live in persistent poverty.

Vertical Diffusion: The dynamic that occurs when one family member initiates a health behavior change and thereby influences another family member to make a similar change.

APPENDIX C

Family Systems Stressor-Strength Inventory (FS³I)*

Karen B. Mischke, RN, WHCNP
Shirley May Harmon Hanson, RN, PMHNP, PhD, FAAN†

INSTRUCTIONS FOR ADMINISTRATION

The Family Systems Stressor-Strength Inventory (FS³I) is an assessment/measurement instrument intended for use with families. It focuses on identifying stressful situations occurring in families and the strengths families use to maintain healthy family functioning. Each family member is asked to complete the instrument on an individual form prior to an interview with the clinician. Questions can be read to members unable to read.

Following completion of the instrument, the clinician evaluates the family on each of the stressful situations (general and specific) and the available strengths they possess. This evaluation is recorded on the family member form.

The clinician records the individual family member's score and the clinician perception score on the Quantitative Summary. A different color code is used for each family member. The clinician also completes the Qualitative Summary, synthesizing the information gleaned from all participants. Clinicians can use the Family Care Plan to prioritize diagnoses, set goals, develop prevention/intervention activities, and evaluate outcomes.

Family Name _____ Date _____

Family Member(s) Completing Assessment _____

Ethnic Background(s) _____

Religious Background(s) _____

Referral Source _____

Interviewer _____

	Family Members	Relationship in Family	Age	Marital Status	Education (highest degree)	Occupation
1.						
2.						
3.						
4.						
5.						
6.						

Family's current reasons for seeking assistance?

_____

_____

_____

* SOURCE: Mischke-Berkey, K. & Hanson, S. M. H. (1991). *Pocket guide to family assessment and intervention.* St. Louis: Mosby – Year Book.
†Respondent to inquiries.

Part I: Family Systems Stressors (General)

DIRECTIONS: Each of the 25 situations/stressors listed here deals with some aspect of normal family life. They have the potential for creating stress within families or between families and the world in which they live. We are interested in your overall impression of how these situations affect your family life. Please circle a number (0 through 5) that best describes the amount of stress or tension they create for you.

Stressors:	Not Apply	Little Stress	Medium Stress	High Stress		Clinician Perception Score
		Family Perception Score				**Clinician Perception**
1. Family member(s) feel unappreciated	0	1	2	3	4	5	_____
2. Guilt for not accomplishing more	0	1	2	3	4	5	_____
3. Insufficient "me" time	0	1	2	3	4	5	_____
4. Self-image/self-esteem/ feelings of unattractiveness	0	1	2	3	4	5	_____
5. Perfectionism	0	1	2	3	4	5	_____
6. Dieting	0	1	2	3	4	5	_____
7. Health/Illness	0	1	2	3	4	5	_____
8. Communication with children	0	1	2	3	4	5	_____
9. Housekeeping standards	0	1	2	3	4	5	_____
10. Insufficient couple time	0	1	2	3	4	5	_____
11. Insufficient family playtime	0	1	2	3	4	5	_____
12. Children's behavior/ discipline/sibling fighting	0	1	2	3	4	5	_____
13. Television	0	1	2	3	4	5	_____
14. Over scheduled family calendar	0	1	2	3	4	5	_____
15. Lack of shared responsibility in the family	0	1	2	3	4	5	_____
16. Moving	0	1	2	3	4	5	_____
17. Spousal relationship (communication, friendship, sex)	0	1	2	3	4	5	_____
18. Holidays	0	1	2	3	4	5	_____
19. In-laws	0	1	2	3	4	5	_____
20. Teen behaviors (communication, music, friends, school)	0	1	2	3	4	5	_____
21. New baby	0	1	2	3	4	5	_____
22. Economics/finances/ budgets	0	1	2	3	4	5	_____

(continued)

Stressors:	Not Apply	Little Stress	Medium Stress	High Stress		Clinician Perception Score
		Family Perception Score				**Clinician Perception**
23. Unhappiness with work situation	0	1	2	3	4	5	_____
24. Overvolunteerism	0	1	2	3	4	5	_____
25. Neighbors	0	1	2	3	4	5	_____

Additional Stressors: _____

Family Remarks: _____

Clinician: Clarification of stressful situations/concerns with family members. Prioritize in order of importance to family members: _____

Part II: Family Systems Stressors (Specific)

DIRECTIONS: The following 12 questions are designed to provide information about your specific stress-producing situation/problem, or area of concern influencing your family's health. Please circle a number (1 through 5) that best describes the influence this situation has on your family's life and how well you perceive your family's overall functioning.

The specific stress-producing situation/problem or area of concern at this time is: _____
_____
_____

Stressors:	Little	Medium	High	Clinician Perception Score
	Family Perception Score			**Clinician Perception**
1. To what extent is your family bothered by this problem or stressful situation? .... 1 2 3 4 5 (e.g., effects on family interactions, communication among members, emotional and social relationships) Family Remarks: _____ Clinician Remarks: _____				_____

	Family Perception Score			Clinician Perception
Stressors:	**Little**	**Medium**	**High**	**Score**

2. How much of an effect does this stressful
   situation have on your family's usual
   pattern of living? .... 1　2　3　4　5　　　_____
   (e.g., effects on lifestyle patterns and
   family developmental task)

   　　Family Remarks: _____

   　　_____

   　　Clinician Remarks: _____

   　　_____

3. How much has this situation affected
   your family's ability to work together as a
   family unit? .... 1　2　3　4　5　　　_____
   (e.g., alteration in family roles, completion
   of family tasks, following through with
   responsibilities)

   　　Family Remarks: _____

   　　_____

   　　Clinician Remarks: _____

   　　_____

Has your family ever experienced a similar concern in the past?
   1. YES　　　If YES, complete question 4
   2. NO　　　If NO, complete question 5

4. How successful was your family in dealing
   with this situation/problem/concern in
   the past? .... 1　2　3　4　5　　　_____
   (e.g., workable coping strategies
   developed, adaptive measures useful,
   situation improved)

   　　Family Remarks: _____

   　　_____

   　　Clinician Remarks: _____

   　　_____

5. How strongly do you feel this current
   situation/problem/concern will affect
   your family's future? .... 1　2　3　4　5　　　_____
   (e.g., anticipated consequences)

   　　Family Remarks: _____

   　　_____

   　　Clinician Remarks: _____

   　　_____

Stressors:	Family Perception Score			Clinician Perception
	Little	**Medium**	**High**	**Score**

6. To what extent are family members able to help themselves in this present situation/problem/concern? 1   2   3   4   5 (e.g., self-assistive efforts, family expectations, spiritual influence, & family resources)

    Family Remarks: _____

_____

    Clinician Remarks: _____

_____

    _____

7. To what extent do you expect others to help your family with this situation/ problem/concern? 1   2   3   4   5 (e.g., what roles would helpers play; how available are extra-family resources)

    Family Remarks: _____

_____

    Clinician Remarks: _____

_____

    _____

Stressors:	Family Perception Score			Clinician Perception
	Poor	**Satisfactory**	**Excellent**	**Score**

8. How would you rate the way your family functions overall? 1   2   3   4   5 (e.g., how your family members relate to each other and to larger family and community)

    Family Remarks: _____

_____

    Clinician Remarks: _____

_____

9. How would you rate the overall physical health status of each family member by name? (Include yourself as a family member; record additional names on back.)

    a. _____   1   2   3   4   5

    b. _____   1   2   3   4   5

    c. _____   1   2   3   4   5

    d. _____   1   2   3   4   5

    e. _____   1   2   3   4   5

    _____
    _____
    _____

Stressors:	Poor	Family Perception Score Satisfactory	Excellent	Clinician Perception Score
10. How would you rate the overall physical health status of your family as a whole?	1	2 3	4 5	_____

Family Remarks: _____

_____

Clinician Perceptions: _____

_____

	Poor	Satisfactory	Excellent	Score
11. How would you rate the overall mental health status of each family member by name? (Include yourself as a family member; record additional names on back.)				
a. _____	1	2 3	4 5	
b. _____	1	2 3	4 5	_____
c. _____	1	2 3	4 5	_____
d. _____	1	2 3	4 5	_____
e. _____	1	2 3	4 5	_____
12. How would you rate the overall mental health status of your family as a whole?	1	2 3	4 5	_____

Family Remarks: _____

_____

Clinician Perceptions: _____

_____

Part III: Family Systems Strengths

DIRECTIONS: Each of the 16 traits/attributes listed below deals with some aspect of family life and its overall functioning. Each one contributes to the health and well-being of family members as individuals and to the family as a whole. Please circle a number (0 through 5) that best describes the extent that the trait applies to your family.

My Family:	Not Apply	Seldom		Usually		Always	Clinician Perception Score
		Family Perception Score					Clinician Perception
1. Communicates and listens to one another	0	1	2	3	4	5	_____
Family Remarks: _____							
Clinician Remarks: _____							
2. Affirms and supports one another	0	1	2	3	4	5	_____
Family Remarks: _____							
Clinician Remarks: _____							
3. Teaches respect for others ..	0	1	2	3	4	5	_____
Family Remarks: _____							
Clinician Remarks: _____							
4. Develops a sense of trust in members	0	1	2	3	4	5	_____
Family Remarks: _____							
Clinician Remarks: _____							
5. Displays a sense of play and and humor	0	1	2	3	4	5	_____
Family Remarks: _____							
Clinician Remarks: _____							
6. Exhibits a sense of shared responsibility	0	1	2	3	4	5	_____
Family Remarks: _____							
Clinician Remarks: _____							

My Family:	Family Perception Score					Clinician Perception
	Not Apply	Seldom	Usually	Always		Score
7. Teaches a sense of right and wrong	0	1	2	3	4	5	_____
Family Remarks: _____						
Clinician Remarks: _____						
8. Has a strong sense of family in which rituals and traditions abound	0	1	2	3	4	5	_____
Family Remarks: _____						
Clinician Remarks: _____						
9. Has a balance of inter-action among members:	0	1	2	3	4	5	_____
Family Remarks: _____						
Clinician Remarks: _____						
10. Has a shared religious core ...	0	1	2	3	4	5	_____
Family Remarks: _____						
Clinician Remarks: _____						
11. Respects the privacy of one another	0	1	2	3	4	5	_____
Family Remarks: _____						
Clinician Remarks: _____						
12. Values service to others	0	1	2	3	4	5	_____
Family Remarks: _____						
Clinician Remarks: _____						
13. Fosters family table time and conversation	0	1	2	3	4	5	_____
Family Remarks: _____						
Clinician Remarks: _____						

| My Family: | Family Perception Score | | | | | | Clinician Perception |
	Not Apply	Seldom	Usually		Always		Score
14. Shares leisure time	0	1	2	3	4	5	_____
Family Remarks:							
Clinician Remarks:							
15. Admits to and seeks help with problems	0	1	2	3	4	5	_____
Family Remarks:							
Clinician Remarks:							
16a. How would you rate the overall strengths that exist in your family?	0	1	2	3	4	5	_____
Family Remarks:							
Clinician Remarks:							

16b. Additional Family Strengths: _____

_____

_____

16c. Clinician: Clarification of family strengths with individual members:

_____

_____

_____

Scoring Summary
Section 1: Family Perception Scores*

Karen B. Mischke, RN, WHCNP
Shirley May Harmon Hanson, RN, PMHNP, PhD, FAAN†

INSTRUCTIONS FOR ADMINISTRATION

The Family Systems Stressor-Strength Inventory (FS³I) Scoring Summary is divided into two sections: Section 1, Family Perception Scores and Section 2, Clinician Perception Scores. These two sections are further divided into three parts: Part I, Family Systems Stressors: General; Part II, Family Systems Stressors: Specific; and, Part III, Family Systems Strengths. Each part contains a Quantitative Summary and a Qualitative Summary.

Quantifiable family and clinician perception scores are both graphed on the Quantitative Summary. Each family member has a designated color code. Family and clinician remarks are both recorded on the Qualitative Summary. Quantitative summary scores, when graphed, suggest a level for initiation of prevention/intervention modes: Primary, Secondary, and Tertiary. Qualitative summary information, when synthesized, contributes to the development and channeling of the Family Care Plan.

Part I Family Systems Stressors (General)

Add scores from questions 1 to 25 and calculate an overall numerical score for Family System Stressors (General). Ratings are from 1 (most positive) to 5 (most negative). The Not Apply (0) responses are omitted from the calculations. Total scores range from 25 to 125.

Family Systems Stressor Score: General

$$\frac{(\quad)}{25} \times 1 =$$

Graph score on Quantitative Summary, Family Systems Stressors: General, Family Member Perception. Color code to differentiate family members.

Record additional stressors and family remarks in Part I, Qualitative Summary: Family and Clinician Remarks.

Part II Family Systems Stressors: Specific

Add scores from questions 1–8, 10, and 12 and calculate a numerical score for Family Systems through Stressors: Specific. Ratings are from 1 (most positive) to 5 (most negative). Questions 4, 6, 7, 8, 10, and 12 are reverse scored.‡ Total scores range from 10–50.

Family Systems Stressor Score: Specific

$$\frac{(\quad)}{10} \times 1 =$$

---

* SOURCE: Mischke-Berkey, K. & Hanson, S. M. H. (1991). Pocket guide to family assessment and intervention. St. Louis: Mosby – Year Book.
†Respondent to inquiries.
‡Reverse Scoring:

Question answered as (1) is scored 5 points
Question answered as (2) is scored 4 points
Question answered as (3) is scored 3 points
Question answered as (4) is scored 2 points
Question answered as (5) is scored 1 point

Graph score on Quantitative Summary: Family Systems Stressor: Specific (Family Member Perceptions). Color code to differentiate family members.

Summarize data from questions 9 and 11 (reverse scored) and record family remarks in Part II, Qualitative Summary: Family and Clinician Remarks

Part III Family Systems Strengths

Add scores from questions 1 to 16 and calculate a numerical score for

Family Systems Strengths. Ratings are from 1 (seldom) to 5 (always). The Not Apply (0) responses are omitted from the calculations. Total scores range from 16 to 80.

$$(\underset{16}{\quad}) \times 1 =$$

Graph score on Quantitative Summary: Family Systems Strengths (Family Member Perception).

Record Additional Family Strengths and Family Remarks in Part III, Qualitative Summary: Family and Clinician Remarks.

Section 2: Clinician Perception Scores*

Part I Family Systems Stressors (General)

Add scores from questions 1 to 25 and calculate an overall numerical score for Family System Stressors (General). Ratings are from 1 (most positive) to 5 (most negative). The Not Apply (0) responses are omitted from the calculations. Total scores range from 25 to 125.

Family Systems Stressor Score: General

$$(\underset{25}{\quad}) \times 1 =$$

Graph score on Quantitative Summary, Family Systems Stressors: General (Clinician Perception).

Record Clinicians' clarification of general stressors in Part I, Qualitative Summary: Family and Clinician Remarks

Part II Family Systems Stressors: Specific

Add scores from questions 1 – 8, 10 & 12 and calculate a numerical score for Family Systems Stressors: Specific. Ratings are from 1 (most

positive) to 5 (most negative). Questions 4, 6, 7, 8, 10, & 12 are reverse scored.* Total scores range from 10 – 50.

Family Systems Stressor Score: Specific

$$(\underset{10}{\quad}) \times 1 =$$

Graph score on Quantitative Summary: Family Systems Stressor: Specific (Clinician Perception).

Summarize data from questions 9 & 11 (reverse order) and record Clinician Remarks in Part II, Qualitative Summary: Family and Clinician Remarks

Part III Family Systems Strengths

Add scores from questions 1 to 16 and calculate a numerical score for Family Systems Strengths. Ratings are from 1 (seldom) to 5 (always).

---

*Reverse Scoring:
Question answered as (1) is scored 5 points
Question answered as (2) is scored 4 points
Question answered as (3) is scored 3 points
Question answered as (4) is scored 2 points
Question answered as (5) is scored 1 point

The Not Apply (0) responses are omitted from the calculations. Total scores range from 16 to 80.

$$(\underset{16}{\quad}) \times 1 = $$

Graph score on Quantitative Sum-

mary: Family Systems Strengths (Clinician Perception).

Record Clinicians' clarification of family strengths in Part III, Qualitative Summary: Family and Clinician Remarks.

Quantitative Summary Family Systems Stressors: General and Specific Family and Clinician Perception Scores

DIRECTIONS: Graph the scores from each family member inventory by placing an "X" at the appropriate location. (Use first name initial for each different entry and different color code for each family member.)

Scores for Wellness and Stability	Family Systems Stressors: General		Scores for Wellness and Stability	Family Systems Stressors: Specific	
	Family Member Perception Score	Clinician Perception Score		Family Member Perception Score	Clinician Perception Score
5.0			5.0		
4.8			4.8		
4.6			4.6		
4.4			4.4		
4.2			4.2		
4.0			4.0		
3.8			3.8		
3.6			3.6		
3.4			3.4		
3.2			3.2		
3.0			3.0		
2.8			2.8		
2.6			2.6		
2.4			2.4		
2.2			2.2		
2.0			2.0		
1.8			1.8		
1.6			1.6		
1.4			1.4		
1.2			1.2		
1.0			1.0		

*PRIMARY Prevention/Intervention Mode: Flexible Line   1.0 - 2.3
*SECONDARY Prevention/Intervention Mode: Normal Line   2.4 - 3.6
*TERTIARY Prevention/Intervention Mode: Resistance Lines   3.7 - 5.0
*Breakdowns of numerical scores for stressor penetration are suggested values

Family Systems Strengths
Family and Clinician
Perception Scores

DIRECTIONS: Graph the scores from the inventory by placing an "X" at the appropriate location and connect with a line. (Use first name initial for each different entry and different color code for each family member.)

Sum of strengths available for prevention/ intervention mode	Family Systems Strengths	
	Family Member Perception Score	Clinician Perception Score
5.0		
4.8		
4.6		
4.4		
4.2		
4.0		
3.8		
3.6		
3.4		
3.2		
3.0		
2.8		
2.6		
2.4		
2.2		
2.0		
1.8		
1.6		
1.4		
1.2		
1.0		

*PRIMARY Prevention/Intervention Mode: Flexible Line   1.0 – 2.3
*SECONDARY Prevention/Intervention Mode: Normal Line   2.4 – 3.6
*TERTIARY Prevention/Intervention Mode: Resistance Lines   3.7 – 5.0

*Breakdowns of numerical scores for stressor penetration are suggested values

Qualitative Summary
Family and Clinician Remarks

Part I: Family Systems Stressors: General

Summarize general stressors and remarks of family and clinician. Prioritize stressors according to importance to family members.

_____
_____
_____

Part II: Family Systems Stressors: Specific

A. Summarize specific stressor and remarks of family and clinician.

_____
_____
_____

B. Summarize differences (if discrepancies exist) between how family members and clinician view effects of stressful situation on family.

_____
_____
_____

C. Summarize overall family functioning.

_____
_____
_____

D. Summarize overall significant physical health status for family members.

_____
_____
_____

E. Summarize overall significant mental health status for family members.

_____
_____
_____

Part III: Family Systems Strengths
Summarize family systems strengths and family and clinician remarks that facilitate family health and stability.

_____
_____
_____

Family Care Plan*

Diagnosis General & Specific Family System Stressors	Family Systems Strengths Supporting Family Care Plan	Goals Family & Physician	Prevention/Intervention Mode		Outcomes Evaluation and Replanning
			Primary, Secondary, or Tertiary	Prevention/Intervention Activities	

*Prioritize the three most significant diagnoses.

The Friedman Family Assessment Model (Short Form)

There are two forms of the Friedman Family Assessment Model: short and long. Only the short form is presented here.

Two words of caution are called for before using the following guidelines in completing family assessments. First, not all areas included below will be germane for each of the families visited. The guidelines are comprehensive and allow depth when probing is necessary. The student should not feel that every subarea needs to be covered when the broad area of inquiry poses no problems to the family or concern to the health worker. Second, by virtue of the interdependence of the family system, one will find unavoidable redundancy. For the sake of efficiency, the assessor should try not to repeat data, but to refer the reader back to sections where this information has already been described.

IDENTIFYING DATA
1. Family name
2. Address and Phone
3. Family Composition
4. Type of Family Form
5. Cultural (Ethnic) Background
6. Religious Identification
7. Social Class Status
8. Family's Recreational or Leisure Time Activities

DEVELOPMENTAL STAGE AND HISTORY OF FAMILY
9. Family's Present Developmental Stage
10. Extent of Developmental Stage Fulfillment
11. Nuclear Family History
12. History of Family of Origin of Both Parents

ENVIRONMENTAL DATA
13. Home Characteristics
14. Characteristics of Neighborhood and Larger Community
15. Family's Geographic Mobility
16. Family's Associations and Transactions with Community
17. Family's Social Support Network

FAMILY STRUCTURE
18. Communication Patterns
    Extent of Functional and Dysfunctional Communication (types of recurring patterns)
    Extent of Affective Messages and How Expressed
    Characteristics of Communication Within Family Subsystems
    Types of Dysfunctional Communication Processes Seen in Family
    Areas of Closed Communication
    Familial and External Variables Affecting Communication
19. Power Structure
    Power Outcomes
    Decision-Making Process
    Power Bases
    Variables Affecting Power
    Overall Family Power
20. Role Structure
    Formal Role Structure
    Informal Role Structure
    Analysis of Role Models (optional)
    Variables Affecting Role Structure

SOURCE: From Family Nursing: Theory and Practice (3rd ed.), by M. M. Friedman, 1992, Norwalk, CT: pp. 409–411, with permission.

21. Family Values
    Compare the family to American or family's reference group values and/or identify important family values and their importance (priority) in family.
    Congruence Between Family's Values and Values of Family's Subsystems As Well As Family's Reference Group and/or Wider Community
    Variables Influencing Family Values
    Are these values consciously or unconsciously held by the family?
    Presence of value conflicts in family.
    Effect of the above values and value conflicts on health status of family.

FAMILY FUNCTIONS

22. Affective Function
    Family's Need – Response Patterns
    Mutual Nurturance, Closeness, and Identification
    Family attachment diagram
    Separateness and Connectedness
23. Socialization Function
    Family Childrearing Practices
    Adaptability of Childrearing Practices for Family Form and Family's Situation
    Who Is (Are) Socializing Agent(s) for Child(ren)?
    Value of Children in Family
    Cultural Beliefs That Influence Family's Childrearing Patterns
    Social Class Influence on Childrearing Patterns
    Estimation About Whether Family Is at Risk for Childrearing Problems and If So, Indication of High-Risk Factors
    Adequacy of Home Environment for Children's Needs to Play
24. Health Care Function
    Family's Health Beliefs, Values, and Behavior
    Family's Definitions of Health-Illness and Their Level of Knowledge

Family's Perceived Health Status and Illness Susceptibility
Family's Dietary Practices
Adequacy of family diet (recommended 24-hour food history record).
Function of mealtimes and attitudes toward food and mealtimes.
Shopping (and its planning) practices.
Person(s) responsible for planning, shopping, and preparation of meals.
Sleeping and Resting Habits
Exercise and Recreation Practices (not covered earlier)
Family's Drug Habits
Family's Role in Self-Care Practices
Family's Environmental Practices
Medically Based Preventive Measures (physicals, eye and hearing tests, and immunizations)
Dental Health Practices
Family Health History (both general and specific diseases — environmentally and genetically related)
Health Care Services Received
Feelings and Perceptions Regarding Health Services
Emergency Health Care Services
Dental Health Services
Source of Medical and Dental Payments
Logistics of Receiving Care

FAMILY COPING

25. Short- and Long-Term Familial Stressors
26. Family's Ability to Respond, Based on Objective Appraisal of Stress-Producing Situations
27. Coping Strategies Utilized (present/past)
    Differences in family members' ways of coping
    Family's inner coping strategies
    Family's external coping strategies
28. Areas/Situations Where Family Has Achieved Mastery
29. Dysfunctional Adaptive Strategies Utilized (present/past)

Answers to Study Questions

CHAPTER 1

1. Each student is asked to consider whom they consider to be their own family as a starting point. Then nurses working with families should ask people whom they consider to be their family and then include those members in health care planning. Hanson & Boyd (in press) defined family as "two or more individuals who depend on one another for emotional, physical, and/or economical support. The members of the family are self-defined."

2. There are many ways to define what is meant by family health. Hanson & Boyd (in press) defined family health as "a dynamic changing relative state of well-being which includes the biological, psychological, spiritual, sociological, and cultural factors of the family system."

3. Any of the following answers: communicates and listens to one another, affirms and supports one another, teaches respect for others, develops a sense of trust in members, displays a sense of play and humor, exhibits a sense of shared responsibility, teaches a sense of right and wrong, has a strong sense of family in which rituals and traditions abound, has a balance of interaction among members, has shared religious core, respects the privacy of one another, values service to others, fosters family table time and conversation, shares leisure time, admits to and seeks help with problem.

4. Definitions may be tailored by the individual nurse to fit their practice. Hanson & Boyd (in press) defined it as "the process of providing for the health care needs of families that are within the scope of nursing practice. Family health care nursing can be aimed at the family as context, the family as a whole, the family as a system, or the family as a component of society."

5. The statements a, b, c, d are all true about family nursing practice.

6. The family as a client centers on the assessment of all individual family members where the family is in the foreground and individuals are in the background. The family is the sum of individual family members with a focus on each and every individual such as one may see in a family medical practice office. The family as system views the family as an interactional systems whereby the interactions between family members become the target for nursing interventions. The nurse focuses on the individual and family simultaneously.

7. Any of the following three roles are identified and discussed. Health teacher. The family nurse teaches about family wellness, family illness, family relations, and parenting.

Coordinator/collaborator/liaison. The family nurse coordinates the care that families may receive, collaborating with the family in the planning of this care.

Deliverer/supervisor of technical care. The family nurse delivers or supervises the actual physical/mental care that families receive in various settings.

Family advocate. The family nurse advocates for families by speaking out for them or by empowering families to speak for themselves.

Consultant. The family nurse consults and advises families or agencies to facilitate family centered care.

Counselor. The family nurse plays a mental health therapeutic role by helping families solve problems or change behavior in coping with health and illness issues.

Case finder/epidemiologist. The family nurse is involved in case finding or a tracker of disease/problems.

Environmental modifier. The family nurse consults with families or other professionals to modify the larger or small environment that impacts family health.

Clarifier-interpreter. The family nurse clarifies and interprets data to family members pertaining to diagnosis, treatment, and prognosis of health and illness conditions.

Surrogate. The family nurse may substitute for another person in the family system.

Researcher. The family nurse identifies practice problems and through the process of scientific investigation, finds solutions.

Role model. The family nurse serves as a role model to other people through her activities.

Case manager. The family nurse provides coordination and collaboration between a group of families and the health care system.

8. The statements a, b, c, d are all true.

9. d

10. False. Family nursing has roots in society from prehistoric times. Most notable of the earlier writings came from Florence Nightingale.

11. Families existed to achieve economic survival.
Families existed to reproduce the species.
Families existed to provide protection from hostile forces.
Families passed along the religious faith (culture).
Families educated their children (socialization).
Families conferred social status to their children.
In modern times, the relationship and health function of families have received more importance.

CHAPTER 2

1. d

2. Answers will vary.

3. Anthropology, sociology, psychology.

4. b, d

5. Economic impact on family. Women in the work force as an impact on family. Diversity of families.

6. Theoretical framework.

7. Mobility of families. Whether data collection will occur with family members together or independently. How children will be included.

CHAPTER 3

1. d 2. d 3. b 4. a 5. b
6. d 7. b 8. c 9. c

CHAPTER 4

1. a 2. c 3. d 4. a 5. d
6. b 7. c 8. a, d 9. b
10. a, b, c, d.

CHAPTER 5

1. a. ii b. iii c. i d. ii.
   e. i f. iii

2. Answers will vary.

3. A faith in God. Family support system that encourages nurturing and affirming relationship. Parenteral responsibility for passing on religious faith.

4. F

5. T

6. F

7. Answers will vary.

CHAPTER 6

1. The family must be visualized in terms of its functions and needs. The family as a unit, and each of its members, must be assessed in terms of the ability to meet the collective needs of the family as well as those of each member. The nurse is dealing with many individuals rather than a single person, and with the multiple relationships which exist between and among the

persons involved. Each step of the nursing process is applied to the unit of care, the family, as well as to particular family members.

2. The NANDA system is currently being used by some nurses in describing the health care concerns of the family. Nursing diagnoses are defined as clinical judgments about responses of the individual, family, or community to actual or potential health problems and/or life processes. NANDA includes the statement that the nurse independently selects the interventions appropriate to the identified problem, and is accountable for the outcomes of interventions. A taxonomy of diagnostic labels has been developed for the use of professional nurses in defining of client problems.

3. The NANDA system is seen by many as having limited usefulness in family health care because the system has only seven diagnosis labels approved for testing that specifically address family health care concerns. Also, it is seen by some as a system that does not address health promotion needs. Only one diagnosis title specifically deals with this area. There is an effort at this time to increase the emphasis on the development and incorporation of health promotion nursing diagnosis labels into the NANDA taxonomy.

4. An ecomap is a diagram of a particular family's relationships, including those between and among its members, and with the environment. Extended family are included, and strengths, weaknesses, and social support systems are shown.

5. Family nursing care is evaluated by monitoring the progress of the family as a

unit, and each of its members as specified, in the achievement of the objectives mutually agreed upon. Specific criteria that will indicate success are identified in consultation and collaboration with the family during the planning process. The achievement of the stated outcome indicates the desired level of functioning has been achieved. Inability to function at the defined level, complete the designated tasks, or demonstrate the particular behaviors indicates satisfactory progress has not been made.

CHAPTER 7

1. b   2. b   3. ii, i, iii, iv

4. d   5. c   6. b   7. a, b, c

8. b, d, e   9. b   10. a

CHAPTER 8

1. e   2. c   3. a   4. b   5. e

6. e

CHAPTER 9

1. Examples are the family home, outpatient clinic, school, industry, nursing home, hospice, and emergency room.

2. Family nursing focuses on all members of the family rather than limiting concerns to a single individual. The context of family nursing involves the broader systems that are a part of that family's daily life such as work, school, neighborhood, church, social organizations, and, certainty, the extended family. The interaction of these systems is important to the nurse's understanding of the family's health needs.

3. Example responses:
Family advocate: the nurse

supports the family in articulating health needs and seeking resources.
Collaborator: the nurse works with the family in a team approach to the family's health care concerns.
Consultant: the nurse provides specialized knowledge and expert clinical information in response to a family's identified needs.
Coordinator: the nurse, with the family's assistance, plans and maintains an organized approach to all systems (including health) interacting with the family.
Facilitator: the nurse identifies the family's strengths and needs and promotes the family's self-help abilities.
Family health educator: the nurse identifies the family's health education needs and provides information and resources.
Leader: the nurse provides direction for the family's health care issues.
Primary caregiver: the family nurse provides entry-level health care and secures specialized resources as needed.
Researcher: the nurse identifies problems, collects data, and develops hypotheses about family health care issues.
Role model: the family nurse serves as a model of positive health behavior.
Health planning: the nurse identifies preventive and health promotion actions with appropriate time lines.
Theory developer: the nurse identifies patterns, relationships, and family structural features that assist in predicting behavior and health outcomes.

4. Urban versus rural setting, population density, geographic features, distinctive climate, industrial or economic features.

5. Is the health care setting ac-

cessible? Does the setting offer appropriate care for the family's health needs? Is the health care affordable? What is the philosophy of care? Does the setting support the family's cultural and religious beliefs?

CHAPTER 10

1. d   2. c   3. d   4. d   5. d

6. a

CHAPTER 11

1. b   2. c   3. a   4. c   5. d

CHAPTER 12

1. d   2. b   3. c   4. d   5. a

6. c   7. b   8. a   9. c

10. d   11. b   12. d

CHAPTER 13

1. c   2. b   3. a   4. c   5. d

6. e   7. a   8. b   9. b   10. c

CHAPTER 14

1. c

2. Retirement of one or both spouses. Onset of physical or cognitive decline. Need for relocation or change in living arrangements. Death of a spouse.

3. Poor health, restricted mobility, limited finances, loss of family/friends due to death or relocation.

4. a.

5. Launching their own children and becoming an "empty nest"; may be expecting more time alone, more leisure, better financial state after college and wedding expenses. Facing their parents' physical decline and increasing need for support and assistance. Facing their own middle age and mortality.

6. c, d

CHAPTER 15

1. a   2. b   3. d   4. c   5. c
6. d   7. c

CHAPTER 16

1. Answers will vary.

2. 1) c 2) a 3) a 4) b 5) c

3. Answers will vary.

4. Answers will vary.

5. Get to know elected officials. Serve on local, regional, state commissions. Become involved in political campaigns.

6. c

7. Increased complexity of care. Shorter hospital stays. More acutely ill individuals in the home setting.

8. a

Index

Numbers followed by an *f* indicate figures; numbers followed by a *t* indicate tabular material.